D1669832

Gastrointestinal Functions

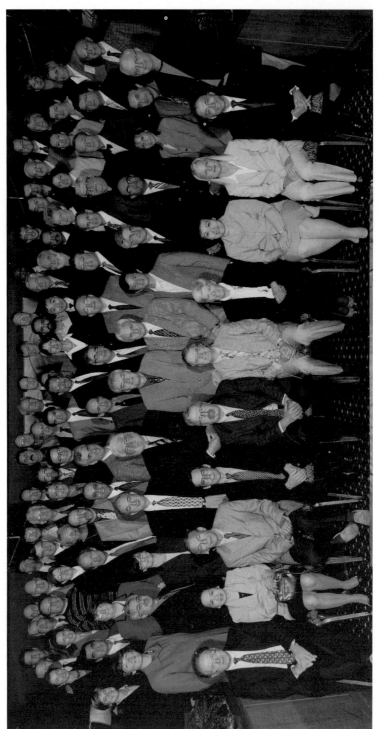

The 46th Nestlé Nutrition Workshop, Gastrointestinal Functions, was held in Montréal, Canada.

Nestlé Nutrition Workshop Series
Pediatric Program Volume 46

Gastrointestinal Functions

Editors

Edgard E. Delvin   *Head, Department of Biochemistry, and Associate Director, Sainte-Justine Hospital Research Center, 3175 Côte Ste. Catherine, Montreal, Québec H3T 1C5, Canada*

Michael J. Lentze *Zentrum für Kinderheilkunde, Adenauerallee 199, D-53113 Bonn, Germany*

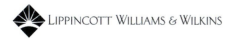

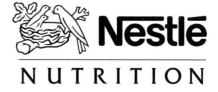

LIPPINCOTT WILLIAMS & WILKINS

Nestlé

NUTRITION

Acquisitions Editor: Beth Barry
Developmental Editor: Carol Field
Production Editor: Melanie Bennitt
Manufacturing Manager: Benjamin Rivera
Compositor: Maryland Composition
Printer: Maple Press

Nestec Ltd, 55 Avenue Nestlé
CH-1800 Vevey, Switzerland
Lippincott Williams & Wilkins,
530 Walnut Street
Philadelphia, PA 19106 USA
LWW.com

© 2001 by Nestec Ltd., and Lippincott Williams & Wilkins. All rights reserved. This book is protected by copyright. No part of this book may be reproduced in any form or by any means, including photocopying, or utilized by any information storage and retrieval system without written permission from the copyright owner, except for brief quotations embodied in critical articles and reviews. Materials appearing in this book prepared by individuals as part of their official duties as U.S. government employees are not covered by the above-mentioned copyright.

Printed in the USA

Library of Congress Cataloging-in-Publication Data

Gastrointestinal functions / editors, Edgard E. Delvin, Michael J. Lentze.
  p. ; cm. — (Nestlé Nutrition workshop series ; v. 46. Pediatric Program)
  Based on the 46th Nestlé Nutrition Workshop.
  Includes bibliographical references and index.
  ISBN 0-7817-3208-5
  1. Pediatric gastroenterology—Congresses. 2. Nutrition disorders in children—Congresses. I. Delvin, Edgard E. II. Lentze, Michael J. III. Nestlé Nutrition workshop series ; v. 46. IV. Nestlé Nutrition workshop series. Pediatric Program.
  [DNLM: 1. Gastrointestinal Diseases—Adolescence—Congresses. 2. Gastrointestinal Diseases—Child—Congresses. 3. Gastrointestinal Diseases—Infant—Congresses. 4. Gastrointestinal System—physiology—Congresses. WS 310 G2557 2001]
  RJ446 .G366 2001
  618.92′33—dc21

00-048145

Care has been taken to confirm the accuracy of the information presented and to describe generally accepted practices. However, the authors, editors, Nestec, and Lippincott Williams & Wilkins are not responsible for errors or omissions or for any consequences from application of the information in this book and make no warranty, expressed or implied, with respect to the currency, completeness, or accuracy of the contents of the publication. Application of this information in a particular situation remains the professional responsibility of the practitioner.

The authors, editors, Nestec, and Lippincott Williams & Wilkins have exerted every effort to ensure that drug selection and dosage set forth in this text are in accordance with current recommendations and practice at the time of publication. However, in view of ongoing research, changes in government regulations, and the constant flow of information relating to drug therapy and drug reactions, the reader is urged to check the package insert for each drug for any change in indications and dosage and for added warnings and precautions. This is particularly important when the recommended agent is a new or infrequently employed drug.

Some drugs and medical devices presented in this publication have Food and Drug Administration (FDA) clearance for limited use in restricted research settings. It is the responsibility of the health care provider to ascertain the FDA status of each drug or device planned for use in their clinical practice.

10 9 8 7 6 5 4 3 2 1

Preface

The subject of gastrointestinal function is topical and extremely complex, as will be appreciated during the next three days.

Physicians caring for children and adolescents are confronted daily by a multitude of chronic or functional gastrointestinal disorders, the nature of which is often poorly understood. Some of these entities are the subject of this workshop.

Over four million infants and children die of diarrhea worldwide each year. In industrialized countries, diarrhea is a major reason for hospital admission (30%) and remains an important cause of infant morbidity and mortality. Diarrhea is by far the most frequent clinical manifestation of a long list of diseases affecting the gastrointestinal tract. The various etiologies range from bacterial, viral, and parasitic agents such as shigellae and enteropathogenic *E. coli*, adenoviruses, rotaviruses, and amoebae, to endocrinopathies (congenital adrenal hyperplasia, hyperthyroidism) and dietary causes (food intolerance, transport defects, protein malnutrition, or overfeeding). Diarrhea is also an important symptom of celiac disease and inflammatory bowel disease. In the above conditions, immune mechanisms are often present in the background.

As our knowledge of cellular biology widens, we become increasingly aware that, in addition to its central function as a digestive organ, the gut plays a key role in the development and maintenance of the host's immune homeostasis. Indeed the intestine is confronted, soon after birth, with a vast array of foreign antigens and microorganisms, armed with only a single epithelial cell layer at the interface between the body and the environment. The intestinal mucosa is thus burdened with the responsibility of generating a physical barrier as well as protective immune response against potential pathogens. The essential role of the gut in protecting the body is well demonstrated in conditions in which the immune function is altered, as seen in congenital or acquired immunodeficiency disorders.

Epidemiological studies clearly indicate that the incidence of ulcerative colitis and Crohn's disease—collectively termed chronic inflammatory bowel disease—has steadily increased to an incidence of 10–20 cases/100,000/year in Canada. Celiac disease, with a prevalence varying from 1/300 to 1/2000 in different countries, is yet another important clinical condition in which the immune system mediates tissue damage. Indeed, excessive production of proinflammatory cytokines (IL-1, IL-6, TNFα) has been documented in young patients with these diseases. These conditions are commonly associated with failure to thrive, resulting from inadequate energy intake because of malabsorption and anorexia.

Although earlier recognition of the diseases results in reduced morbidity, their diagnosis is often delayed or missed owing to the lack of sensitive and specific diagnostic tools. However, recent advances in serology are producing assays that may be of significant value for the diagnosis of both Crohn's disease and ulcerative colitis. Nevertheless, these conditions remain a diagnostic challenge for the physician as many cases pass unnoticed because of the subtlety of their presentation. All the diseases briefly mentioned above are associated with alterations in gastrointestinal cell proliferation, differentiation, and/or apoptotic processes. A better understanding of the cell biology of the enterocyte will thus improve our ability to diagnose and treat these patients.

In this Workshop, renowned investigators in their respective fields highlight recent advances in various gastrointestinal conditions and discuss in detail the different animal and cell models currently employed to resolve some of the enigmas with which we are confronted. Among the clinical topics addressed are the management of intractable diarrhea, esophageal dysfunction, gut motility disorders, and inflammatory bowel disease. To further our understanding of the pathophysiology of these conditions, recent data and concepts are presented on the mechanisms involved in the assembly of brush border membranes, the role of extracellular matrix proteins in intercellular interactions and the differentiation of enterocytes, the structure-function relation of intestinal disaccharidases, and the early development and the role of the gastric epithelium.

This volume reflects the state-of-the-art in the field of gastroenterology, presented by a panel of internationally renowned clinical and biomedical investigators. It will be a reference work for the upcoming generation of researchers.

Professor Edgard E. Delvin, Montreal, Canada
Professor Michael J. Lentze, Bonn, Germany

Foreword

As a primary organ in direct contact with the environment, the gastrointestinal tract plays a major role in the nutrition and health of infants and children.

A previous Nestlé Nutrition Workshop covered some aspects of gastrointestinal tract function. However, during the past decade considerable knowledge has been compiled and this volume updates the recent progress made in this field. The program of this workshop, proposed by Professor Edgard Delvin and Professor Michael Lentze, covers the most relevant developmental aspects of the structure and functions of the gastrointestinal tract.

One of the most striking features of the gastrointestinal epithelium is the rapid, continuous cellular differentiation and renewal occurring in this organ. Although structural studies permit a better understanding of cellular activity, molecular biology now opens new perspectives on how the organization and function of the intestinal epithelium may be controlled.

As presented and discussed in this volume, some basic understanding of control mechanisms is now available, at least in the normal intestine. The complexity of the relation between structure and function becomes evident in diseases such as celiac disease and chronic inflammatory bowel disorders. However, despite considerable research, the development of these diseases remains enigmatic.

We thank the chairmen and speakers for their invaluable contribution to the program, as well as all the participants for their discussions. Nestlé Canada hosted the 46th Nestlé Nutrition Workshop and we thank them for the excellent organization and warm hospitality.

PROFESSOR FERDINAND HASCHKE M.D.
DR. ANNE-LISE CARRIÉ-FÄSSLER
Nestec Ltd.
Vevey, Switzerland

Contents

Contributing Authors

Speakers

David H. Alpers
William B. Kountz Professor of Medicine
Department of Internal Medicine;
Assistant Director
Center for Human Nutrition
Washington University School of
  Medicine
660 S. Euclid Avenue, Box 8124
St. Louis, Missouri 63110
USA

Jean-François Beaulieu
Professor and Chair
Department of Anatomy and Cell Biology
University of Sherbrooke
Faculty of Medicine
3001, 12ᵗʰ Avenue North
Sherbrooke, Québec
Canada J1H 5N4

Per Brandtzaeg
Professor and Chairman
Institute of Pathology
Head, Group for Laboratory Medicine
Medical Faculty, University of Oslo;
Head, Laboratory for
  Immunohistochemistry and
  Immunopathology (LIIPAT)
Department of Pathology
Rikshospitalet N-0027 Oslo
Norway

Hans A. Büller
Department of Pediatrics
Sophia Children's Hospital
P.O. Box 2060
NL – 3000 CB Rotterdam
The Netherlands

Edgard E. Delvin
Head
Department of Biochemistry
Associate Director
Ste-Justine Hospital Research Center
3175 Côte Ste Catherine
Montreal, Québec H3T 1C5
Canada

Yvo Ghoos
Professor
Department of Pathophysiology
Catholic University of Leuven
Chief
Laboratory "Digestion–Absorption"
UZ Gasthuisberg E 462
Herestraat, 49
B – 3000 Leuven
Belgium

Olivier Goulet
Professor
Department of Pediatrics
University of Paris – Necker;
Department of Gastroenterology
Hôpital Necker-Enfants Malades
149, rue de Sèvres
75743 Paris Cedex 15
France

Michael J. Lentze
Zentrum für Kinderheilkunde
Adenauerallee 119
D-53113 Bonn
Germany

Stanislas Lyonnet
Département de Génétique et
  Unité INSERM U-393
Hôpital Necker-Enfants Malades
149, rue de Sèvres
75743 Paris Cedex 15
France

Markku Mäki
Professor
Department of Pediatrics
Tampere University Hospital;
Professor
Institute of Medical Technology
University of Tampere
P.O.B. 2000
FIN 33014 Tampere
Finland

Charles M. Mansbach
Professor of Medicine and Physiology
Department of Gastroenterology
University of Tennessee William F. Bowld
  Hospital
University of Tennessee Health Science
  Center
951 Court Avenue, Room 555 Dobbs
Memphis, Tennessee 38163
USA

Daniel Ménard
Professor
Department of Anatomy and Cell Biology
University of Sherbrooke
Faculty of Medicine
3001, 12th Avenue North
Sherbrooke, Québec
Canada J1H 5N4

Peter Milla
Gastroenterology Unit
Institute of Child Health
30, Guilford Street
London, WC1N 1EH
United Kingdom

Jean Morisset
Professor
Department of Medicine
University of Sherbrooke
3001, 12th Avenue North
Sherbrooke, Québec
Canada J1H 5N4

Hassan Y. Naim
Professor
Department of Physiological Chemistry
School of Veterinary Medicine, Hannover
Buenteweg 17
D-30559 Hannover
Germany

N. Nanda Nanthakumar
Department of Pediatric Gastroenterology
  and Nutrition
Massachusetts General Hospital
149 13th Street, Room 3404
Charlestown, Massachusetts 02129
USA

Sylvie Robine
Director of Research
CNRS UMR 144
Institut Curie
26, rue d'Ulm
75231 Paris
France

Yvan Vandenplas
Head
Department of Pediatrics
Academy Hospital and Faculty of
  Medicine
Vrije Universiteit Brussel (A.Z.VUB)
Laarbeeklaan 101
B-1090 Brussels
Belgium

Ernest M. Wright
Professor
Department of Physiology
UCLA School of Medicine
650 Charles Young Drive North,
53-213 CHS
Los Angeles, California 90095
USA

Nicholas A. Wright
Head, Histopathology Unit
Imperial Cancer Research Fund
Deputy Principal
Imperial College School of Medicine
Hammersmith Hospital
Du Cane Road
London W12 ONN
United Kingdom

Session Chairmen

D. G. Gall / *Canada*
S. Zlotkin / *Canada*
E. Lévy / *Canada*
E. Seidman / *Canada*
C. Roy / *Canada*

Invited Attendees

M. B. de Morais / *Brazil*
A. Celso Calçado / *Brazil*
J. V. Spolidoro / *Brazil*

P. Janeva / *Bulgaria*
G. A. Bruce / *Canada*
A. Griffiths / *Canada*
J. R. Hamilton / *Canada*
R. Issenman / *Canada*
S. Moroz / *Canada*
A. Otley / *Canada*
H. Parsons / *Canada*
R. Schreiber / *Canada*
Ph. Sherman / *Canada*
L. J. Smith / *Canada*
M. Ste-Marie / *Canada*
Ch. Xu / *China*
B. L. Salle / *France*
H. Böhles / *Germany*
J. Henker / *Germany*
S. Koletzko / *Germany*
F. M. Rümmele / *Germany*
I. Bjarnason / *Great Britain*
J. Panagiotou-
  Angelakopoulou / *Greece*
D. Chun Yuen Lau / *Hong
  Kong*
P. Bodi / *Hungary*
E. Solyom / *Hungary*
G. Iacono / *Italy*

P. Lionetti / *Italy*
A. Marini / *Italy*
G. Salvioli / *Italy*
G. Zoppi / *Italy*
Y. Yamashiro / *Japan*
C. Vella / *Malta*
S. Jayaramdas / *Oman*
I. A. Memon / *Pakistan*
Z. Naeem / *Pakistan*
R. Castro / *Philippines*
J. Sio / *Philippines*
K. Fyderek / *Poland*
J. Ksiazyk / *Poland*
P. M. Mahalhães Ramalho / *Portugal*
G. Al Thani / *Qatar*
C. Ulmeanu / *Romania*
D. F. Wittenberg / *South Africa*
D. Infante Pina / *Spain*
I. Villa-Elizaga / *Spain*
I. Jakobsson / *Sweden*
P. Baehler / *Switzerland*
Ch. P. Braegger / *Switzerland*
J. Spalinger / *Switzerland*
P. Jirapinyo / *Thailand*
Ph. Mai Tran Thi / *Vietnam*

Nestlé Representatives

Giorgio Albertini	Nestlé Italiana, S.P.A., Milano, Italy
Richard Black	Nestlé Canada Inc., Ontario, Canada
Paulina Bravo	Nestlé Chile, S.A., Santiago, Chile
Anne-Lise Carrié-Fässler	Nestec Ltd., Vevey, Switzerland
Wolf Th. Endres	Nestlé Alete GmbH, Munich, Germany
Bianca-Maria Exl	Nestlé Suisse SA, Vevey, Switzerland
Lajos Hanzel	Nestlé Hungaria, Kft., Budapest, Hungary
Evan Kaloussis	Nestec Ltd., Vevey, Switzerland
Gabriella Metzger	Nestlé Italiana, S.P.A., Milano, Italy
Marie-Josephe Mozin	Nestlé Belgilux S.A., Belgium
Marie-Christine Secretin	Nestec Ltd, Vevey, Switzerland
Philippe Steenhout	Nestec Ltd, Vevey, Switzerland
Heidi Storm	Nestlé USA, Deerfield, IL, USA
Peter Van-Dael	Nestlé Research Centre, Lausanne, Switzerland

Nestlé Nutrition Workshop Series
Pediatric Program

Gastrointestinal Functions

Gastrointestinal Functions, edited by Edgard E. Delvin and Michael J. Lentze. Nestlé Nutrition Workshop Series, Pediatric Program, Vol. 46, Nestec Ltd., Vevey/Lippincott Williams & Wilkins, Philadelphia © 2001.

The Development of the Crypt–Villus Axis

Nicholas A. Wright

Histopathology Unit, Imperial Cancer Research Fund; Imperial College School of Medicine, Hammersmith Hospital, London, UK

The epithelium of the small intestine is fashioned to produce *crypts* (tubular structures containing the proliferating cells of the system) and *villi* (finger-shaped projections covered with cells that perform the absorptive functions of the gut). It is a model that has been extensively used to study epithelial proliferation and differentiation. The intestinal crypts contain the epithelial *stem cells*, which are considered to have multipotential properties and give rise to all the epithelial cell lineages in the mucosa—the Paneth cells, the mucin-secreting goblet cells, the endocrine cells, and the secreting and absorptive columnar epithelial cells. Cell production is confined to these crypts, and cells lose the capacity to divide before migrating to emerge onto the villus epithelial surface. Once there, they continue to migrate up the side of the villus in tight cohorts of cells disposed in straight lines and quickly acquire a whole range of differentiated properties that allow them to perform their absorptive functions. Finally, as epithelial cells approach the villus tip, it is now recognized that they are lost by a process of apoptosis rather than by simple extrusion.

From a developmental viewpoint, the small intestine is probably the best studied organ in the gastrointestinal tract; and our understanding of its ontogeny is well in advance of that of other parts. As noted above, for epithelial biology generally, the organization of the intestine in terms of its crypt–villus structure, regional differences in development, and high rate of cell proliferation makes it an attractive model for the study of development. This has been seized on by many investigators in recent years at several different levels. In *Drosophila*, recent work has shed light on the earliest phase of gut development, as here endoderm differentiates under the influence of mesoderm. In the mouse, progress has been made in our understanding of the generation of the crypt–villus unit, and mechanisms of cytodifferentiation of gut epithelium have been elucidated. Because of problems in tissue access and the limits of human experimentation, the focus in humans has been somewhat more narrow.

HOX GENES AND GUT DEVELOPMENT

A major finding in recent years has been the characterization of a group of genes whose products serve to specify positional identity throughout the longitudinal axis of the *Drosophila* embryo. This group, termed the *homeotic complex*, possesses highly conserved counterparts in higher organisms, including mice and humans (1). Its members, which include the *Antennapedia* and *Ultrabithorax* genes, are important in gut development because they appear to have a role at the earliest stage of gut ontogeny in specifying regional differences in the developing gastrointestinal tract, and also in maintaining these differences in those tissues in the adult. Moreover, a distinct possibility exists that, when the gastrointestinal mucosa undergoes damage such as ulceration, these genes are modulated in some way to interfere with the regional specification; thus, intestinal metaplasia accompanies chronic atrophic gastritis and Barrett's esophagus.

These gene products influence programs of differentiation, and their profound effects on the morphology of the developing embryo are thought to be mediated through the coordinated control of many genes at the transcriptional level. Their expression domains in development are tightly regulated and follow simple rules: anteroposterior gradient for maternal genes, parasegmental boundaries for homeotic genes, stripes for pair-rule genes, and so on. The characteristic of this gene family is the conserved *homeobox* sequence that encodes for a DNA binding *homeodomain*, a 60-amino acid helix-loop-helix motif containing the most highly conserved residues and which is directly involved in DNA binding, recognizing a core TAAT motif in double-stranded DNA.

In early *Drosophila* development, two ectodermal invaginations from the anterior and posterior pole of the embryo grow toward each other and fuse to form a continuous tube which develops into the foregut and midgut. This tube has a mesodermal and an endodermal cell layer—the precursors of the gut epithelium and mesenchyme. The foregut gives rise to the mouth, buccal cavity, pharynx, and esophagus, whereas in the midgut three constrictions occur, dividing it up into four morphologically distinct chambers which correspond to segments within the ectodermal layer of the developing embryo (2).

In *Drosophila*, genes specifying the characteristics of the body segments—the homeotic selector genes—are clustered into two complexes called together the *HOM* genes. They consist of the *Antennapedia* and *Bithorax* complexes, which appear in mammals as four paralogous groups called the *Hox* complexes. Homeobox genes are also present outside the *Hox* cluster in the *Parahox* cluster. Gain and loss of function studies have shown that *Hox* genes determine positional specification in both ectodermal and mesodermal structures.

Expression domains of members of the homeotic complex have been defined for visceral mesoderm in *Drosophila* (3). *Antp*, *Ubx*, and *abd-A* are all expressed in adjacent parasegmental domains, the boundaries of which depend on regulatory interactions between these genes, but this pattern of *Hox* gene expression is not observed in the overlying endoderm. Instead, a homeotic gene, *lab*, is expressed in the latter stages of midgut development within the endodermal cell layer. Induction of *lab* might thus be under the control of the underlying segmented mesoderm mediated by a diffusible factor. St. Johnston and Gelbart (4) showed that expression domains coincided for *Ubx* and *decapentaplegic* (*dpp*): *dpp* encodes a protein-sharing homology with the *TGFβ* gene family. Subsequently, it was shown that expression of *dpp* is abolished in the absence of *Ubx* (2,5), and the same applies for *Antp*, which is expressed one parasegment down from *Ubx*, and *wg*, which is related to the mammalian proto-oncogene *int-1* or *wnt-1*. Appropriate expression of *lab* depends on normal function of all four of the aforementioned genes in a clear hierarchy.

Thus, an important conclusion is that positional information is supplied by the segmented mesoderm to a nonsegmented endoderm early on in development, through diffusible factors under the control of *Hox* genes. Longitudinal gradients of expression of genes such as *lab* may play a role in the histogenesis of specialized tissues longitudinally along the gastrointestinal tract, with a transcriptional hierarchy leading to the terminally differentiated state. Moreover, cell lineage determination may also be influenced by *Hox* genes, as expression of *lab* is strictly required for formation of a highly specialized cell type within the larval midgut, the *copper cell* (6).

In the mouse, foregut and hindgut first appear from endoderm on embryonic day 7 (E7), and are followed by midgut a day later. Proliferation of the epithelium takes place after E10, and between E15 and E18 a proximal-to-distal wave of cytodifferentiation takes place to convert the solid endodermal rod into an epithelial tube lined with a simple columnar epithelium. Villi become apparent toward late gestation owing to upward growth of mesenchyme at the core of each villus. At this stage, intestine-specific gene expression occurs. True crypts develop from the flat sheet of intervillus epithelium just after birth, and between the second and third week, their number increases by a process of crypt fission. Comparable expression domains for genes of the homeotic complex have been established (1). The zinc finger transcription factor HNF-4, which is expressed in early primary embryonic endoderm, is a marker for future endodermal differentiation in the implanting blastocyst, occurring later in pancreas, stomach, and intestine (7). Knocking out the *HNF-4* gene is lethal in HNF-4 $-/-$ homozygotes, with no embryos surviving beyond E11; cell death occurs in the embryonic ectoderm at E6.5, when this tissue normally initiates gastrulation, but so little embryonic tissue of any kind developed that no conclusions were possible about later effects on gut development. The heterozygotes, on the other hand, appeared normal (8).

Considerable interest is seen in members of the *Cdx* family of *Hox* genes. The homologue of *Cdx*-1 in *Drosophila* is *caudal* or *cad*; it belongs to the hexapeptide class of homeobox genes, as do the *Antennapedia* genes. Loss of maternal and zygotic *cad* gene product causes shortening of the posterior portions of larvae with loss of posterior segments. The mammalian homologue of *cad*, *Cdx*1, although distributed widely in embryogenesis, is also seen in the posterior gut mesoderm. *Cdx*1 shows conserved linkage with *Pdx*1, found in the duodenal and pancreatic mesoderm, and both belong to the *ParaHox* cluster. The expression of a further *cad* homologue, *Cdx*2, is later confined to the posterior gut mesoderm and is also present here postnatally. *Cdx*2 appears to affect the expression of proteins involved in cell-cell and cell-matrix interactions and of molecules that mark enterocytic differentiation. Although

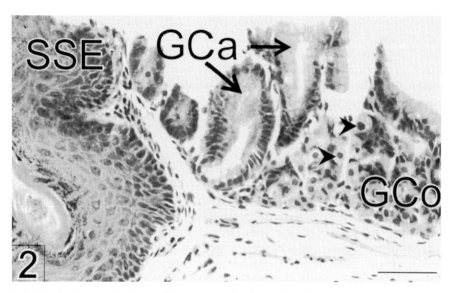

FIG. 1. A colonic polyp from a *Cdx*± mouse showing stratified squamous epithelium, gastric cardia, and gastric corpus with characteristic parietal cells (courtesy of Prof. Felix Beck).

$Cdx2 -/-$ animals fail to implant, perhaps because $Cdx2$ is strongly expressed in the trophectoderm at implantation, $Cdx2 +/-$ animals show a variety of interesting phenotypic changes, including an anterior homeotic shift involving the cervical and thoracic spines (9,10). From the viewpoint of our present interest, $Cdx2 +/-$ animals show multiple polyps in the colon, most often in the proximal colon, which is the site of maximal expression of the $Cdx2$ gene in the adult animal; indeed, lesions were seen only in the small intestine and colon and not in the esophagus, stomach, or rectum, where $Cdx2$ is not seen in development. These lesions show a fascinating appearance (Fig. 1), with areas of stratified squamous epithelium, cardiac corpus and pyloric gastric mucosa, and small intestinal and normal colonic mucosa appearing sequentially, with all cell lineages usually present in these epithelia being found.

A possible sequence of events here is that a proliferating (?stem) cell in the proximal colon, where $Cdx2$ levels are normally high, gives rise to a clone of cells in which $Cdx2$ levels are too low to promote the induction of the normal colonic phenotype. This lack of a ''colon differentiating signal'' will result in the differentiation of a more proximal epithelial phenotype, such as fore- or glandular stomach. The small intestinal and gastric pylorus between the forestomach and the colon results from the process of intercalation, possibly caused by differentiation down a gradient of positional information. In this respect, it is interesting to note that the intercalated small intestine is positive for $Cdx2$ expression, whereas the gastric derivatives are negative, perhaps supporting this gradient proposal. These important observations give insight into the possible ways in which regional specification occurs in the gut, and also how, when the gut is damaged, abnormal regeneration in the form of metaplasia occurs. It is reasonable to propose that damage to stem cells which determine cell fate and morphology in a specific part of the gut might change the differentiation pathway of that stem cell and give rise to epithelium of different characteristics.

It is becoming clear that the Tcf/Lef (T-cell factor/lymphoid enhancing factor) family of HMG box transcription factors is important in gut development: these are found downstream in the Wingless/Wnt pathway in *Xenopus* and *Drosophila*. Essential to this signaling pathway is the formation of β-catenin/Tcf nuclear complexes, with β-catenin providing an essential transactivation domain. The gene *Tcf7l2* encodes Tcf-4, a mammalian homolog seen in the central nervous system and the intestine. In the mouse, expression occurs at E13.5, immediately before the conversion of the endoderm to an epithelial sheet, and *Tcf7l2* is then present throughout life. Targeted disruption of this gene yields homozygotes that die in the first few days of life, even though milk is present in the stomachs of the animals (11). At E16.5, a reduction in villus height occurs with reduced numbers of cells in the intervillous ridges, and although goblet cells and enterocytes are seen, endocrine cells are absent. In fact, no cell proliferation occurs in the intervillous ridges and lower villus epithelium, as in seen in wild-type animals at E16. Hence, Tcf-4 is required to establish the stem cell phenotype in nascent crypts, only in the small intestine but not in the colon, where another gene, *Tcf7l1*, may provide redundancy. The target of Tcf-4/β-catenin in the nucleus is none other than the proto-oncogene c-*myc* (12). Incidentally, these findings show the importance of keeping β-catenin out of the nucleus: normally APC and GSK3b (glycogen synthetase kinase, a serine/threonine kinase) and axin (conductin) bind β-catenin, leading to its degradation through a ubiquitin–proteosome complex. Mutated APC (Adenomatous Polyposis Coli) allows β-catenin into the nucleus where active complexes with Tcf-4 are seen; such cells will possess stem cell characteristics and live much longer. We have emphasized above the role of the underlying mesenchyme in inducing gut development; here, it is likely that the stroma is responsible for maintaining the stem cell compartment by the secretion of soluble factors relayed by Tcf-4.

Other mediators of epithelial-mesenchymal cross talk include the winged helix transcription factor Forkhead homologue 6, which is also present in the intestinal mesoderm of the mouse. *Fkh6*−/− mice show delayed mesodermal invagination of the endoderm and blunted villi, with large numbers of proliferating cells in abnormal situations (13). Postnatally, surviving animals have elongated villi, hyperproliferative crypts, and goblet cell hyperplasia; thus, *Fkh6* might well be a negative regulator of cell proliferation. *Hlx* is another *Hox* gene expressed in mouse visceral mesoderm, which when knocked out, gives nonviable animals that die with gut hypoplasia at E15 (14). Sonic hedgehog (*Ssh*), found throughout the mouse intestinal endoderm, may be involved in endoderm-mesoderm signaling, as ectopic expression of *Ssh* in pancreatic endoderm leads to the induction of intestinal-like mesoderm, complete with interstitial cells of Cajal, and the pancreas undergoes a partial intestinal differentiation program, with goblet cell differentiation (15).

THE CRYPT–VILLUS UNIT

In the adult mouse, as in all mammals, the crypt–villus unit is well established, with numbers of crypts furnishing cells to a single villus. Moving down the small intestine from the duodenum to the ileum, differences are seen in crypt–villus relationships, with some 14 crypts per villus in the proximal intestine, but only 5 in the ileum. Similarly, the size of villi is reduced, with some 8,000 cells clothing duodenal villi, compared with 2,000 in the ileum. Cells migrate from the crypts to the villus tip, which takes between 2 and 5 days in the mouse (16).

An important advance in our knowledge of the development of the crypt–villus unit has come from the use of allophenic tetraparental mice: two strains of mice are selected, one of which bears a marker specific for the tissue of interest, and fertilized zygotes from each strain are combined to form a single zygote. Introduction of these chimeric zygotes into the uterus of pseudopregnant females gives offspring that are chimeras of the two strains selected (17). A polymorphism in lectin binding capacity exists in the intestine in the *Dlb*-1 locus, carried on chromosome 1, and thus mice of the C57Bl strains bind the lectin *Dolichos biflorus* agglutinin (DBA), which selectively binds to the *N*-acetylgalactosamine residues present on blood group markers on the cell surfaces. Mouse strains such as RIII/Lac-*ro* and DDK do not bind the lectin in the intestinal epithelium (18).

Staining the small intestine and colons of such mice with DBA shows that the crypts are either positive or negative—never mixed (18). Mixed crypts were not detected in *adult* mice after observing tens of thousands of crypts. The important conclusion is that each crypt forms a *clonal population*. Crypts are each derived, ultimately, from a single cell: goblet cells and Paneth cells share in this clonality (Fig. 2). Note also that the villi are polyclonal, as they are supplied by cells from more than one crypt, which of course may be positive or negative for the *DBA* marker. The study of whole mounts, or of three-dimensional reconstructions, shows that cells traverse the villus in discrete straight lines and little or no mixing of the cell progeny occurs from supplying crypts.

Using this chimeric model, Schmidt et al. investigated the process of crypt formation in neonatal mice (19). Before differentiation of crypts, the intervillous epithelium is polyclonal. After birth, within the intestine, patches of staining were seen indicating *DBA*-positive crypts. At the boundaries of these patches, mixed crypts were observed, indicating a mixed clonal origin for that crypt. From day 2 to day 14, the number of mixed crypts, expressed as a percentage of crypts at patch boundaries, fell from 50% to close to zero, indicating a process in which *crypt monoclonality* is gradually established in early postnatal life. Thus, it appears that in development, crypts are *pleoclonal* or *polyclonal* (i.e., multiple stem cells form individual crypts, but, by an obscure process, these crypts sort themselves out to become monoclonal). Possible mechanisms for "cleansing" of these crypts include either overgrowth and extrusion of one stem cell lineage by the other or the possibility of segregation of the lineages because of the extremely active replication of crypts by fission at this point. The system also gives insight into the commitment of intestinal stem cells

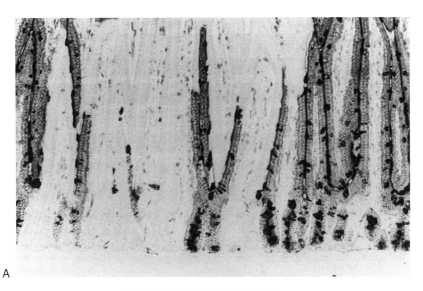

A

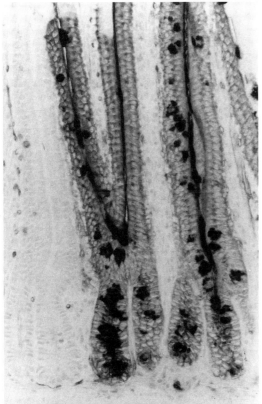

B

FIG. 2. A section from the jejunal mucosa of a tetraparental allophenic mouse stained with the lectin *Dolichos biflorus* agglutinin, which differentiates between the two types of cells present in the chimera. Note in (**A**), and confirm in (**B**) (at high power), that crypts are either totally positive or totally negative, indicating that each crypt was originally the progeny of a single cell, or group of cells, of the same type, and supporting the concept of a clonal origin of crypts. The polymorphism is also shown in the endothelial cells (photographed from a preparation made available through the courtesy of Professor B. Ponder).

before the formation of crypts: using mice that are homozygous for the *Dlb*-1 marker, a mutation can be induced in stem cells that causes loss of that marker using the mutagen ethylnitrosourea (ENU). These mutations show up as patches of *Dlb*-1 negative crypts in early adult life. When ENU is given early in embryogenesis (at E7), the size of the patches is large (~3,200 crypts). However, when the ENU is given later (at E11), patches reduced in size (~310 crypts) appear with greater frequency. These experiments indicate that the embryonic gut contains precursor cells that can give rise to gut stem cells; and, as commitment of these cells proceeds, their proliferative potential is reduced although their number might increase.

The concept of the monoclonal crypt implies a single multipotential stem cell giving rise to all contained crypt cell lineages. Theoretically, however, cells from each partner in the chimera could segregate independently in development, so that apparently monoclonal crypts are nothing more than *monophenotypic*. On the other hand, mice who are heterozygous for a defective glucose-6-phosphate dehydrogenase (*G6PD*), a gene carried on the X chromosome, show crypts which, as a result of lyonization, have a crypt restricted pattern of G6PD histochemical staining (20). In these animals, the crypts are also monophenotypic, with no mixed crypts appearing; this confirms the conclusion that crypts are derived from a single stem cell, in this case either showing normal *G6PD* expression or lacking it.

It is currently believed that the stem cell is the progenitor of every epithelial cell within a given crypt, including the enteroendocrine, Paneth's, and goblet cells. Experiments where expression of the *Dlb*-1 gene product is knocked in by a mutagen have shown that stem cells do not directly give rise to differentiating progeny such as goblet cells, but these arise from long-lived committed precursor cells housed in the lower crypt (21).

Thus, the important conclusion remains that crypts *develop* as clonal structures from a single stem cell laid down in embryonic life and giving rise to all contained cell lineages, whereas villi are polyclonal, being supplied from a number of crypts. But how are these crypts maintained in the adult animal: as clonal progeny of stem cells? A model in which stem cell behavior can be studied has been exploited by Winton and Ponder (22), Williams et al. (23), and Park et al. (24). When mice heterozygous for the *Dlb*-1 gene (*Dlb*-1 +/−) are given a single dose of mutagen and crypts are stained for *DBA*, or if G6PD is used as the marker, in the weeks that follow, crypts appear that are apparently composed of cells with a different, mutated phenotype. In these experiments an induction of a rapid but transient increase in crypts is seen, showing a partial, or segmented, mutated phenotype (Fig. 3); later on, an increase occurs in the frequency of crypts showing a completely or wholly mutated phenotype, an increase that levels off at the same time that partially or segmented crypts disappear.

Interestingly, the small intestine and colon show a major difference in the timing of these events: the plateau is reached at between 5 and 7 weeks in the colon (24) but not until some 12 weeks in the small intestine. The emergence of the partially mutated crypts, and their replacement by wholly mutated crypts, can be explained by a mutation at the *Dlb*-1 or G6PD locus in the single stem cell from which all

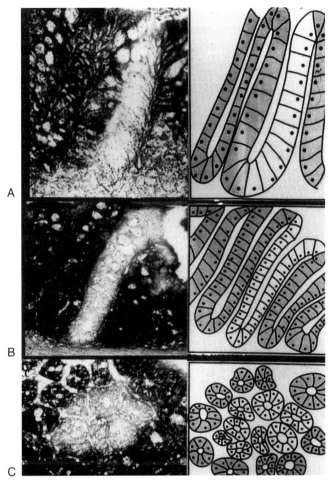

FIG. 3. Sections from the colon of a mouse treated with a single injection of a mutagen (ethylnitrosourea, ENU), and histochemically stained for glucose-6-phosphate dehydrogenase activity. (**A**) A partially negative crypt, where only a portion of the crypt is positive; (**B**) a wholly negative crypt without any positive cells; (**C**) a patch of negative staining cells (courtesy of Dr. Hyun Sook Park).

lineages are derived. Thus, a partially mutated crypt is a crypt in the process of being colonized by progeny from the mutated stem cell; this crypt will ultimately develop into a wholly mutated crypt. Alternatively, some of these partially mutated crypts could derive from mutations in nonstem proliferative cells, and these, of course, would disappear as the mutated clone was lost through migration out of the crypt.

These experiments again indicate that a single stem cell can give rise to all crypt lineages in both the colon and small intestine. The reasons for this difference in the timing of this process between the small intestine and the colon could be explained by different durations of the stem cell cycle time (22), the present of a stem cell "niche" with differences in the number of stem cells between the two tissues (23), and the possibility that crypt fission plays an important part in the genesis of the wholly mutated phenotype (24). Loeffler et al. (25) have also formulated a model that explains this phenomenon stochastically, on the basis of several indistinguishable stem cells per crypt, which can replace each other.

In humans, such experimental maneuvers are not possible, but making use of certain "natural experiments" has cast some light on the development of the crypt–villus unit. Approximately 9% of the white population secrete sialic acid lacking in *O*-acetyl substituents, in which case colonic goblet cells stain with the mild periodic acid Schiff (mPAS) technique and negatively, or weakly, with techniques that show *O*-acetyl sialic acid, such as the periodate-borohydride/potassium hydroxide saponification/PAS (PB/KOH/PAS) method. This is explained by genetic variability in the expression of the enzyme *O*-acetyl transferase (OAT) (26). This 9% of the population is homozygous for inactive OAT genes: OAT$-$/OAT$-$. The Hardy–Weinberg equilibrium then predicts that some 42% of the population are heterozygous (OAT$-$/OAT$+$), but *O*-acetylation proceeds as there is one active OAT gene. Loss of this gene converts the genotype to OAT$-$/OAT$-$. In heterozygotes, this shows as crypt-restricted mPAS staining in a negative background (Fig. 4). Indeed, this is seen in

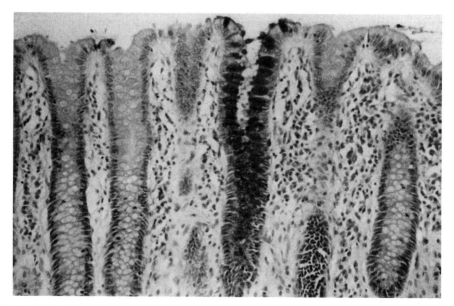

FIG. 4. A section from the human colon stained with the mild periodic acid Schiff method for nonacetylated sialomucin; note that the loss of acetylation is confined to single crypt, *crypt restricted*, and that all goblet cells in the crypt are stained (courtesy of Dr. Fiona Campbell).

approximately 42% of the population, and again is most simply explained by a mutation or loss of the gene by non-disjunction in the single crypt stem cell and the colonization of this crypt by the clonal progeny of the mutated stem cell. This unicryptal loss of heterozygosity occurs randomly, is increased by age, as would be expected (27), and is also increased in individuals who have received pelvic irradiation (28). These observations indicate that the repertoire of human colonic stem cells includes goblet cells in the colonic crypt, but of course reveals nothing about the other contained cell lineages, the columnar cells and the endocrine cells. Here, we must look to a different natural experiment.

Such an experiment was noted by Novelli et al. (29), who described a very rare individual who showed the genotype XO/XY, a phenotypic male of short stature but with no other stigmata of Turner's syndrome. By coincidence, this individual also had familial adenomatous polyposis, for which he had undergone a prophylactic total colectomy at 32 years of age, from which material was available for analysis. A combination of karyotyping and fluorescent *in situ* hybridization (FISH) on the patient's peripheral blood lymphocytes showed the Y chromosome to be dicentric; the karyotype was 45,X/46,Xdic(Y) (Ypter→cen→Yq11.23::Yp11.3) and approximately 20% of peripheral blood lymphocytes were XO.

Using nonisotopic *in situ* hybridization on histologic sections of small and large intestine, with Y chromosome–specific probes, intestinal crypts were seen to be composed exclusively of either XY or XO cells (Fig. 5a). The patches of XO crypts were irregular in shape with widely varying patch size (mean patch width 1.85 crypts, range 1–14 crypts). Crypts examined at patch borders showed no mixed XO/XY cellularity, and all indigenous epithelial cell lineages could be directly visualized as XO or XY, including columnar cells, goblet cells (Fig. 5b), and endocrine cells (Fig. 5c). Human intestinal crypts are also clonal populations, each derived ultimately from a single multipotential stem cell. Small intestinal crypts showed the same clonal architecture; and, as seen in the mouse, villi from the ileum showed a polyclonal structure, again reflecting that multiple crypts supply a single villus. From the thousands of crypts examined, four *mixed* crypts were seen in otherwise pure XY patches, similar to the partial loss of *O*-acetylated sialomucins described in human colonic crypts (27) and in mice given mutagens (22–24). Hence, occasional mixed crypts probably occur from non-disjunction, with loss of the Y chromosome, in a crypt stem cell. Whether the developing human intestinal crypts show the polyclonal structure seen in the mouse is not yet known.

For some time, it has been clear that crypt fission is an important mechanism determining crypt number in the small intestine and colon (30); initial studies indicated its pivotal position in two processes: the massive increase in crypt number occurring in the postnatal period (31), and during the recovery of the intestine from irradiation (32) and cytotoxic chemotherapy (33). In many instances, crypt fission begins as an indentation in the base of the crypt, and advances through a vertical split in the crypt, which continues until two new crypts are produced. In some instances, the process begins asymmetrically with respect to the crypt axis, a process

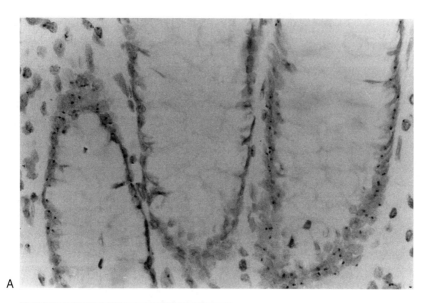

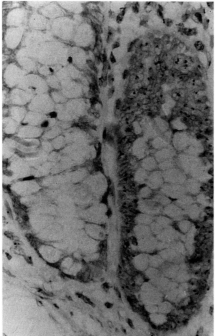

FIG. 5. Sections from a patient with the XO/XY phenotype, with the XY cell demonstrated by *in situ* hybridization. (**A**) All cells are positive or negative for the Y chromosome; (**B**) goblet cell clonality; (**C**) sections stained with chromogranin A for endocrine cells (red), showing clonal derivation; (**D**) a hemicrypt that has lost nuclear staining for the Y chromosome. (From Novelli MR, Williamson JA, Tomlinson IPM, *et al.* Polyclonal origin of colonic adenomas in an XO/XY patient with FAP. *Science* 1996; 272: 1187–90; with permission).

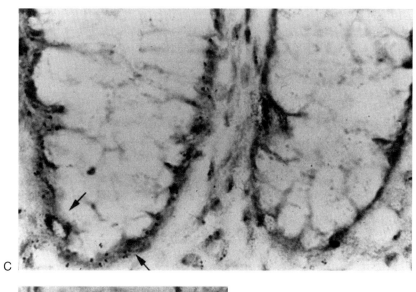

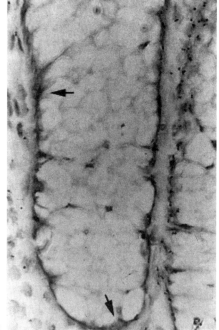

FIG. 5. (Continued)

called "budding," which can be seen in apparently normal human colonic mucosa. However, this is more common in precancerous states such as familial adenomatous polyposis and rat colonic mucosa after systemic treatment with carcinogens such as 1,2-dimethylhydrazine. In some situations, notably after irradiation, multiple buds can be seen coming off the same crypt (32).

The dynamics of crypt fission have been described in a series of seminal papers by Bjerknes et al. (34–36), whose studies led to the concept of the crypt cycle. Crypts, born by fission, gradually increase in size; in the mouse, after about 108 days, the crypt undergoes fission, a process that takes about 12 hours. Measurements of crypt volume or size showed that crypts at the upper end of the crypt size distribution initiated fission, suggesting that crypts have to attain a certain size before fission begins. This introduces the concept of a threshold size for the number of stem cells above which crypt fission is initiated. In the human colon, the fraction of crypts in fission, the crypt fission index (f_i), is small—of the order of 0.003%—and calculations indicate a crypt cycle time of 17 years. Although not as clear as in the mouse, a tendency is seen for larger crypts to undergo fission.

Attention has been focused on the stem cell number and the nature of stem cell divisions in the control of crypt fission; a simple concept is that the threshold for triggering crypt fission is a doubling of the stem cell number (37). Although studies of the distribution size of crypts about to divide indicated that crypt population size was perhaps the stimulus for crypt fission, the incidence of crypt fission in animals treated with the mitogen epidermal growth factor (EGF), which increases crypt size, showed no increase in crypt fission. However, animals given dimethylhydrazine, a colonic carcinogen, showed no increase in crypt size but raised crypt fission indices (38). These studies indicate that specific actions on the patterns of stem cell division may be important in the control of crypt fission.

The aforementioned changes that occur in the intestinal crypts of mice treated with mutagens (e.g., ENU or DMH) have been followed, and they show the gradual emergence of crypts that are partially and wholly negative for G6PD (Fig. 3**A**, 3**B**). Significantly, with time, an increase is seen in the number of negative patches, defined as a group of negative crypts exceeding 1 (Fig. 3**C**); an increase also occurs in the size of the patches, particularly in the colon. *It is therefore clear that the mechanism for expansion of these mutated clones is crypt fission.*

In ulcerative colitis, it is by no means unusual for dysplasia to occur as a developing stage for the carcinoma known to complicate the condition. In colonic dysplasia, crypt architecture is preserved, but these crypts are populated by cells of malignant phenotype. Using fluorescent antibody cell sorting (FACS) analysis on single cell suspensions from these cases, it has been shown that considerable areas of colonic mucosa (> 9 cm in length) contain crypts that have been colonized by the same aneuploid stem line (39–41). In Fig. 3**C** a single mutated clone (i.e., a crypt that contains a mutation at the G6PD locus) that has enlarged to a group of eight mutated crypts by crypt fission is seen. Thus, this observation could readily be extrapolated to apply to the situation in ulcerative colitis, concluding again that mutated clones in the human colon also spread by crypt fission. Additionally, it is also clear that the main mode of growth of colonic adenomas in familial adenomatous polyposis is by crypt fission, this time of the adenomatous crypts (42), a further example of a mutated clone spreading by the fission process.

How the crypt–villus unit is maintained, and the mechanism of migration of villus cells, are interesting questions. The crypt and villus epithelial cells are held firmly together by homotypic E-cadherin molecules to form a cohesive sheet. E-cadherin also binds to β-catenin: expression of β-catenin with an amino terminal 89 residue deletion, which does not bind to GSK3b in chimeric mice, increases crypt cell proliferation but slows migration, although villus size remains normal, owing to increased apoptosis (43). Interestingly, E-cadherin expression was increased, as the mouse E-cadherin gene has a binding site for Lef/Tcf. Thus, this increase in E-cadherin is probably caused by increased transcription. In turn, the epithelial cells are anchored to the underlying extracellular matrix (ECM) by integrins and their receptors, which vary according to the level in the crypt–villus unit. The localization of the stem cell and the different migration kinetics of the several cell lineages could well be dependent on this, as has been shown for the localization of the epidermal stem cell (44). Paneth cells, for example, do not migrate in the general escalator; they remain in the crypt base, and the turnover of endocrine cells is longer than for other epithelial cells. Such differential migration kinetics are likely to be related to epithelial-ECM interactions; additionally, gut endocrine cells express P-cadherin (placental cadherin), which might also play a part in their differential migration.

The migration kinetics of cells as they emerge from the mouth of the crypt onto the villus is interesting. It has been known for some time that cells move up the villus in a tight cohort in straight lines. Bjerknes and Cheng (21) have pointed out that it is impossible to continuously deform a circle into a line segment—the output of a crypt is circular and, of course, the villus forms a plane. Hence, at least one cell must break contact with its neighbors as it migrates onto the villus. This can be seen in chimeric animals or in animals where administration of mutagens deletes or expresses a marker such as the *Dlb*-1 gene product. Thus, crypts can be seen to supply two villi, the emergent flow from one crypt forms more than one stripe on the villus, or the flow can even wind around an adjacent crypt on its way to the villus to be supplied with cells.

EPITHELIUM AND STROMA

In gut development, signals appear to derive from the stroma, which controls epithelial cell changes; thus, an important question with regard to the process of gut development has been to determine to what extent differentiation of the gut epithelium is genetically programmed, and to what extent it is determined by factors within the gut lumen. An experimental model that examines this issue directly involves the transplantation of segments of fetal small intestine into the subcutaneous tissues of young adult nude mice (45–47). Pregnant mice at E15 or E16 are killed and the embryos dissected to give two intestinal "halves," proximal (duodenum/jejunum) and distal (ileum). Each part, with the ends clipped, is implanted in the subcutaneous fascia of a young adult nude mouse (CBY/B6) and, 4 to 6 weeks after engraftment, each intestinal segment is removed and examined. Intestinal and liver fatty acid binding proteins and a variety of peptides expressed in enteroendocrine cells show an appropriate pattern of region-specific differentiation. Whether this spatial information is irreversibly imprinted at a discrete period in development or whether it requires continuous expression of a particular gene is a separate question. Although transcriptional activation of *L-fabp* does not occur in the fetal intestine until E17 in the jejunum, and in the ileum 2 days later, the nature of the positional information that the intestine uses to implement this is currently a matter for speculation and, in any case, may well form part of a hierarchy.

CONCLUSIONS

A growing knowledge of the way the epithelium develops in the small intestine is setting the scene for a better understanding of stem cell origins and cell cycle control within the intestinal crypt. This should provide insights into the mechanisms of carcinogenesis within the gastrointestinal tract. A coupling of advances in gene therapy with increased knowledge of the mechanisms of intestinal epithelial gene regulation could lead to new therapeutic avenues in specific disease states (e.g., specific enzyme deficiency and short bowel syndrome), and such interventions in these conditions might be at hand.

ACKNOWLEDGMENTS

It is a pleasure to record the assistance of Charles Shaw-Smith in the writing of this chapter. Work from our laboratory was supported by the Imperial Cancer Research Fund.

REFERENCES

1. McGinnis W, Krumlauf R. Homeobox genes and axial patterning. *Cell* 1992; 68: 283–302.
2. Reuter R, Panganiban GE, Hoffmann FM, Scott MP. Homeotic genes regulate the spatial expression of putative growth factors in the visceral mesoderm of *Drosophila* embryos. *Development* 1990; 110: 1031–40.
3. Tremml G, Bienz M. Homeotic gene expression in the visceral mesoderm of *Drosophila* embryos. *EMBO J* 1989; 8: 2677–85.
4. St Johnston RD, Gelbart WM. Decapentaplegic transcripts are localized along the dorsal-ventral axis of the *Drosophila* embryo. *EMBO J* 1987; 6: 2785–91.
5. Immergluck K, Lawrence PA, Bienz M. Induction across germ layers in *Drosophila* mediated by a genetic cascade. *Cell* 1990; 62: 261–8.

6. Hoppler S, Bienz M. Specification of a single cell type by a Drosophila homeotic gene. *Cell* 1994; 76: 689–702.

7. Duncan SA, Manova K, Chen WS, *et al.* Expression of transcription factor HNF-4 in the extraembryonic endoderm, gut, and nephrogenic tissue of the developing mouse embryo: HNF-4 is a marker for primary endoderm in the implanting blastocyst. *Proc Natl Acad Sci USA* 1994; 91: 7598–602.

8. Chen WS, Manova K, Weinstein DC, *et al.* Disruption of the HNF-4 gene, expressed in visceral endoderm, leads to cell death in embryonic ectoderm and impaired gastrulation of mouse embryos. *Genes Dev* 1994; 8: 2466–77.

9. Beck F, Chawengsaksophak K, Swaring P, Playford R, Burness JB. Reprogramming of intestinal differentiation and intercalary regeneration in *Cdx2* mutant mice. *Proc Natl Acad Sci USA* 1999; 96: 7318–23.

10. Tamai Y, Nakajima R, Ishikawa T, *et al.* Colonic hamartoma development by anomalous duplication in *Cdx2* knockout mice. *Cancer Res* 1999; 59: 2965–70.

11. Korinek V, Barker N, Moerer P, *et al.* Depletion of epithelial stem cell compartments in the small intestine of mice lacking Tcf-4. *Nat Genet* 1998; 19: 379–82.

12. He T-C, Sparkes AB, Rago C, *et al.* Identification of c-myc as a target of the APC pathway. *Science* 1999; 281: 1509–11.

13. Kaestner KH, Silberg DG, Traber PG, Schutz G. The mesenchymal winged helix transcription factor Fkh6 is required for the control of gastrointestinal proliferation and differentiation. *Genes Dev* 1997; 11: 1583–95.

14. Hentsch B, Lyons I, Li R, *et al.* Hlx homeobox gene is essential for an inductive tissue interaction that drives expansion of liver and gut. *Genes Dev* 1996; 10: 70–9.

15. Apelqvist A, Ahlgren U, Edlund H. Sonic hedgehog directs specialised mesoderm differentiation in the intestine and pancreas. *Curr Biol* 1997; 7: 810–14.

16. Wright NA, Alison MR. *The biology of epithelial cell populations*, Vol 2. Oxford: Clarendon Press, 1984.

17. Mintz B. Experimental genetic mosaicism in the mouse. In: *Pre-implantation stages of pregnancy* (CIBA Foundation Symposium). London: Churchill, 1965: 194–216.

18. Ponder BAJ, Schmidt GH, Wilkinson MM, *et al.* Derivation of mouse intestinal crypts from a single progenitor cell. *Nature* 1985; 313: 689–91.

19. Schmidt G, Winton DJ, Ponder BAJ. Development of the pattern of cell renewal in the crypt–villus unit of the chimaeric mouse small intestine. *Development* 1988; 103: 785–90.

20. Griffiths DF, Davies SJ, Williams D, Williams GT, Williams ED. Demonstration of somatic mutation and crypt clonality by X-linked enzyme histochemistry. *Nature* 1988; 333: 461–3.

21. Bjerknes M, Cheng H. Clonal analysis of mouse intestinal epithelial progenitors. *Gastroenterology* 1999; 116: 7–14.

22. Winton DJ, Ponder BAJ. Stem cell organisation in mouse intestinal epithelium. *Proc R Soc Lond B Biol Sci* 1990; 241: 13–18.

23. Williams ED, Lowes AP, Williams D, Williams GT. A stem cell niche theory of intestinal crypt maintenance based on a study of somatic mutation in colonic mucosa. *Am J Pathol* 1992; 141: 773–6.

24. Park HS, Goodlad RG, Wright NA. Crypt fission in the small intestine and colon: a mechanism of the emergence of transformed crypts after treatment with mutagens. *Am J Pathol* 1995; 147: 1416–27.

25. Loeffler M, Birke A, Winton DJ, Potten CS. Somatic mutation, monoclonality and stochastic models of stem cell organisation in the intestinal crypt. *J Theor Biol* 1993; 162: 471–91.

26. Jass JR, Robertson AM. Colorectal mucin histochemistry in health and disease: a critical review. *Pathol Int* 1994; 44: 487–504.

27. Fuller CE, Davies RP, Williams GT, Williams ED. Crypt-restricted heterogeneity of goblet cell mucus glycoprotein in histologically normal human colonic mucosa; a potential marker of somatic mutation. *Br J Cancer* 1990; 61: 382–4.

28. Campbell F, Fuller CE, Williams GT, Williams ED. Human colonic stem cell mutation frequency with and without irradiation. *J Pathol* 1994; 174: 175–82.

29. Novelli MR, Williamson JA, Tomlinson IPM, *et al.* Polyclonal origin of colonic adenomas in an XO/XY patient with FAP. *Science* 1996; 272: 1187–90.

30. St. Clair WH, Osborne JW. Crypt fission and crypt number in the small and large bowel of adult rats. *Cell Tissue Kinetics* 1985; 14: 467–77.

31. Maskens AP, Dujardin L. Kinetics of tissue proliferation in colorectal mucosa during postnatal growth. *Cell Tissue Kinetics* 1981; 14: 467–77.
32. Cairnie AB, Millen BH. Fission of crypts in the small intestine of the irradiated mouse. *Cell Tissue Kinetics* 1975; 8: 189–96.
33. Wright NA, Al-Nafussi AI. The kinetics of villus cell populations in the mouse small intestine. II. Studies on growth control after death of proliferative cells induced by cytosine arabinoside, with special reference to negative feedback mechanisms. *Cell Tissue Kinetics* 1982; 15: 611–21.
34. Totafurno J, Bjerknes M, Cheng H. The crypt cycle: evidence for crypt and villus production in the adult mouse small intestine. *Biophys J* 1987; 52: 279–94.
35. Bjerknes M. The crypt cycle and the asymptomatic dynamics of the proportion of differently sized mutant crypt clones in the mouse intestine. *Proc R Soc Lond B Biol Sci* 1995; 260: 1–6.
36. Bjerknes M. Expansion of mutant stem cell populations in the human colon. *J Theor Biol* 1996; 178: 381–5.
37. Loeffler M, Bratke T, Paulus U, Li Y-Q, Potten CS. Clonality and life cycles of intestinal crypts explained by a state-dependent stochastic model of epithelial stem cell organisation. *J Theor Biol* 1997; 186: 41–54.
38. Park H-S, Goodlad RA, Ahnen DJ, *et al*. The effects of epidermal growth factor and crypt fission in the colon: cell proliferation and crypt fission are controlled independently. *Am J Pathol* 1996; 151: 125–36.
39. Ahnen D. Abnormal DNA content as a biomarker of large bowel cancer risk and prognosis. *J Cell Biochem Suppl* 1992; 16G: 143–50.
40. Levin DS, Rabinovitch PS, Haggitt RC, *et al*. Distribution of aneuploid cell populations in ulcerative colitis with dysplasia or cancer. *Gastroenterology* 1991; 101: 1198–210.
41. Burner GC, Rabinovitch PS, Haggitt RC, *et al*. Neoplastic progression in ulcerative colitis: histology, DNA content, and loss of a p53 allele. *Gastroenterology* 1992; 103: 1602–11.
42. Wasan HS, Park H-S, Liu KC, *et al*. APC in the regulation of crypt fission. *J Pathol* 1998; 185: 246–55.
43. Wong MH, Rubinfield B, Gordon JI. Effects of forced expression of an N-terminal truncated β-catenin on mouse epithelial homeostasis. *J Cell Biol* 1998; 141: 765–77.
44. Jensen UB, Lowell S, Watt FM. The spatial relationship between stem cells and their progeny in the basal layer of human epidermis: a new view based on whole mount labelling and lineage analysis. *Development* 1999; 26: 2409–18.
45. Rubin DC. Spatial analysis of transcriptional activation in fetal rat jejunal and ileal gut epithelium. *Am J Physiol* 1992; 263: G853–63.
46. Rubin DC, Swietlicki E, Roth KA, Gordon JI. Use of fetal intestinal isografts from normal and transgenic mice to study the programming of positional information along the duodenal-to-colonic axis. *J Biol Chem* 1992; 267: 15122–33.
47. Rubin DC, Swietlicki E, Gordon JI. Use of isografts to study proliferation and differentiation programs of mouse stomach epithelia. *Am J Physiol* 1994; 267: G27–39.

DISCUSSION

Dr. Zoppi: In a clinical situation such as celiac disease, where the crypts and villi are profoundly damaged, what happens when the cause of the damage is removed?

Dr. N. Wright: We studied this many years ago. What appears to happen is that if a patient is put on very strict gluten-free diet, within a few days the height of the enterocytes increases. Very quickly after, remodeling of the mucosa begins, with villogenesis but with reduction in crypt size and cellular output, so there is a return toward what looks like a partial villous atrophy situation. Tom MacDonald, from St. Bartholomew's Hospital in London, has been looking at the molecules involved in remodeling in celiac disease. A very active growth factor for the epithelium is keratinocyte growth factor KGF7; but, in this case, a wholesale remodeling of the connective tissue occurs, and metalloproteinases are very active at this stage as well. So when gluten is withdrawn, a condition that looks like embryogenesis ensues.

Dr. Ghoos: Has the lamina propria any role in maintaining the structure and organization of this differentiation?

Dr. N. Wright: I would say the lamina propria is of critical importance in maintaining epithelium continuity and differentiation. I showed a photograph where around each crypt is seen a very tight sheath of fibroblasts. These cells contain smooth muscle-actin, so they are really myofibroblasts. I think what probably happens is that, although the *Hox* genes are expressed in the epithelium, they will actually activate genes within the lamina propria, because the lamina propria contains cells that produce factors that act at very short range to induce differentiation within these cells. In any sort of gut cell line, differentiation can be induced; thus, when undifferentiated epithelial cells are placed onto myofibroblasts they will differentiate toward either the small bowel or colon, depending on the origin of the myofibroblasts.

Dr. Seidman: In relation to your studies of the BAG retrovirus and grafting endoderm into nude mice, we are interested in the role of cytokines in immune cell–epithelial cell interactions. Of course, in the nude mice recipient there would be very little input from the immune system, and I was wondering whether these tissues undergo normal differentiation and apoptosis.

Dr. N. Wright: Our method involves taking rat or mouse intestines at about day 10 or 11, and treating them with a proteinase and a collagenase. Then if they are incubated for a short time, the endoderm can be slid out as a kind of solid rod. If that is wrapped in type I collagen and grafted into a nude mouse, within 12 days it will differentiate into fully formed small intestine. What is interesting about it is that, although the epithelial cells come from the donor and are entirely free of any mesenchyme, the endoderm induces differentiation in the subcutaneous tissues of the nude mouse. So if rat endoderm is inserted, the epithelial cells are rat, but the lamina propria, the muscularis mucosa, and the muscularis propria are all induced from the mouse. So again, epithelial-mesenchymal interaction occurs.

The way we have used this is to take the BAG retrovirus and drive Lac-Z with the LTR, but if bigger genes were desired, a promoter could be inserted. Then, a high titer retrovirus results, and when the endoderm or isolated crypts are incubated, the result is a very stable transfection with the reporter gene. It is interesting to note that this reporter gene is not transcribed in the crypts, but it is on the villi. As cells move out of the crypt and onto the villus, intense transcriptional machinery is seen at the base of the villus. So, this retrovirus is being transcriptionally regulated by the villus epithelial cells. I think this could be a very valuable model for overexpressing cytokines, growth factors, and so forth, without going to the bother of actually making a formal overexpression transgene.

Dr. Brandtzaeg: I am confused about the gastric mucosa. Where did the parietal cell come from, and can you explain intestinization of the gastric mucosa with intestinal metaplasia?

Dr. N. Wright: A very important series of papers by Karam and Leblond (1), show how they worked out the cell lineage patterns for the gastric gland. There is certainly a stem cell there, which goes through a series of precursors before achieving differentiation. Their well-established technique—pulsing with tritiated thymidine, making thin sections, and then watching differentiation—shows with certainty that a preparietal cell goes on to become a parietal cell. They have worked out a whole lineage map. Some of the findings are surprising; for example, they showed that the chief (peptic) cells actually come from the mucous neck cells. So, the pre-neck cell goes on to give rise to a mucous neck cell, which then becomes a chief cell. This is a surprising cell lineage for me, but nevertheless, it has been worked out. So, I think that is how the parietal cells work. The only problem is that one would expect that if there was a single stem cell as seen in the intestinal crypt, gastric glands should be clonal populations. And certainly, the picture of the male/female chimera Mary Thompson published in *Development* a few years ago (2) shows that the antral glands appear to be clonal. But the recent paper by Tan in *Developmental Biology* shows that when the animals are born, most of the gastric glands have at least two populations of cells within them (3). As the animal matures, the number of mixed glands goes right down, but even at 6 months 10% of the glands are polyclonal. This means they have more than one stem cell in them, and what these cells are doing I have no idea. Whether there is some sort of reserve for damage, or whether they can perhaps undergo more fission and produce more glands, I have no idea. Looking at the polymorphisms of the human androgen receptor gene, Nomura showed in 1996 that, although antral glands are clonal, gastric glands in the fundus had this very complex clonal structure (4), as though each gastric gland had more than one stem cell in the human. So, I am beginning to believe that the gastric gland is a very complex system with multiple stem cells.

So far as intestinization goes, I have a better idea. I think what happens is that regional specification within the intestine and the stomach is via the *Hox* genes. When *Helicobacter pylori* induces atrophic gastritis, cytokines and nitrates and all manner of nasty things are produced that damage the stem cell. Mutations then occur within the stem cell, and these will occasionally be within a *Hox* gene, knocking out the *Hox* gene that makes gastric specification. The *Hox* gene that has intestinal specification may also be mutated and gain a function. Then intestinal differentiation begins. This intestinal differentiation spreads through the mucosa by a process of crypt fission, so it spreads like a carpet across the gastric mucosa. That is my hypothesis, which I think is reasonable. But I cannot explain or understand multiple stem cells in the gastric neck.

Dr. Koletzko: You suggest that the metaplasia occurring with *H. pylori* infection may trigger a mutation in the *Hox* gene and then these mutated clones expand over time. With infection clearance, this metaplasia is reversible both in the stomach and in the duodenum. Do you know anything about whether these clones disappear completely, or will they reactivate later with another trigger?

Dr. N. Wright: Approximately 14 studies have looked at whether intestinal metaplasia is reversible. Seven of these say it is, and seven say it is not. The problem in looking at the reversibility of intestinal metaplasia is its focal nature and the very small numbers of patients involved in the studies (between 7 and 12), with a follow-up time of only about 18 months. I think it is premature to say that intestinal metaplasia is reversible. It is becoming clear that in intestinal metaplasia mutations in p53, loss of heterozygosity for APC, and changes in tumor suppressor genes and oncogenes are found, even in the absence of dysplasia. If a stem cell change occurs, intestinal metaplasia should be clonal, and it should not be reversible.

Dr. Lentze: How is a balance achieved between the cell clones? Why do we not get an excess of endocrine clones or goblet cell clones?

Dr. N. Wright: I do not think anybody can answer that question. Bjerknes and Cheng found that when they gave a mutagen, ethylnitrosourea, they knocked in the DBA, and very soon they could see little goblet cell clones halfway up the crypt (5). So, they had mutated a cell which divided into two goblet cells, although these disappeared quite quickly. Far fewer endocrine cells were found, but they did find endocrine clones and columnar cell clones. Then, they also found stem cell clones, which remained in the crypt for a long period of time. So, they had actually mutated the stem cell.

So that is the model. Now, what determines lineage specification is a question which all gut stem cell biologists would like to answer. By interpolation from the bone marrow, there will be growth factors with lineage-specific functions. We cannot investigate this in the gut yet, because we do not have the equivalent long-term cultures to enable us to dissect the way in which lineage specification is done. However, an important paper just out in *Gastroenterology* describes clonal growth *in vitro* of mouse crypt epithelial cells (6). So, we may soon begin to understand what it is that actually makes this differentiation. It is very interesting that the mouse homologs of notch and delta are present in the stem cell zone of a mouse crypt. It may be that genes such as notch and delta are responsible for lineage commitment, but at present this is just hand waving. I really do not know what determines stem cell commitment within the crypt.

Dr. Yamashiro: How do M cells differentiate from crypt cells? Is there any key factor known to be involved?

Dr. N. Wright: I am the wrong person to answer that question. Can Dr. Brandtzaeg answer this?

Dr. Brandtzaeg: Two ways exist to obtain what we call an "M cell." The first is that any epithelial cell can be transformed into an M cell if it comes into contact with B cells and certain cytokines from B cells. So, that is a kind of adaptive transformation; it can acquire the function of picking up antigens and transporting them into the underlying lymphoid cells. The other way is through a special cell lineage from down in the crypt area, which can migrate up toward the tip of the dome where it undergoes apoptosis. Which is the most important pathway, I do not know. This has not been resolved.

Dr. Mansbach: I am interested in the apoptotic mechanism. What induces these cells to become apoptotic?

Dr. N. Wright: I have no idea what switches on apoptosis. It is only recently that we have begun to believe that this is an active process. Until recently, we believed that cells were moved up the escalator and just dropped off the top by a process of extrusion; there were even villus extrusion zones. Now, however, we know an active process of apoptosis occurs, although not what induces it.

Dr. Mäki: Do stem cells divide symmetrically or asymmetrically? And do we have stem cells around in the gut during our whole life?

Dr. N. Wright: Osgood laid down the principles of symmetry and asymmetry in stem cell division in 1957 (7). Asymmetry is not supposed to occur in the gut, because no mechanism exists for this, although statistically, all stem cell divisions eventually are asymmetric. What is now quite clear is that stem cell division is polarized. Each stem cell division is a polarized division giving rise to one stem cell and one daughter cell. We have no way of looking at that in the gut, but at least now we should be used to the idea that stem cells have the ability to divide asymmetrically. A hypothesis called the "immortal strand hypothesis" relates to the persistence of stem cells. The stem cells one has in the intestine at birth have to last until one dies; one is not going to get any other stem cells, so they are very important. The proposal is that when a mutation in a stem cell occurs, a mechanism exists whereby the damaged DNA is segregated into the daughter cell, which then moves away allowing the mutation to be lost. If stem cell biologists are asked about the polarity of these divisions, they will say they probably are asymmetric divisions.

REFERENCES

1. Karam SM, Leblond CP. Dynamics of epithelial cells in the corpus of the mouse stomach. Identification of proliferative cell types and pinpointing of the stem cell. *Anat Rec* 1993; 236: 269–79.

2. Thompson M, Fleming K, Evans D, Wright NA. Gastric endocrine cells share a clonal origin with other gastric cell lineages. *Development* 1990; 110: 477–81.
3. Nomura S, Esumi H, Job C, Tan S-S. Lineage and clonal development of gastric glands. *Dev Biol* 1998; 204: 124–35.
4. Nomura S, Kaminishi M, Sugiyaya K, Oohara T, Esumi H. Clonal analysis of single fundic and pyloric glands of stomach using X-linked polymorphism. *Biochem Biophys Res Commun* 1996; 226: 385–90.
5. Bjerknes M, Cheng H. Clonal analysis of mouse intestinal epithelial progenitors. *Gastroenterology* 1999; 116: 7–14.
6. Whitehead RH, Demmler K, Rochmann SP, Watson NK. Clonogenic growth of epithelial cells from normal colonic mucosa from both mice and human. *Gastroenterology* 1999; 117: 858–65.
7. Osgood EG. A unifying concept of the etiology of the leukemias, lymphomas and cancers. *J Natl Cancer Inst* 1957; 18: 155–66.

Gastrointestinal Functions, edited by Edgard E. Delvin and Michael J. Lentze. Nestlé Nutrition Workshop Series, Pediatric Program, Vol. 46, Nestec Ltd., Vevey/Lippincott Williams & Wilkins, Philadelphia © 2001.

Assembly and Disassembly of Brush Borders Driven by Villin, a Unique Bundling/Severing Actin-Binding Protein

Sylvie Robine, Evelyne Ferrary, Alexandre Lapillonne, and Daniel Louvard

CNRS UMR 144, Institut Curie, Paris, France

Digestive processes involve several organs composed of highly specialized epithelial cells. Despite a great diversity of function, all epithelial cells along the digestive tract have certain common structural and functional features. These cells display a unique organization that reflects their particular specialized roles in transport, endocytosis, or transcytosis. These functions contribute to the generation of steep concentration gradients of nutrients and electrolytes between the external and the internal milieus of the body. The ability of this epithelium to create an asymmetric chemical gradient between the fluid bathing its luminal membrane and the basolateral membrane in contact with the internal milieu can be explained by an asymmetric distribution of membrane-bound enzymes and transporting systems between these membranes. The cellular architecture that contributes to the functional polarity of these cells implies the existence of distinct domains of the plasma membrane and a specialized cytoskeletal matrix associated with membrane domains. The polarized distribution of cellular components is achieved in the course of terminal differentiation and is maintained after this event.

At their apical borders facing the external milieu, epithelial intestinal cells possess a unique organelle, the brush border. The brush border provides a greatly expanded surface that facilitates absorption of digestion products. It is composed of thousands of stiff microvilli containing bundles of microfilaments made of actin, associated with actin-binding proteins (ezrin, fimbrin, brush border myosin I, espin, and villin). Among these proteins, villin shows special features suggesting that it plays a key role in the dynamics of the brush border.

In this chapter recent advances in the understanding of the brush border assembly and the role of villin in the reorganization of this organelle are described.

ORGANIZATION OF THE BRUSH BORDER CYTOSKELETON

Proteins of the Brush Border Cytoskeleton

The brush border of absorptive epithelial cells is composed of the microvilli and the terminal web (Fig. 1). In the core of each microvillus is a bundle of 20 specialized

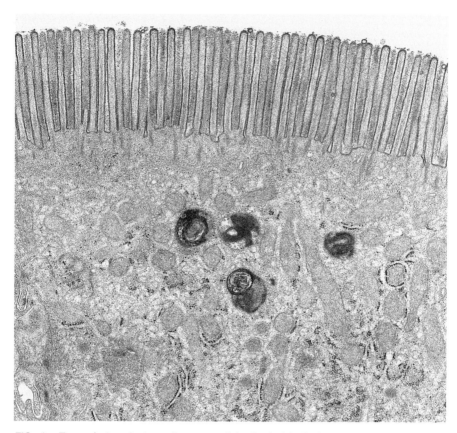

FIG. 1. Transmission electron microscopy of the luminal half of an epithelial cell of mouse small intestine, ×16,000. (Micrograph obtained from G. Pehau-Arnaudet, UMR 144, CNRS-Institut Curie, Paris, France.)

actin filaments that play a structural role, maintaining the shape of the microvillus. The (+) ends of these microfilaments point toward the site of membrane insertion at the tip of the microvillus in a dense structure that is not well characterized (1) (Fig. 2). The rootlets of the bundles are connected to the terminal web by another actin complex that also contains myosin II and nonerythroid spectrin proteins (2).

The microvillus core bundles are assembled by a specific set of proteins that are important in generating their rigid structure. Each microvillar protein belongs to a family of proteins (Table 1). Many of the component proteins have been identified and cloned, and their function *in vitro* has been studied in detail. These proteins can be classified as proteins that cross link actin filaments to form bundles (villin, I-fimbrin, and espin) or proteins that link actin filaments to the plasma membrane (brush border myosin I, and ezrin) (Fig. 2, Table 1).

The protein villin is one the major proteins that cross links the actin filaments to form bundles in a ratio of one villin molecule to 10 actin monomers. This protein,

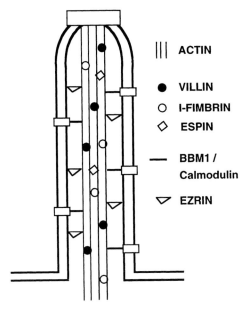

FIG. 2. Schematic localization of the major proteins of the brush border cytoskeleton.

which bundles actin filaments in a Ca^{++}-dependent manner, is described in detail below. The effect of Ca^{++} on the length of the microvillar core is thought to be physiologically important. As an actin cross-linking protein, fimbrin also forms tightly packed parallel actin bundles by binding actin filaments in a ratio of one fimbrin molecule to 10 actin monomers. Among the three isoforms of fimbrin (L-, T-, and I-fimbrin), intestinal epithelial cells express a unique fimbrin isoform, I-fimbrin (3). Espin, a recently discovered third actin-bundling protein, is estimated to be present in a ratio of one espin molecule for every 130 actin monomers (4).

Another actin-binding protein, brush border myosin I, forms in association with calmodulin the cross bridges that tether actin bundles to the inner surface of the plasma membrane. Ezrin distribution is not restricted to cells with well-organized brush borders, differing in this respect from villin, brush border myosin I, and I-fimbrin. Together with radixin and moesin, ezrin belongs to the ERM (ezrin/radixin/moesin) subfamily of the band 4.1 protein superfamily. Thus, it has been proposed that ezrin plays a role in linking the microfilaments to the plasma membrane (5).

All these proteins that are involved in the organization of the brush border cytoskeleton are highly conserved among species. They are all expressed in the brush border of mature enterocytes but have different patterns of expression during embryogenesis.

Assembly of the Intestinal Microvilli

During differentiation of the intestine, the epithelium undergoes a transition from a simple epithelium, the surface of which is sparsely covered by short and irregular

TABLE 1. *Properties of microvillar cytoskeletal proteins of intestinal cells*

Protein	Molecular weight (kd)	*In vitro* activities	Ligands	Family proteins	Localization
Villin	92.5	Capping Nucleating Severing Bundling	F/G Actin Ca^{++} PiP2	Advillin Supervillin Protovillin Quail gene product Dematin Gelsolin Severin Fragmin	Epithelial cells of the urogenital and digestive tracts
I-fimbrin	68	Bundling	F-actin Ca^{++}, Mg^{++}	L/T-fimbrin/plastin Dystrophin Spectrin/fodrin α-actinin Filamin ABP 120	Brush borders of intestinal and kidney cells
BBM1	110	Mechano enzyme	F-actin Mg^{++} ATP Phospholipids Calmodulin	Myosins Iα	Brush borders of absorptive cells
Ezrin	67	Linking the microfilaments to the plasma membrane	F-actin PiP2 CD44/rho-GDI CD43 I-CAM PKA EBP50 RhoGDI	Radixin Moesin Merlin/schannomin EM 1PTPH1 PTPase MEG Band 4.1 Talin	Epithelial cells
Espin	30	Bundling	F-actin	Espin 110 kd Forked protein	Brush borders of intestinal and kidney cells

BBMI, brush border myosin I.

microvilli, to a mature epithelium covered by the densely packed microvilli of the brush border. This morphologic change is essential for the highly efficient absorptive function of the intestine. Assembly of the brush border initially occurs during villus morphogenesis. In human fetuses, short and irregularly placed microvilli cover the epithelial cells during the late second and early third fetal months (6,7). Subsequently, short and regular microvilli fill the apical surface. Although the course of microvillus assembly has not been carefully examined in human fetal intestines, it has been studied in detail in developing mouse and chicken intestine (2). It is likely that human brush borders are generated in the same manner.

How are these different components assembled to form a microvillus? Analysis of the pattern of gene expression encoding for these proteins and of the proteins during embryogenesis and, in the adult, along the crypt–villus axis reveals that this structure is not autoassembled. Assembly of the microvillus core is strictly regulated, both spatially and temporally (8–14). All proteins are present in the cytoplasm before being localized to the apical surface of the cells. Ezrin is already produced in oocyte and is present throughout preimplantation of the embryo, long before a rudimentary gut is formed. Before compaction, ezrin is located at the cell cortex. It becomes restricted to the apical microvilli of the outer cells and remains there until after cell stages 8-16 (15). Thus, ezrin localization to the microvilli is correlated with cell polarization. During mouse embryogenesis, intestinal epithelium maturation is characterized by a transition from a thick pseudostratified structure to simple columnar cells (from embryo day 11 to day 15, depending on the intestinal segments). Ezrin has already appeared in the pseudostratified epithelium by day 10 (Fontaine JJ, personal communication, 1998). The apical localization of ezrin precedes that of villin. Villin localizes at the apex of cells when rudimentary microvilli appear on the surface at 12.5 days (8,10–13). Fimbrin isoforms are sequentially switched on and off during development (14). L- and T-fimbrin, the two nonintestinal epithelial cell isoforms, are first produced by 10.5 days. Whereas T-fimbrin is predominantly

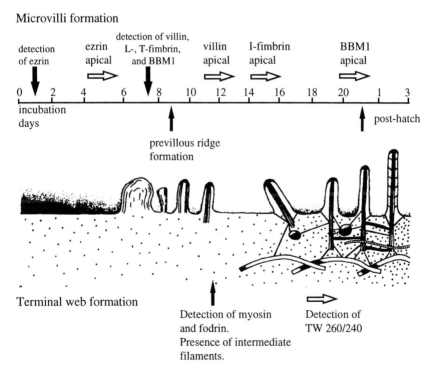

FIG. 3. Diagram depicting the major morphologic events and the time course of protein appearance during chicken brush border development. BBM1, brush border myosin I. (Adapted from Arpin M, Friederich E. Cytoskeletal components in intestinal brush border morphogenesis: an evaluation of their function. In: Fleming TP, ed. *Epithelial organization and development.* London: Chapman & Hall, 1992.)

located at the apex of the cells, L-fimbrin is found at the basal surface of the epithelial cells. I-fimbrin is synthesized at 14.5 days and has an apical localization by 16.5 days, which coincides with the appearance of well-organized microvilli and with the disappearance of L- and T-fimbrin isoforms. As a result, the rudimentary microvilli observed at the earlier stage of development are organized by villin and T-fimbrin (14). Brush border myosin I is the last of the major proteins to localize in the microvilli, which corresponds with the final maturation step of this structure (8) (Fig. 3). No data are available concerning espin during development.

ROLES OF VILLIN IN THE BRUSH BORDERS

Specific Properties of Villin

In contrast to other actin-binding proteins, villin displays original features that confer its specific properties. Villin is composed of six repeats, each containing about 150 residues, which together constitute the core domain, followed by the carboxy terminal domain, the headpiece (Fig. 4). Villin has structural features that are also found in gelsolin, scinderin, fragmin, and severin. These proteins can sever, nucleate, and cap actin filaments in a calcium-dependent manner (17). The carboxy terminal headpiece domain of villin that is not present in the other members of the family is required for actin filament bundling. This F-actin binding site is calcium independent (18–21). Recently, several proteins homologous to villin have been identified, which all contain a villinlike headpiece: supervillin (22), advillin (23),

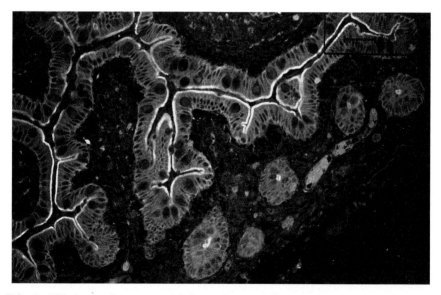

FIG. 4. Villin immunofluorescence labeling on ileum paraffin-embedded section from a 4-year-old child. The brush border at the apex of the enterocytes is heavily labeled. Notice the cytoplasmic staining in all the epithelial cells in the crypt region as well as along the villus (×200).

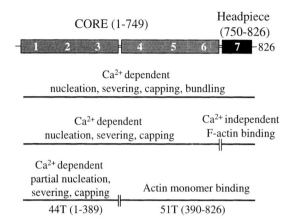

FIG. 5. Domain organization of the primary structure of villin (*filled boxes*) and *in vitro* activities of chicken wild-type villin, and villin-derived fragments obtained by limited proteolysis of villin. Repeats forming the core domain are numbered from 1 to 6. Domain 7 corresponds to the headpiece domain. Numbers given in brackets correspond to residue positions of the wild-type villin sequence. The positions of hinge regions between core and headpiece or between domains 1–3 and domains 4–7 are indicated (*black lines*). Wild-type villin caps, nucleates, severes, and bundles actin filaments in a Ca^{++}-dependent manner. Whereas the core domain retains Ca^{++}-dependent capping, nucleating, and severing activity, the headpiece binds to F-actin in a Ca^{++}-independent manner. The *in vitro* activity of the villin fragment termed "44T" (domain 1–3) is similar to that of the core with the difference that nucleating activity is highly reduced. The carboxy terminal fragment named "51T" (domains 4–7) binds actin monomers in a Ca^{++}-dependent manner (27). (Adapted from Friederich E, Vancompernolle K, Louvard D, Vandekerckhove J. Villin function in the organisation of the actin cytoskeleton: correlation of *in vivo* effects to its biochemical activities *in vitro. J Biol Chem* 1999; 274: 26751–60.)

protovillin (24), quail (25), and dematin (26). These proteins share some common properties with villin. Nevertheless, their *in vivo* properties have not been yet defined.

Villin is not a ubiquitous protein; it displays strict tissue-specific expression, restricted to epithelial cells that develop a brush border—the epithelial cells of the intestine mucosa, gall bladder, kidney proximal tubule, and testis afferens tubule. It is also present in some epithelia that lack a brush border but which are derived from embryonic gut: the duct cells of the exocrine pancreas and the biliary cells of the liver. In all these tissues, villin is concentrated in the apical part of the cell, either in the brush border or in the apical cytoplasm (Fig. 5).

Villin production has been analyzed during intestinal cell maturation. The intestinal mucosa epithelium is continually renewed during adult life, turning over every 3 to 4 days in the human. Cells migrate from the intestinal crypts to the tip of the villi. Villin can be detected in the immature precursors of the crypts, and its production increases when enterocytes differentiate during their migration along the crypt–villus axis. Thus, villin is a marker of endodermic cells in the primitive gut and later becomes a marker of intestinal differentiation.

During development, villin is already present in the visceral endoderm of the yolk sac (9). Its synthesis continues until the end of gestation. In the intestinal tube, villin is detectable as soon as the tube is formed, at which time the epithelium is composed of immature, multistratified cell layers (8,10–13,28–30). Later in development, it becomes monostratified and differentiates as villin synthesis increases and villin concentrates at the apical pole of the epithelial cells.

In Vitro Activities of Villin

Villin activities on actin polymerization and organization of actin filaments have been determined using *in vitro* assays, including viscosimetry and sedimentation methods, measurement of actin polymerization kinetics with fluorescent actin, and electron microscopic analysis. Villin contains at least three actin-binding sites, two of which are Ca^{++}-dependent and located on the core domain. The third, situated on the headpiece domain, is Ca^{++}-independent. The approximate kd values of the F-actin binding sites located in the core and in the headpiece domain are 7 μM and 0.3 μM, respectively (31). At high Ca^{++} concentrations (0.2–1.0 mM), villin severs F-actin into short filaments. The severing activity of villin is inhibited in the presence of phosphoinositol-2-phosphate (PIP2) (32). At lower Ca^{++} concentration (10–100 nM), villin caps the fast growing end of actin microfilaments, thereby preventing elongation. At the same Ca^{++} concentration, villin nucleates microfilament growth when added to actin monomers. In the absence of Ca^{++}, villin has no effect on actin polymerization but bundles actin filaments. Villin is the only member of the gelsolin family that has all four of these *in vitro* activities. Tropomyosin I, an actin-binding protein present in the terminal web of the brush border, competes with villin for the same binding site on F-actin, thereby inhibiting actin bundling by villin. Functional domains of villin have been mapped by testing the activities of villin fragments obtained by limited proteolytic digestion. The 90-kd villin core domain retains the Ca^{++}-dependent severing and capping activities but does not induce bundling of actin microfilaments. Capping activity requires the N-terminal domain (14T), whereas severing activity is retained by domains 1 and 2, and partial nucleation activity by domains 1, 2, and 3 of the core. The headpiece domain, which is required for F-actin bundling, binds to F-actin in a Ca^{++}-independent manner and has no activity on actin polymerization (Fig. 4).

A role for villin in the assembly of the microvillus core bundle has been determined by reconstitution experiments *in vitro* (33). Addition of villin and fimbrin, one of the other actin-bundling proteins associated with the microvillar core, to homogeneous F-actin is sufficient for the formation of bundles with a basic structure similar to that of the *in vivo* brush border microvilli.

Villin Functions in Transfected Cells

Villin overproduction or villin mRNA ablation in cultured cells also suggests that villin supports assembly of the actin core bundle of microvilli (34–36). Fibroblastlike cells transfected with a full-length complementary DNA (cDNA) encoding villin

(34) or microinjected with villin protein (35) are covered by long microvilli containing bundles of actin filaments to which villin is associated. Mutational analysis of villin showed that these morphologic modifications require the first half of the core, also named villin 44T, and the headpiece domain (34,37). When cells are transfected with villin cDNA and treated with low concentrations of cytochalasin D, the growth of microvilli is inhibited, suggesting that the microvillus actin filaments are not capped by villin (38). The capacity of villin to induce microvilli growth in cells correlates with its ability to bundle F-actin *in vitro* but not with its nucleating activity (39). The headpiece domain of human villin contains at its carboxy terminus a cluster of predominantly basic residues (KKEK) that is essential for the morphogenic activity of villin in transfected cells (38). Experiments *in vitro*, using a 22 amino acid synthetic peptide composed of this cluster of amino acids, have confirmed that this motif is part of an actin-binding site (38). Additional residues in the villin headpiece that define the F-actin binding site have been identified by cysteine scanning mutagenesis (40). The second repeat of the core domain (V2) is composed of a stretch of basic residues (31) that is important for the severing activity of the 44T villin subdomain (41). Substitutions of these basic residues impairs villin activity in cells and reduces its binding to F-actin in the absence of Ca^{++}, as well as its bundling and severing activities *in vitro* (39). Moreover, permanent downregulation of the endogenous villin messenger by antisense dramatically affects brush border assembly in the human adenocarcinoma cell line CaCo2. This effect is reversed by transfection with a cDNA encoding a partial sense villin RNA (36).

Role of Villin in Membrane Protein Regulation

Several observations suggest that signals originating from receptors located at the basolateral surface of cells can act on microvillar membrane proteins through cytoskeletal proteins. Such an interaction has recently been demonstrated in ileal absorptive cells after carbachol stimulation for villin, showing that villin is a substrate of tyrosine kinase (42). On binding to its basolateral membrane receptor, this cholinergic agonist inhibits Na^+ absorption and induces endocytosis of the brush border Na^+/H^+ exchanger. Activation of the muscarinic receptors leads to an increase in the calcium and diacylglycerol concentrations with the translocation of active protein kinase C and phospholipase C (PLC-γ1) onto the brush border (43–46). This process activates a tyrosine kinase. Carbachol induces tyrosine phosphorylation of a small amount of villin, which has been shown to be associated with PLC-γ1 in a detergent-soluble fraction. This suggests that villin might be implicated in the trafficking of membrane proteins such as the Na^+/H^+ exchanger through changes in actin filament organization.

IN VIVO ROLE OF VILLIN

The aforementioned structural and functional characteristics have been the origin of the efforts made to disrupt the villin gene in mice. This has been achieved by a classical homologous recombination process, inserting a neomycin resistance gene in the second exon of the villin gene. Surprisingly, these mice are viable and fertile; no obvious pathology was observed (47,48), and no digestive or general pathology was found in them up to 2 years of age. In addition, blood indices (Na, K, Cl, glucose, creatinine, proteins, cell count) were unchanged in the villin null mice (48).

The intestinal cells of these villin null mice display a brush border structure—as seen by scanning and transmission electron microscopy—that is indistinguishable from that of wild-type animals (47,48). Analysis of the crystalline hexagonal brush border structure by Fourier transform did not show any significant difference. No noticeable changes were observed in the localization and expression of the actin-binding proteins (I-, L-, T-fimbrin isoforms, espin, ezrin) of the brush border, which suggests either redundancy or compensation for the villin-bundling property. Indeed, it can be assumed that known actin-bundling proteins (e.g., I-fimbrin) are sufficient to assemble actin filaments in a well-organized structure. Alternatively, compensation can be achieved by expression of another yet unknown villinlike protein that remains to be characterized.

On the other hand, the *in vivo* severing property of villin might not be either compensated for or redundant. Our experiments support the view that villin is the major protein capable of controlling Ca^{++}-induced actin fragmentation in brush borders. We have shown that the response to raised intracellular Ca^{++} mainly differs between mutant and normal mice. In wild-type animals, isolated brush border preparations were disrupted by the addition of Ca^{++}, whereas Ca^{++} had no effect in villin null isolates. In anesthetized wild-type animals, serosal carbachol or mucosal Ca^{++} ionophore A23187 applications—both of which are supposed to increase the intracellular Ca^{++} concentration—resulted in the disappearance of F-actin phalloidin labeling. These data show that *in vivo* the Ca^{++}-dependent severing of F-actin filaments in brush borders requires the presence of villin. This F-actin disruption has also been observed in physiologic fasting and refeeding experiments. In contrast, analysis of the villin null mice using the same protocols failed to show any alteration of the F-actin labeling.

With respect to these results, pathophysiologic conditions in which actin severing might be implicated (e.g., infections, lesions, stress, or diet) remain to be investigated in detail. With this goal in mind, by giving dextran sulfate sodium (DSS) in drinking water, we have induced experimental colitis in both wild-type and villin null mice. This agent is known to cause colonic epithelial injury by modification of the intestinal flora. In wild-type animals, colonic epithelial lesions were observed in a limited area, whereas, in villin null mice, large mucosal lesions were observed. This treatment also caused a higher probability of death in mice lacking villin compared with wild-type mice (70% vs. 36% after 13 days of DSS treatment, $p = .008$).

These results (48) show that *in vivo* the bundling activity of villin is dispensable (i.e., redundant or compensated), but that villin remains necessary for the actin reorganization elicited by various signals (Fig. 6). It can be postulated that this property might be involved in cellular plasticity related to cell injury.

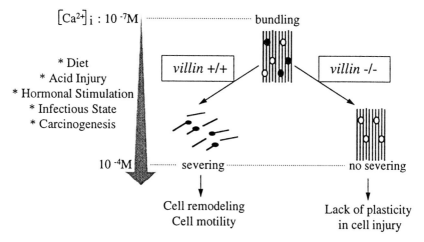

FIG. 6. Dynamics of F-actin microfilaments driven by villin in cell shape remodeling and cell motility. This diagram schematizes the possible *in vivo* consequences of villin expression considering the different states of actin polymerization and organization as a function of Ca^{++} concentration (48). At low Ca^{++} concentration, in presence or absence of villin, bundles of F-actin filaments are observed in the brush borders of enterocytes. When increased Ca^{++} concentration is achieved by physiologic or pathologic conditions, two situations are observed: (*a*) in the wild-type villin $+/+$ animal, the F-actin phalloidin labeling disappears, indicating fragmentation of actin that allows cell remodeling and cell motility; and (*b*) in the villin $-/-$ animal, the bundle of F-actin is not modified, indicating the absence of severing activity. This stable structure might be responsive for the lack of plasticity in cell injury. Filled circles, villin; empty circles, I-fimbrin; black line, actin filaments.

CONCLUSIONS

Important progress has been made in understanding the development and organization of the intestinal brush border over the last decade. However, neither the mechanism by which assembly of the brush border is carried out nor the signals initiating its formation is currently known. Microvillar cytoskeletal proteins can integrate various signals through different pathways. Changes in actin organization can modulate the activity of different membrane proteins (e.g., ion channels and exchangers). Conversely, these membrane proteins might modulate actin microfilament organization. Studies in villin null mice illustrate the importance of villin in these pathways.

REFERENCES

1. Mooseker MS, Tilney LG. Organization of an actin filament-membrane complex. Filament polarity and membrane attachment in the microvilli of intestinal epithelial cells. *J Cell Biol* 1975; 67: 725–43.
2. Heintzelman MB, Mooseker MS. Assembly of the intestinal brush border cytoskeleton. *Curr Top Dev Biol* 1992; 26: 93–122.
3. Lin C-S, Shen W, Chen ZP, Tu Y-H, Matsudaira P. Identification of I-plastin, a human fimbrin isoform expressed in intestine and kidney. *Mol Cell Biol* 1994; 14: 2457–67.
4. Bartles JR, Zheng L, Li A, Wierda A, Chen B. Small espin: a third actin-bundling protein and potential forked protein ortholog in brush border microvilli. *J Cell Biol* 1998; 143: 107–119.

5. Arpin M, Crepaldi T, Louvard D. Cross-talk between apical and basolateral domains of epithelial cells regulates microvillus assembly. In: Birchmeier W, Birchmeier C, eds. *Epithelial morphogenesis in development and disease*. Amsterdam, The Netherlands: Harwood Academic Press, 1999: 95–116.
6. Lev R. Morphological development of fetal small intestine. In: Lebenthal E, ed. *Textbook of gastroenterology and nutrition*. New York: Raven Press, 1981: 57–75.
7. Montgomery RK, Mulberg AE, Grand RJ. Development of the human gastrointestinal tract: twenty years of progress. *Gastroenterology* 1999; 116: 702–31.
8. Shibayama T, Carboni J, Mooseker M. Assembly of intestinal brush border: appearance and redistribution of microvillar core proteins in developing chick enterocytes. *J Cell Biol* 1987; 105: 335–44.
9. Maunoury R, Robine S, Pringault E, *et al.* Villin expression in the visceral endoderm and in the gut anlage during early mouse embryogenesis. *EMBO J* 1988; 7: 3321–9.
10. Maunoury R, Robine S, Pringault E, Léonard N, Gaillard JA, Louvard D. Developmental regulation of villin gene expression in the epithelial cell lineages of mouse digestive and urogenital tracts. *Development* 1992; 115: 717–28.
11. Ezzell RM, Chafel MM, Matsudaira PT. Differential localization of villin and fimbrin during development of the mouse visceral endoderm and intestinal epithelium. *Development* 1989; 106: 407–19.
12. Heintzelman MB, Mooseker MS. Assembly of the brush border cytoskeleton: changes in the distribution of microvillar core proteins during enterocyte differentiation in adult chicken intestine. *Cell Motil Cytoskeleton* 1990; 15: 12–22.
13. Heintzelman MB, Mooseker MS. Structural and compositional analysis of early stages in microvillus assembly in the enterocyte of the chick embryo. *Differentiation* 1990; 43: 175–82.
14. Chafel MM, Shen W, Matsudaira P. Sequential expression and differential localization of I-, L-, and T-fimbrin during differentiation of the mouse intestine and yolk sac. *Dev Dyn* 1995; 203: 141–51.
15. Louvet S, Aghion J, Santa-Maria A, Mangeat P, Maro B. Ezrin becomes restricted to outer cells following asymmetrical division in the preimplantation mouse embryo. *Dev Biol* 1996; 177: 568–79.
16. Arpin M, Friederich E. Cytoskeletal components in intestinal brush border morphogenesis: an evaluation of their function. In: Fleming TP, ed. *Epithelial organization and development*. London: Chapman & Hall, 1992.
17. Friederich E, Pringault E, Arpin M, Louvard D. From the structure to the function of villin, an actin-binding protein of the brush border. *Bioessays* 1990; 12: 403–8.
18. Glenney JRJ, Kaulfus P, Weber K. F-actin assembly modulated by villin: Ca^{++}-dependent nucleation and capping of the barbed end. *Cell* 1981; 24: 471–80.
19. Bazari WL, Matsudaira PT, Wallek M, Smeal J, Jakes R, Ahmed Y. Villin sequence and peptide map identify six homologous domains. *Proc Natl Acad Sci USA* 1988; 85: 4986–90.
20. Arpin M, Pringault E, Finidori J, *et al.* Sequence of human villin: a large duplicated domain homologous with other actin-severing proteins and a unique small carboxy-terminal domain related to villin specificity. *J Cell Biol* 1988; 107: 1759–66.
21. Hartwig JH, Kwiatkowski DJ. Actin-binding proteins. *Curr Opin Cell Biol* 1991; 3. 87–97.
22. Pestonjamasp KN, Pope RK, Wulkuhle JD, Luna EJ. Supervillin (p205): a novel membrane associated, F-actin-binding protein in the villin/gelsolin superfamily. *J Cell Biol* 1997; 139: 1255–69.
23. Marks PW, Arai M, Bandura JL, Kwiatkowski DJ. Advillin (p92): a new member of the gelsolin/villin family of actin regulatory proteins. *J Cell Sci* 1998; 111: 2129–36.
24. Hofmann A, Noegel AA, Bomblies L, Lottspeich F, Schleicher M. The 100 kDa F-actin capping protein of Dictyostelium amoebae is a villin prototype (protovillin). *FEBS Lett* 1993; 328: 71–6.
25. Mahajan-Miklos S, Cooley L. The villin-like protein encoded by the drosophila quail gene is required for actin bundle assembly during oogenesis. *Cell* 1994; 78: 291–301.
26. Rana AP, Ruff P, Maalouf GJ, Speicher DW, Chishti AH. Cloning of human erythroid dematin reveals another member of the villin family. *Proc Natl Acad Sci USA* 1993; 90: 6651–5.
27. Janmey PA, Matsudaira PT. Functional comparison of villin and gelsolin. Effects of Ca^{++}, KCl, and polyphosphoinositides. *J Biol Chem* 1988; 263: 16738–43.
28. Mackay D, Esch F, Furthmayr H, Hall A. Rho- and Rac-dependent assembly of focal adhesion complexes and actin filaments in permeabilized fibroblasts: an essential role for ezrin/radixin/moesin proteins. *J Cell Biol* 1997; 138: 927–38.
29. Sachs M, Weidner KM, Brinkmann V, *et al.* Motogenic and morphogenic activity of epithelial receptor tyrosine kinases. *J Cell Biol* 1996; 133: 1095–107.
30. Haarer BK, Lillie SH, Adams AE, Magdolen V, Bandlow W, Brown SS. Purification of profilin from *Saccharomyces cerevisiae* and analysis of profilin-deficient cells. *J Cell Biol* 1990; 110: 105–14.
31. Pope B, Way M, Matsudaira PT, Wedds A. Characterization of the F-actin binding domain of villin: classification of F-actin binding proteins into two groups according to their binding sites on actin. *FEBS Lett* 1994; 338: 58–62.

32. Janmey PA, Lamb J, Allenn PG, Matsudaira PT. Phosphoinositides binding peptides derived from the sequences of gelsolin and villin. *J Biol Chem* 1992; 267: 11818–23.
33. Coluccio LM, Bretscher A. Reassociation of microvillar core proteins: making a microvillar core *in vitro*. *J Cell Biol* 1989; 108: 495–502.
34. Friederich E, Huet C, Arpin M, Louvard D. Villin induces microvilli growth and actin redistribution in transfected fibroblasts. *Cell* 1989; 59: 461–75.
35. Franck Z, Footer M, Bretscher A. Microinjection of villin into cultured cells induces rapid and long-lasting changes in cell morphology but does not inhibit cytokinesis, cell motility, or membrane ruffling. *J Cell Biol* 1990; 111: 2475–85.
36. Costa de Beauregard M-A, Pringault E, Robine S, Louvard D. Suppression of villin expression by antisense RNA impairs brush border assembly in polarized epithelial intestinal cells. *EMBO J* 1995; 14: 409–21.
37. Finidori J, Friederich E, Kwiatkowski DJ, Louvard D. *In vivo* analysis of functional domains from villin and gelsolin. *J Cell Biol* 1992; 116: 1145–55.
38. Friederich E, Kreis TE, Louvard D. Villin-induced growth of microvilli is reversibly inhibited by cytochalasin D. *J Cell Sci* 1993; 105: 765–75.
39. Friederich E, Vancompernolle K, Louvard D, Vandekerckhove J. Villin function in the organisation of the actin cytoskeleton: correlation of *in vivo* effects to its biochemical activities *in vitro*. *J Biol Chem* 1999; 274: 26751–60.
40. Doering DS, Matsudaira P. Cysteine scanning mutagenesis at 40 of 76 positions in villin headpiece maps the F-actin binding site and structural features of the domain. *Biochemistry* 1996; 35: 12677–85.
41. de Arruda MV, Watson S, Lin C-S, Leavitt J, Matsudaira P. Fimbrin is a homologue of the cytoplasmic phosphoprotein plastin and has domains homologous with calmodulin and actin gelation proteins. *J Cell Biol* 1990; 111: 1069–79.
42. Khurana S, Arpin M, Patterson R, Donowitz M. Ileal microvillar protein villin is tyrosine-phosphory-lated and associates with PLC-γ1. *J Biol Chem* 1997; 272: 30115–21.
43. Donowitz M, Cohen ME, Gould M, Sharp GWG. Elevated intracellular Ca^{++} acts through protein kinase C to regulate rabbit ileal NaCl absorption. *J Clin Invest* 1989; 83: 1953–62.
44. Cohen ME, Wesolek J, McCullen J, *et al.* Carbachol- and elevated Ca^{++}-induced translocation of functionally active protein kinase C to the brush border of rabbit ileal Na+ absorbing cells. *J Clin Invest* 1991; 88: 855–63.
45. Kabsch W, Mannherz H, Suck D, Pai E, Holmes K. Atomic structure of the actin: DNAse I complex. *Nature* 1990; 347: 37–43.
46. Khurana S, Kreydiyyeh S, Aronzon A, *et al.* Asymmetric signal transduction in polarized ileal Na+-absorbing cells: carbachol activates brush-border but not basolateral-membrane PIP2-PLC and translocates PLC-γ1 only to the brush border. *Biochem J* 1996; 313: 509–18.
47. Pinson KI, Dunbar L, Samuelson L, Gumucio DL. Targeted disruption of the mouse villin gene does not impair the morphogenesis of microvilli. *Dev Dyn* 1998; 200: 109–21.
48. Ferrary E, Cohen-Tannoudji M, Pehau-Arnaudet G, *et al. In vivo*, villin is required for Ca^{++} dependent F-actin disruption in intestinal brush-borders. *J Cell Biol* 1999; 146: 819–29.

DISCUSSION

Dr. Lentze: With regard to congenital microvillus atrophy, which of these proteins might be defective in this disorder?

Dr. Robine: With the villin gene, perhaps a more subtle mutation—a point mutation or something of the kind—occurs. This would be interesting to look at now that we have a better insight of the *in vivo* function of the gene.

Dr. Nanthakumar: Villin is expressed in the crypts as well as in the microvilli; however, in patients with microvillus inclusion disease, the crypts are normal, so it seems unlikely that villin plays a role. The disease is precipitated at birth, so something happens around that time that only affects the small and large intestine. It is unlikely to be a structural defect; it must be something in the lumen rather than defective brush border assembly or defect in any other function.

Dr. Naim: When treating CaCo2 cells with villin antisense RNA, a very dramatic effect is seen on the brush border membrane. What happens to the targeting and assembly of typical brush border proteins?

Dr. Robine: We observed that sucrase-isomaltase was no longer released at the apical pore. It appeared to be retained as a vesicle in the cytoplasm of the cell.

Dr. Naim: Sorting, therefore, could depend on the presence of villin?

Dr. Robine: No way is currently available to address this question using the villin gene, because the whole structure has disappeared. From knowledge of the other proteins, it seems more likely that brush border myosin is implicated in targeting vesicular structures to the apical pole rather than the villin gene.

Dr. Büller: It was a great surprise that the villin knockout survived. There appeared to be an inflammatory response when DSS was given. What kind of inflammation was it? Was it a leaking epithelium that makes everything go wrong? You had epithelial function until the moment that the DSS was given. So villin is not important under normal conditions when the epithelium functions. But when you put stress on the epithelium, it appears to become chaotic.

Dr. Robine: We would like to analyze this type of experiment in more detail, and in particular to look at less severe lesions. This has not yet been done.

Dr. N. Wright: If villin is involved in cell migration, it would be expected to affect epithelial restitution rather than regeneration. The DDS model of colitis causes very severe damage, so if looking at restitution, which is the way in which epithelial cells move over an intact basement membrane, the correct model would be to induce, for instance, hyperosmolar damage, just to knock off some villous enterocytes and see if migration is affected.

Dr. Büller: Going back to Dr. Lentze's question, the interesting clinical aspect is those children who do not recover from infections or who have difficulty in recovering. If this is a model that functions normally until a stress of some kind is provided, then it clearly is not difficult to come up with diseases in pediatrics in which affected children sometimes do not recover from a "normal" intestinal infection. Is that because of villin that is only marginally functional? Is there any more information about whether the villin, in fact, was unable to cover the epithelium and realign it?

Dr. Robine: Not as yet.

Dr. Marini: With the very high levels of calcium in the medium and the damage that occurred, was an attempt made to lower the calcium level or to block calcium entry with a calcium blocking drug?

Dr. Robine: Such experiments have been planned, but they have not been done yet.

Dr. Alpers: The early stages of repair seem to involve the mitogen-activated protein (MAP) kinase pathway, so is villin involved in any way in the early signaling portion of this pathway? A number of cell systems have been used to study spreading and early repair where antisense mRNA could be used (1).

Dr. Robine: A very small part of villin can be phosphorylated, but up to now no data exist on how this interacts with MAP kinase.

Dr. Alpers: So other than saying that the cell might repair, how might villin be working in this situation?

Dr. Robine: This will be difficult to study in the animal directly, so two different approaches are being used. First, an attempt is being made to immortalize the cells from the knockout, and second, now Madin-Darby canine kidney (MDCK)-inducible cells are available that either express villin or do not express villin. Both approaches may allow analysis of the repair pathway.

Dr. Goulet: Have the effects described in renal tubular cells been reproduced?

Dr. Robine: Apart from a very short experiment with ischemia, the kidney has not yet been investigated. This is an interesting question and it could be useful to look at what happens in the kidney. So far, the focus of interest has been on the intestine.

Dr. N. Wright: Have migration rates in the knockout animals been examined, and are they normal?

Dr. Robine: After looking at proliferation and the numbers of crypts and villi in the normal situation with no treatment and with BrdU bromodesoxyuridine (BRDU) and so on, no major differences were detected.

Dr. N. Wright: What about the migration rate? Migration in the villus is an active process.

Dr. Robine: Perhaps that should be evaluated in more detail.

Dr. Delvin: In your model, it can be seen that villin is associated with actin, but this protein is also associated with other structural proteins. In the knockout model, are there any differences in expression of those other proteins, so as to compensate for the loss of villin which was alluded to?

Dr. Robine: This was looked into extensively, but the only difference found—and that was very small—was with espin expression. Another approach is now being pursued, which is to extract the cytosolic fraction from the brush border and to analyze the protein pattern in this, comparing wild-type with knockout. This may show that some proteins are expressed in the knockout but not in the wild-type. Perhaps this will provide a clue about how this structure is assembled in the absence of villin. But it is also possible that fimbrin or I-fimbrin is sufficient to build the brush border without needing to be overexpressed.

Dr. Ghoos: The term ''cellular plasticity'' was mentioned. Has villin any influence on tight junction structure and permeability?

Dr. Robine: There appears to be an effect. For example, in the knockout mouse, the EPEC (enteropathogenic *Escherichia coli*) infection does cross the epithelial barrier, although it is not known how, and this is not the case in normal wild-type mice. It is not known whether they cross through the tight junction because it is loosened, or whether they cross beneath the epithelial cell. But knowing this may provide some clues to the function of this gene.

Dr. Marini: Did the knockout mice die after birth?

Dr. Robine: No, these mice are viable, they reproduce, and no phenotypic effect occurs when they are reared in a normal animal house without infection or stress.

Dr. Lentze: In the antisense experiment, normal brush border enzymes or proteins do not find their way to the microvillus. In the villin knockout mouse, did they find their way into the brush border?

Dr. Robine: Yes.

Dr. Lentze: Then how do you explain the difference?

Dr. Robine: It is always a problem to explain the difference between cell culture models and the results obtained with live animals. All the cell models use cells from carcinoma cell lines and might introduce some differences; of course, in the animal all the changes that occur with development that can compensate for certain functions are found. The results clearly show that important morphogenetic effects observed *in vitro*, as has been shown for villin expression in a CV1 cell, may not affect the function of the gene *in vivo*.

Dr. Alpers: CaCo2 are not normal cells, they are cancer cells; they act like fetal ileal cells, and they are partially colonocytes.The fact that two different results occur may just mean that CaCo2 is not the right cell model.

Dr. Robine: However, it is difficult to produce an intestinal model that is not derived from colonocytes.

Dr. Alpers: That is understood, but it would be of most help if CaCo2 cells were used to study physiologic events that are actually reproduced in the *in vivo* situation; when they are not, the results are interesting, but now a CaCo2 cell is being studied!

Dr. Nanthakumar: In the experiment done with zero calcium, it was shown that in the wild-type mouse everything in the brush border disassembles, but not in the knockout mice. How was zero calcium concentration obtained? Was this experiment done with EDTA?

Dr. Robine: Yes, EDTA was used. The conditions used were strictly those used by Burgess and Prum who described vesiculization of the brush border preparation in normal animals (2).

Dr. Nanthakumar: Various studies have been done on polarized membranes and the assembly of the tight junction. When the calcium level is brought down, the cadherins disappear with the breakdown of the tight junction, but they reform when the calcium is replaced. What is surprising in your experiment is that in the knockout mice even with zero calcium everything looks as though it is completely intact in the brush border.

Dr. Robine: Let me make it clear that these experiments were done on a brush border preparation. The cells are separated from each other and there are no tight junctions.

REFERENCES

1. Dieckgraefe BK, Weems DM. Epithelial injury induces egr-1 and fos expression by a pathway involving protein kinase C and ERK. *Am J Physiol* 1999; 276: G322–30.
2. Burgess DR, Prum BE. Reevaluation of brush border motility: calcium induces core filament solution and microvillar vesiculation *J Cell Biol* 1982; 94: 97–107.

Gastrointestinal Functions, edited by Edgard E. Delvin and
Michael J. Lentze. Nestlé Nutrition Workshop Series, Pediatric
Program, Vol. 46, Nestec Ltd., Vevey/Lippincott Williams &
Wilkins, Philadelphia © 2001.

Regulation of Functional Development of the Small Intestine

N. Nanda Nanthakumar

*Department of Pediatric Gastroenterology and Nutrition, Massachusetts General Hospital,
Charlestown, Massachusetts, USA*

The gastrointestinal tract is responsible for acquisition of energy and nutrients to sustain life. The small intestine, an important tissue of this organ, is responsible for the terminal stages of digestion and absorption (1–3). Diseases that disrupt the function of this tissue are rare and usually incompatible with life. However, any disease that directly affects the gut presents a significant challenge to the physician to prevent disruption of digestion and absorption (4). If specific nutrients are not digested because of malabsorption, diarrhea ensues. Diagnosing the cause of symptoms requires a complete understanding of small intestinal function and its development.

Understanding development is important, especially for physicians caring for immature infants and adults with short bowel syndrome (4,5). Medical advances have resulted in increased survival of premature infants with an underdeveloped gastrointestinal tract (7). To ensure the survival and growth of a premature infant, special attention must be paid to nutritional intake (8). Thus, understanding the functional development of the small intestine is critical (9). The immature gut responds inappropriately when exposed to nutrients and microbes in diseased conditions such as necrotizing enterocolitis (NEC) (10). However, the use of prenatal cortisone in the prevention of hyaline membrane disease resulting from lack of lung development has also fortuitously produced significant reductions in the incidence of NEC (11,12). These observations suggest that steroids can stimulate development of the human gut. Glucocorticoids have a profound effect on all aspects of the developing gastrointestinal tract in rodent models, thereby facilitating the transition from milk to a solid food (13). Apart from precociously inducing digestive and absorptive functions, glucocorticoids are responsible for the important process of gut closure that results in the transient increase in permeability of the gut to large molecules such as antibodies and growth factors that are found in colostrum and milk (4,14,15). This is the way in which the infant acquires passive immunity from the mother. Whether steroid treatment in premature infants alters the ontogeny of this process is not completely understood at present. Thus, it is important to understand the role of glucocorticoids in normal and precocious development of the gut. Understanding the cellular and molecular mechanisms by which glucocorticoids alter functional development of the small intestine will help gastroenterologists to devise strategies to provide appropriate supplements to mother's milk or formula that will enhance the growth of the infant but will also prevent the onset of NEC. This will also help physicians care for mucosal dysfunction in trauma patients and after extensive bowel resection.

ORGANIZATION OF THE SMALL INTESTINE

Most of the final digestive and absorptive functions are carried out by the differentiated enterocytes of the small intestine (16,17). In the mature epithelium, the absorptive enterocytes make up 93% to 95% of cells (18,19). The remaining differentiated epitheliums consist of mucus-secreting goblet cells (20–22), gastrointestinal hormone–producing enteroendocrine cells (18,23,24), and defensin-producing Paneth's cells. With the exception of Paneth's cells (21,22,25,26), these differentiated cells migrate on to tonguelike projections called villi. Each villus is surrounded by a number of pitlike structures called crypts of Lieberkühn. The proliferative and undifferentiated cells reside in the crypts and they continuously supply enterocytes, goblet cells, and enteroendocrine cells to the villi (18,20,27). As cells leave the proliferative phase, they undergo cytodifferentiation in a lineage-specific manner. Thus, a continuous state of cellular proliferation, differentiation, and migration occurs along the crypt–villus axis, discussed extensively in Chapter 1 (18,20). During development, the ontogenic changes are superimposed on a constant proliferation and differentiation within this epithelium.

In adults, a single stem cell (18,21), which is located at the lower half of each crypt, produces all differentiated cells after a strict program of hierarchical proliferation (27–30). Most of the cells differentiate as enterocytes as they leave the crypts (20). The vertical migration of these cells from crypts to villi takes 2 to 3 days in adult rats and mice (31,32) and 5 to 6 days in humans (32,33). As enterocytes leave the crypts, a burst of transcriptional activation of differentiation markers occurs. However, accumulation of differentiated markers decreases as the cells migrate toward the villus tip where they undergo apoptosis (20). The nature of the stem cell and the mechanism of lineage differentiation are still a poorly understood area in intestinal epithelial biology.

Enterocytes increase their apical surface by the presence of microvilli, also known as the brush border (20,34,35). The digestive enzymes and absorptive transporters, which are anchored in the microvilli, provide an excellent tool for the study of cellular differentiation and intestinal development. Among these, the disaccharidases are widely used markers because of ease of assay and tissue specificity. The disaccharidases are lactase, sucrase, maltase, and trehalase, which are responsible for terminal digestion of carbohydrates (34,36); enzyme complexes occur, which include lactase–phlorizin hydrolase, sucrase–isomaltase, and maltase–glucoamylase (34). These enzymes are synthesized as a single polypeptide, glycosylated, anchored on the apical membrane, and cleaved by pancreatic proteases into two subunits, which remain together noncovalently as a dimeric enzyme complex (34). The disaccharidases are synthesized from a single copy gene through a single species of mRNA.

The expression of sucrase–isomaltase and lactase–phlorizin hydrolase is intestinal specific, whereas the other two enzymes are also expressed in the brush border of proximal tubules in the kidney (34).

The small intestinal mucosa displays a gradient of morphologic and functional characteristics along the duodenal–ileal (longitudinal) axis. The villus height decreases from the duodenum to ileum (20) and, consequently, the time spent by each cell on the villus before being shed decreases (31). The proliferative rate of the crypt does not change (each crypt produces on average 13–16 new cells/h) (27,28,31), but the average number of cells in each crypt decreases along the gut (18,28). Also, the number of crypts supplying each villus decreases along the longitudinal axis (28). Therefore, the surface area for absorption is maximal in the proximal gut. Morphologic differences in enterocytes along the longitudinal axis include changes in microvillus density (37) and fluidity, because of changes in the protein to lipid ratio (38). The expression of disaccharidases and other intestinal markers displays distinct gradients along the duodenal–ileal axis. Goblet cells are found with increasing frequency (39) and the Paneth's cells increase in number (21) from the duodenum to ileum. Also, various subsets of enteroendocrine cells producing peptide hormones have a distinct distribution along the length of the gut (18).

The polarized epithelium is separated by a thin continuous basement membrane from the underlying lamina propria (35,40). Both epithelial cells and the underlying fibroblasts (35,41) contribute components of the extracellular matrix. The sheet of fibroblasts present beneath the crypt epithelium proliferates and migrates along the villi in the matrix, along with the epithelium (40,42). It has been suggested that migrating subepithelial fibroblasts deposit different matrix components along the proliferative compartment and then along the differentiation compartment, and that these different matrices signal the differentiating epithelium to switch from proliferation to differentiation (43). The significance of the epithelial–mesenchymal interaction during cellular differentiation along the crypt–villus axis has been well established (35,41) and will be discussed in the next chapter.

DEVELOPMENT OF THE SMALL INTESTINE

Both in rodents and humans, the functional development of the small intestine is carried out in two phases. The first phase of maturation follows organogenesis, where the initial enterocyte-specific differentiation is established (Fig. 1). In humans, the first phase of functional development coincides with the beginning of the second trimester and in rodents just before birth. However, our knowledge of intestinal development is incomplete for the period after 22 weeks of fetal human development until birth because of a lack of access to human tissue (9,32). Fortunately, the development of the rat and mouse small intestine is well characterized, and comparisons can be made of the similarities between rodent and human gut development to illustrate salient developmental features (1,20,33). Several characteristics are functionally conserved from *Drosophila* to mice to humans (43), which should not be surprising as the genetic control of gastrointestinal development is conserved from worms to *Drosophila* to mice. However, a few differences are seen between these two mammalian species, which will be noted as the ontogeny of the gut is discussed.

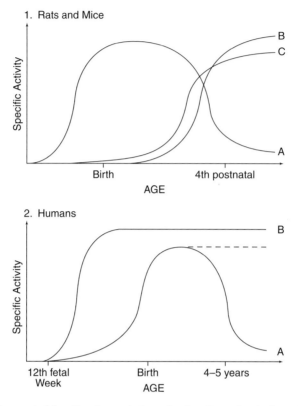

FIG. 1. Development of the digestive and absorptive functions of rodents and humans. The onset of enterocytic differentiation that results in digestive and absorptive properties of the intestinal mucosa and the resulting phenotypes is illustrated during development. (Summarized from data in references 1–4, 9, 13, 16–20.)

In rodents (rats and mice), gestation is 21 days (1,20), whereas in humans it is 40 weeks (9,32). During this period, embryonic and fetal development are completed and at birth the small intestine is ready to digest both milk and solid food in humans, but only milk (1) in rodents. Functional maturation coincides with the end of organogenesis as the epithelium becomes a polarized monolayer. As the columnar cells appear, they begin to express the first set of developmental markers (e.g., alkaline phosphatase and a few disaccharidases), initiating the first phase of functional development of the small intestine (1,16,17,44). Just before birth, in rodents and by 12 weeks of gestation in humans, well-developed crypts are formed (27,45). By the terminal stage of functional development, the crypt–villus architecture is established and the enterocytes begin to express the second set of developmental markers and the adult markers (13,16). This phase of development is initiated during the third trimester of human gestation and during the third week of postnatal development in rodents. These two phases of functional development can be defined using differentiation-specific enterocyte markers.

Disaccharidases are classical developmental markers. These enzymes provide excellent tools for delineating functional development because they can be quantified by a reproducible, sensitive assay. They are first detected by initial cytodifferentiation of the enterocytes, but the levels of disaccharidases vary according to species (29,36,40). In humans, lactase remains very low *in utero* but sucrase is very high, equivalent to levels found in infants, whereas in rodents sucrase is undetectable and lactase is raised to maximal activity. The level of maltase is low during this phase of development and reaches adult level by the terminal stage of development. However, trehalase is expressed in a similar manner to sucrase. At the end of the first phase of functional development, rodents are ready to digest and absorb only milk carbohydrates, whereas humans can digest solid food as well.

The final phase of functional development, often referred to as "terminal maturation," is initiated during the third trimester in humans and during weaning (third postnatal week) in rats and mice. In rodents, the expression of sucrase, trehalase, glucoamylase, and maltase activities increases to adult levels (13,16). At the same time, adult markers begin to establish their gradients along the duodenal–ileal axis (16,18,46). During this period, lactase activity rapidly declines to the lower levels seen in adult rodents. Terminal maturation of the small intestine temporally coincides with weaning, and the enzymatic changes reflect the adaptive processes necessary for survival of rat and mouse pups in the absence of maternal milk (16). It is apparent from this brief discussion of development that rodent animal models have been important in our understanding of late gestational changes in humans and early neonatal small intestinal development.

In mice, during the first phase of development, more than one stem cell is present in each crypt (i.e., the crypt is pluripotent). Just before the next phase of development, crypts become monoclonal (i.e., each crypt contains a single stem cell) (27,28,45, 47). However the timing of clonality and the nature of stem cells are not known in humans and may have an important significance on age viability of preterm infants in the extrauterine environment.

REGULATION OF INTESTINAL DEVELOPMENT

The transition from the first to the terminal phase of functional development is regulated by various factors. To unravel the complex mechanisms of development, extensive studies have been done in the rodent model. Owing to the inaccessibility of human tissues and an adequate model system, few data are available on human gut development. Therefore, studies from rodents are summarized in this section as a guide to presumed human gut development. The regulators of intestinal development can be either *extrinsic* (luminal) factors (e.g., amniotic fluid, diet, and microbial flora), or *intrinsic* factors (e.g., circulating growth factors such as glucocorticoids, thyroids, insulin, epidermal growth factor [EGF], and so on), intrinsic timing mechanisms (a biological clock), and epithelial–mesenchyme interactions. The roles of these possible regulators are briefly discussed below.

Extrinsic (Luminal) Factors

Mother's milk is a complex biological fluid that contains many substances including proteins such as casein, micelles, membranes, membrane bound globules, and viable cells. A complete citation of the macro- and micronutrients in milk is published in a recent review (48). However, detailed discussion of the role of the factors present in breast milk is beyond the scope of this chapter. Numerous growth factors and hormones are present in physiologic quantities (Table 1) and their roles are being defined in the context of intestinal development (4,49,50). Other factors in human milk such as lactoferrin are also helpful in modulating luminal protein digestion and maintaining an appropriate luminal pH, both processes being poorly developed in the newborn human gastrointestinal tract (51). As "knockout mice" models become available, the role of growth factors alone or in combination is being defined in intestinal development.

In rodents, terminal maturation of the small intestine coincides with dietary changes associated with spontaneous weaning of the pup. During the third week of life, the diet of the pup changes from high fat, low carbohydrate milk to low fat, high carbohydrate solid food. Therefore, the temporal relationship of the dietary changes could be a causal factor for the maturation of the small intestine. However,

TABLE 1. *Hormones and growth factors in human breast milk that may promote gatrointestinal maturation*

Hormones	Growth factors
Cortisol	Epidermal growth factor
Thyroxine	Nerve growth factor
Calcitonin	Insulin-like growth factor I
Insulin	Insulin-like growth factor II
Prolactin	Transforming growth factor-
Somatostatin	Transforming growth factor-
Fibroblast growth factor	
Melatonin	Hormone-like substances
Oxytocin	Erythropoietin
Growth hormone-releasing factor	Bombesin
Gonadotrophin releasing	Neurotensin
hormone	Vasoactive intestinal peptides
Thyrotrophin releasing hormone	
Thyroid-stimulating hormone	Others
Estrogen	Transferrin
Progesterone	Lactoferrin
Contraceptives	Prostaglandins
	Nucleotides
	cAMP
	cGMP

cAMP, cyclic adenosine monophosphate; cGMP, cyclic guanosine monophosphate.
Adapted from Sanderson IR, Walker WA. Uptake and transport of macromolecules by the intestine: possible role in clinical disorders (an update). *Gastroenterology* 1993; 104: 622–9; Xanthou M, Bines J, Walker WA. Human milk and intestinal host defense in newborns: an update. *Adv Pediatr* 1995; 42: 171–208; Koldovsky O, Thornburg W. Hormones in milk. *J Pediatr Gastroenterol Nutr* 1987; 6: 172–96.

experimental evidence is contrary to this view. When pups are prevented from weaning, the ontogenic changes that occur during the third postnatal week still occur (1,17). The conflicting data from early weaning experiments are difficult to interpret. In these experiments, pups were stressed by early weaning and as a result endogenous glucocorticoid secretion increased, which may be a potent modulator of the ontogenic changes of the gut (see below). This hypothesis was later supported by studies in which early weaning induced the maturational changes that normally occur during the third week in the intact pup but not in adrenalectomized rats (16,52). Therefore, despite the temporal relationship, it is unlikely that a primary causal relationship exists between the dietary changes of weaning and the final phase of the developing small intestine.

Other studies support the conclusion that a change in diet does not play a direct role in the terminal maturation of the rat small intestine. When sucrose was fed to artificially reared rat pups, precocious appearance of sucrase activity and increased cell proliferation was observed, but not in adrenalectomized pups (53). These results indicate that precocious induction of the artificially reared pups was caused by a stress-induced increase in glucocorticoid secretion resulting from the altered diet rather than as a direct dietary or weaning response. Studies using intestinal loop diversion from the luminal stream showed that direct changes in the luminal contact with food had no role in developmental induction of sucrase and maltase activities (52,54). Furthermore, *in vitro* studies with intestinal explants from the small intestine of suckling pups have shown no influence of nutrients in the media on the initiation of adult enzyme markers (52).

At the time of weaning, a major change occurs in the composition of microbial flora in the intestine. Thus, is it possible that the changes in microbial flora and their products could influence functional development during this period. To answer this question, experiments were carried out in germ-free rats (55,56). This study showed no difference in ontogenic changes in the small intestine when compared with conventional animals. However, developmental changes in the proliferation rate of crypt cells and migration in the adult germ-free animals were very similar to those of suckling animals. These studies suggest that changing microbial flora at the time of weaning can have a causal role in crypt cell proliferation and migration. When the germ-free animals were placed in a normal environment, gradual microbial colonization occurred in the small intestine, which was accompanied by a change in the epithelial transit time from 4 to 2 days, similar to the ontogenic changes that are known to occur during the third postnatal week (16,55–57). Therefore, maturation of the small intestine at weaning, an event similar to changes in the human at birth, is a complex process involving secondary hormonal changes and alteration in microbial flora.

Intrinsic Factors

Several intrinsic factors have been implicated as potential regulators in the functional development of the small intestine. Among these are circulating growth factors, a putative intrinsic timing mechanism, and epithelial–mesenchymal interaction. These three intrinsic factors are discussed in detail below.

Circulating Growth Factors

To establish a circulating growth factor as a candidate regulator of the developing small intestine (13) four important criteria must be satisfied: (*a*) early administration should initiate the developmental changes precociously; (*b*) the circulating level of this factor should increase just before the ontogenic changes; (*c*) this should directly induce the same maturational events *in vitro*; and (*d*) removal of the organ secreting this before its rise in the circulation should prevent the functional development of the gut.

Several factors have thus far been implicated as potential growth factors regulating the development of the rodent small intestine (1,13,17). Among these, only glucocorticoids meet all the above criteria and, thus, are discussed in detail below. The other factors that have been studied are thyroxine, insulin, gastrin, EGF, prostaglandin, transforming growth factor α (TGF-α), TGF-β, and cholecystokinin.

The pioneering work by Moog (58) initially demonstrated the role of the pituitary–adrenal axis in postnatal development of the mouse small intestine using alkaline phosphatase as a marker. Later, Doell and Kretchmer (59) identified glucocorticoids as potential regulators of developmental induction of sucrase activity in the developing rat small intestine *in vivo* and *in vitro*. Both exogenous and endogenous glucocorticoids could induce a precocious rise in various digestive enzymes and absorptive transporters in the small intestine (1,60,61). To meet the second criterion for a candidate circulatory factor modulating the ontogeny of the gut, circulating levels of free and total glucocorticoids were measured, along with jejunal lactase and sucrase activities in the same animal during the first 4 weeks of postnatal life (62). This study showed a developmental surge of circulating levels of corticosterone at the end of the second week, just 2 days before the ontogenic changes of both enzyme activities. Thus, glucocorticoids could play a role in regulating the development of the terminal maturation. *In vitro* studies, either with suckling or fetal intestinal explant cultures, confirmed that the glucocorticoids act directly on the immature intestine to elicit precocious maturation (1,16,52,61). These experiments strongly suggest that the glucocorticoids regulate the functional maturation of the small intestine. To establish the instructive role of endogenous glucocorticoids, adrenalectomy was performed in suckling animals before circulating levels of corticosterone rose (63,64). Adrenalectomy did not abolish the developmental changes that characterize the terminal maturation of the rat and mouse small intestine. However, it did retard the rate of increase of adult markers and delay the decline of lactase. This observation was in agreement with a study in which glucocorticoid antagonists did not totally abolish the changing pattern of enzyme activities during the third week (65). Therefore, glucocorticoids are not absolutely necessary for the final stage of functional development, but do play a critical role in regulating the rate of transition from one phase to another.

An attempt was made to determine the site of glucocorticoid action along the crypt–villus axis (66,67). Expression of differentiated villus enterocytes at the time of treatment was unaffected by steroids. After 24 hours, markers such as sucrase activity and mRNA were detected at the crypt–villus junction, and then, as time progressed, the activity was extended along the villi at a rate consistent with that of cellular migration. As the undifferentiated cells, in turn, differentiate and replace the villus epithelium, they begin to express adult markers such as sucrase and trehalase activity, immunoreactive protein, and mRNA (68). These results suggest that glucocorticoids act on newly divided crypt cells. However, direct action of this hormone in undifferentiated crypt epithelium has not been demonstrated. Furthermore, elegant co-culture experiments have proved the role of mesenchyme in normal and precocious glucocorticoid-induced developmental changes (see below) (35,41). Therefore, the targets of glucocorticoids could be mesenchymal cells as well (40).

The effect of glucocorticoids in suckling rodents is not confined to the small intestine, but also influences the terminal maturation of the entire gastrointestinal tract (1). Either exogenous glucocorticoids or endogenous glucocorticoids increased by corticotropin before day 10 have been shown to cause precocious induction of salivary amylase, gastrin receptor, pancreatic amylase, ileal bile salt transport, hepatic pyruvate kinase, hepatic tryptophan oxygenase, and hepatic ornithine aminotransferase, as well as to accelerate the ontogenic decline of ileal lysosomal enzymes, jejunal and ileal pinocytosis, and hepatic production of α-fetoprotein (1,16,52). Thus, glucocorticoids may act on a pathway widely used by these circulating hormones.

Glucocorticoids also play a role in changing epithelial proliferation and the migration of intestinal epithelium during the terminal phase of functional development. Crypt cell proliferation and migration, as measured by the transit time of labeled cells from the crypt to the villus tip, were dramatically increased, along with changing epithelial markers of the developing small intestine (27,31,68–70). However, these changes could be precociously induced by treatment with glucocorticoids in suckling rodents (67,68). Adrenalectomy before the rise in circulating corticosteroids prevents the developmental changes in the proliferation rate (64). Therefore, glucocorticoids play an important role not only in the terminal maturation of the digestive and absorptive function of the gut, but also in epithelial proliferation and migration. However, the mechanism by which steroids affect the cell cycle, differentiation, and migration is not known.

Noncirculating autocrine or paracrine factors may also affect the ontogeny of the intestine (13,26). New factors have been identified (71) that may play a role in human epithelial differentiation and intestinal development; however, their roles in autocrine or paracrine control of the intestinal epithelia have yet to be established (71). Direct evidence for their role in the maturation of the gut is not available because of the lack of a suitable *in vitro* system to study the developing small intestine (72,73). As *in vitro* models and human intestinal cell lines are established, the additive role of growth factors in conjunction with glucocorticoids can be determined. This information may provide a better understanding of gut development and also be used in gut repair after resection or vascular insufficiency.

An Intrinsic Timing Mechanism (a Biological Clock)

Several investigators have sought to determine the intrinsic factors controlling the terminal maturation of the rodent small intestine (74,75). Removal of endogenous glucocorticoids (in adrenalectomized animals) delays the ontogenic changes, but does not abolish them (52,63), suggesting that the timing of transition to the terminal phase of development is not dependent on hormones. To study the ontogenic changes *in vitro* was not possible, because of lack of availability of a model system (76). Explant culture is an alternative method, but such a model maintains reliable mucosal morphology only for a short period, depending on the age of the gut (74,77–80). Ménard used this model extensively to study developing gastric function and these studies will be discussed in a later chapter. As an alternative approach to determining the intrinsic capabilities of maturation in the small intestine, isograft and bypassed intestinal loops provide useful *in vivo* model systems. The studies performed using these techniques with fetal and suckling small intestine suggest that an intrinsic timing mechanism or a biological clock initiates the functional development of the gut. The existence of a "hot-wired local trigger" mechanism in the small intestine has been suggested (54) and a similar hypothesis for other intrinsic timing mechanisms has been proposed in other systems (30). However, the cellular basis and the molecular nature of this clock are unknown and remain to be elucidated.

Epithelial–Mesenchyme Interactions

The importance of epithelial–mesenchymal interactions during development and crypt–villus differentiation has been noted using various inter- and intraspecies hybrids as *in vivo* grafts or *in vitro* co-cultures (74,81). In all of these studies, functional development, as well as differentiation in response to mesenchyme, was assessed by species- and region-specific markers. The formation of the three-dimensional structure of crypts and villi was determined by scanning electron microscopy, and the timing and establishment of all cellular lineages were determined by enzyme markers.

The pioneering work by Le Douarin (82) has established the role of epithelial–mesenchymal interaction in the developing gut. Using interspecies recombinants composed of chick–rat and chick–human intestinal anlagans, a specific role for mesenchyme in epithelial differentiation and cytodifferentiation was established. Both epithelium and mesenchyme are necessary for proper development; however, the epithelium has an instructive role and the mesenchyme has a permissive role in epithelial cytodifferentiation of the small intestine. Furthermore, species-specific epithelial expression of disaccharidases indicates that mesenchyme cannot switch epithelial differentiation toward the species from which it was derived but can stimulate epithelial differentiation inherent to the epithelial species. A few exceptions, however, have been reported (81), indicating the inductive properties of small intestinal mesenchyme on heterologous endoderm derived from other parts of the digestive tract.

The proliferative sheath of subepithelial fibroblasts and their migration along with epithelium may contribute to epithelial differentiation (40). To establish a role for fibroblast cells in epithelial differentiation, experiments were carried out using an IEC-17 cell line, an immortalized, undifferentiated rat crypt epithelial cell (76). The

IEC-17 cells were then associated either with cultured submucosal fibroblast cells (35) in intact mesenchymal sheath (83), or with skin fibroblast cells previously cultured with primary epithelial cells from the intestine (43). The results clearly show that IEC-17 cells could complete cytodifferentiation with all four major epithelial cell types with enterocytes expressing differentiated markers. Furthermore, the inductive capacity of skin fibroblasts to differentiate IEC-17 cells only when previously cultured with primary enterocytes clearly establishes that the primary instructive signal originates from the epithelium. Similarly, differentiating primary crypt cells could induce fibroblasts to develop into muscle layers (83–85). However, the IEC-17 cells do not differentiate when cultured alone or with untreated skin fibroblasts, suggesting that these cells have the capability to differentiate only if they are co-cultured in a proper environment and with mesenchymal cells.

As stated, glucocorticoids are well established as a factor in the development of the gut. When intact or heterologous epithelial and mesenchymal recombinants were grafted in a poor hormonal environment (chicken embryo), development was arrested at the first phase (86), whereas complete maturation was observed when they were grafted into the strong hormonal environment of the adult rat (87). Furthermore, hybrid intestine in co-culture experiments showed similar results when the *in vitro* culture medium was supplemented with glucocorticoids (86), suggesting that their action may be mediated through epithelial–mesenchymal interactions. However, no direct evidence exists for the site of action of glucocorticoids in the functional maturation of small intestine.

On the basis of these studies, it has been suggested that the mesenchymal cells are the actual mediators of glucocorticoid action. As endodermal cells are not capable of differentiating in the absence of corresponding mesenchymal cells, it is difficult to delineate the actual mechanism. It has been postulated that glucocorticoids may affect cell-to-cell communication through the extracellular matrix components (43) or through soluble factors that activate surface receptors (88,89). When intestinal cells were cultured appropriately with mesenchymal cells of different species, the expression of enterocyte-specific markers and hormonal responsiveness appeared to be independent of the mesenchymal origin (74), suggesting that the dominant signal has to be intrinsic to the epithelium.

The mechanism by which the mesenchyme is able to transmit signals to the epithelium remains to be determined. Changes in receptor expression for the extracellular matrix components on epithelial cells are another possible explanation for the regulating mesenchymal influence. Currently, several investigators have begun to show evidence for a crucial change in the extracellular matrix during postnatal development (76,90–94). The mesenchymal interaction could also be mediated by (*a*) an "epithelial signal" inducing the formation of receptors in the adjacent mesenchyme, as demonstrated in the mammary gland (95); (*b*) production of one or more factors which, in turn, trigger a response in the epithelial cells, as in the fetal lung (96) or fetal liver (97); or (*c*) a combination of both types of signaling mechanism. Even a putative biological clock, responsible for the precise events leading to final maturation, could be one of these signals, rather than being a cellular component of specific tissue.

Various recent studies may have shed light on mediators of epithelial–mesenchymal interaction. The soluble protein "sonic hedgehog" (shh) is expressed by the endodermal cells (88) and determines positional information along the anteroposterior (AP) axis of the developing embryonic gut (89,98), except for the region that is destined to be pancreas. These secreted proteins induce BMP-4 (a member of the TGF-β family), which is implicated in the proper development of visceral mesoderm (89), and members of the Abd-B class of *Hox* genes (known regulators of body pattern) in the surrounding mesoderm of the mid- and hindgut (99). BMP-4 is a another soluble factor, and its inappropriate expression in the foregut mesenchyme may convert foregut into midgut development (89). However, the role of these factors in glucocorticoid-mediated intestinal development is not known. From the information presently available, the initiation of these markers or of hormonal action could either be manifested directly by factors such as shh at the epithelial cells (which appear to have an instructive property), or when cultured with appropriate mesenchyme or factors such as BMP-4 at the mesenchymal cells (which seem to play a permissive role), or by a combination of both in the development of the gut. Elucidation of molecular action of shh, BMP-4, and various *Hox* genes provides a better understanding of the role of mesenchymal–epithelial interaction in developing small intestine. SMADs are cytosolic proteins responsible for the signal transduction of BMP-4 and other factors involved in TGF-β signaling (72,100), and the *Smad* gene has been shown to be a tumor suppressor gene in colon and pancreatic cancer (73,100). Therefore, understanding the mechanism of epithelial–mesenchymal interaction in gut development may lead to prevention of the premalignant state or to the identification of early cancer markers for gut malignancy.

In the investigations of intestinal differentiation or development, the lack of a suitable *in vitro* system has severely hampered any further understanding of the role of mesenchyme at the molecular level. However, new techniques such as immortalized, nonmalignant human cell lines may help answer this question.

SUMMARY AND CONCLUSIONS

The current understanding of morphologic appearance and cytodifferentiation of the intestinal epithelium and the development of the small intestine have been summarized in this chapter. The development of the human gastrointestinal tract may be different from the extensively studied rodent model. However, emphasis has been on the similarity between rodents and humans, so that studies in animal models could be correlated with the developing human small intestine, or at least provide a starting point to begin *in vitro* studies in human intestinal models (cell lines, organ culture, and so on). This review was purposefully devoted only to the functional development of the gut. Another important aspect of the gut ontogeny is the development of mucosal immunity, which is extensively reviewed elsewhere (10,14,101, 102), and in a subsequent chapter by Brandtzaeg in this text.

The morphologic and functional development of the small intestine is divided into two distinct phases, and some of the factors important for these developmental changes are currently being elucidated in gene knockout mice models. As these ontogenic programs are conserved from worms to insects to mice (103), it is likely that some of the fundamental components will be the same in human development as well. Knowledge of the function of these important genes will be critical for the treatment of early preterm infants with digestive disorders and adults after extensive bowel resection. As the survival of humans depends on the proper function of the gut, the care of disrupted function in the intestine of a child or an adult will depend on the developing knowledge of the gastrointestinal tract. A better understanding of development will also help in our approach to identifying the premalignant state and malignant degeneration.

ACKNOWLEDGMENTS

I thank the members of the Developmental Gastroenterology Laboratory for their encouragement during the course of the work and Dr. Nancy Lewis for critically reading the manuscript. This work was supported by the NIH Grants R37 HD-12437, HD-31852, and PO31 DK-33506, and a pilot feasibility study by the Center for the Study of Inflammatory Bowel Disease at Massachusetts General Hospital.

REFERENCES

1. Henning SJ. Functional development of the gastrointestinal tract. In: Johnson LR, ed. *Physiology of the gastrointestinal tract*, 2nd ed. New York: Raven Press, 1987: 285–300.
2. Koldovsky O. Ontogeny of digestion and absorption as related to perinatal changes in food composition of the infants. *Acta Paediatr Suppl* 1989; 35: 7–12.
3. Lebenthal E, Leung Y-K. Alternative pathways of digestion and absorption in the newborn. In: Lebenthal E, ed. *Textbook of gastroenterology and nutrition in infancy*, 2nd ed. New York: Raven Press, 1989: 3–7.
4. Sanderson IR, Walker WA. Uptake and transport of macromolecules by the intestine: possible role in clinical disorders (an update). *Gastroenterology* 1993; 104: 622–9.
5. Scolapio JS, Fleming CR. Short bowel syndrome. *Gastroenterol Clin North Am* 1998; 27: 467–79.
6. Lykins TC, Stockwell J. Comprehensive modified diet simplifies nutrition management of adults with short-bowel syndrome. *J Am Diet Assoc* 1998; 98: 309–15.
7. Marchand V, Baker SS, Baker RD. Enteral nutrition in the pediatric population. *Gastrointest Endosc Clin N Am* 1998; 8: 669–703.
8. Redel CA, Shulman RJ. Controversies in the composition of infant formulas. *Pediatr Clin North Am* 1994; 41: 909–24.
9. Grand RJ, Watkins JB, Torti FM. Development of the human gastrointestinal tract. A review. *Gastroenterology* 1976; 70: 790–810.
10. Insoft RM, Sanderson IR, Walker WA. Development of immune function in the intestine and its role in neonatal diseases. *Pediatr Clin North Am* 1996; 43: 551–71.
11. Bauer CR, Morrison JC, Poole WK, *et al.* A decreased incidence of necrotizing enterocolitis after prenatal glucocorticoid therapy. *Pediatrics* 1984; 73: 682–8.
12. Israel EJ. Neonatal necrotizing enterocolitis, a disease of the immature intestinal mucosal barrier. *Acta Paediatr Suppl* 1994; 396: 27–32.
13. Henning SJ, Rubin DC, Shulman RJ. Ontogeny of the intestinal mucosa. In: Johnson LR, ed. *Physiology of the gastrointestinal tract*, 3rd ed. New York: Raven Press, 1994: 571–610.
14. Neutra MR. Current concepts in mucosal immunity. V. Role of M cells in transepithelial transport of antigens and pathogens to the mucosal immune system. *Am J Physiol* 1998; 274: G785–91.
15. Teichberg S, Wapnir RA, Moyse J, Lifshitz F. Development of the neonatal rat small intestinal

barrier to nonspecific macromolecular absorption. II. Role of dietary corticosterone. *Pediatr Res* 1992; 32: 50–7.

16. Henning SJ. Postnatal development: coordination of feeding, digestion, and metabolism. *Am J Physiol* 1981; 241: G199–214.

17. Traber PG, Wu GD. Intestinal development and differentiation. In: Rustgi AK, ed. *Gastrointestinal cancers: biology, diagnosis and therapy*. Philadelphia: Lippincott-Raven, 1995: 21–43.

18. Gordon JI. Intestinal epithelial differentiation: new insights from chimeric and transgenic mice. *J Cell Biol* 1989; 108: 1187–94.

19. Cheng H, Leblond CP. Origin, differentiation and renewal of the four main epithelial cell types in the mouse small intestine. I. Columnar cell. *Am J Anat* 1974; 141: 461–80.

20. Leblond CP. Life history of cells in renewing systems. *Am J Anat* 1981; 160: 113–58.

21. Ouellette AJ, Greco RM, James M, *et al.* Developmental regulation of cryptdin, a corticostatin/defensin precursor mRNA in mouse small intestinal crypt epithelium. *J Cell Biol* 1989; 108: 1687–95.

22. Cheng H. Origin, differentiation and renewal of the four main epithelial cell types in the mouse small intestine. II. Mucous cell. *Am J Anat* 1974; 141: 481–502.

23. Cheng H, Leblond CP. Origin, differentiation and renewal of the four main epithelial cell types in the mouse small intestine. III. Entero-endocrine cell. *Am J Anat* 1974; 141: 503–20.

24. Solica E, Capella C, Buffa R, *et al.* Endocrine cells of the digestive system. In: Johnson LR, ed. *Physiology of the gastrointestinal tract*, 2nd ed. New York: Raven Press, 1987: 111–30.

25. Chwalinski S, Potten CS, Evans G. Double labelling with bromodeoxyuridine and [^{3}H]-thymidine of proliferative cells in small intestinal epithelium in steady state and after irradiation. *Cell Tissue Kinetics* 1988; 21: 317–29.

26. Podolsky DK. Peptide growth factors and regulation of growth in the gastrointestinal tract. In: Rustgi AK, ed. *Gastrointestinal cancers: biology, diagnosis and therapy*. Philadelphia: Lippincott-Raven, 1995: 45–64.

27. Wright NA, Alison M. *The biology of the epithelial cell population*. Oxford: Clarendon Press, 1984.

28. Potten CS, Loeffler M. A comprehensive model of the crypts of the small intestine of the mouse provides insight into the mechanisms of cell migration and the proliferation hierarchy. *J Theor Biol* 1987; 127: 381–91.

29. Meinzer HP, Sandblad B. Evidence for cell generation controlled proliferation in the small intestinal crypt. *Cell Tissue Kinetics* 1986; 19: 581–90.

30. Wood WG, Bunch C, Kelly S, Gunn Y, Breckon G. Control of haemoglobin switching by a developmental clock? *Nature* 1985; 313: 320–3.

31. Klein RM, McKenzie JC. The role of cell renewal in the ontogeny of the intestine. I. Regulation of cell proliferation in adult, fetal, and neonatal intestine. *J Pediatr Gastroenterol Nutr* 1983; 2: 10–43.

32. Lipkin M. Proliferation and differentiation of normal and diseased gastrointestinal cells. In: Johnson LR, ed. *Physiology of the gastrointestinal tract*, 2nd ed. New York: Raven Press, 1987: 255–84.

33. Klein RM, McKenzie JC. The role of cell renewal in the ontogeny of the intestine. II. Regulation of cell proliferation in adult, fetal, and neonatal intestine. *J Pediatr Gastroenterol Nutr* 1983; 2: 204–28.

34. Semenza G. Anchoring and biosynthesis of stalked brush border membrane proteins: glycosydase and peptidase of enterocytes and renal tubuli. *Annu Rev Cell Biol* 1986; 2: 255–313.

35. Haffen K, Kedinger M, LaCroix B. Cytodifferentiation of the intestinal villus epithelium. In: Desnuelle P, Sjostrom H, Noren O, eds. *Molecular and cellular basis of digestion*. Amsterdam: Elsevier, 1986: 311–22.

36. Hauri H-P. Biosynthesis and transport of plasma membrane glycoproteins in the rat intestinal epithelial cell: studies with sucrase-isomaltase. In: *Brush border membranes*. London: Pitman Books (Ciba Foundation Symposium 95), 1983: 132–49.

37. Kurokawa M, Lynch K, Podolsky DK. Effects of growth factors on an intestinal epithelial cell line: transforming growth factor β inhibits proliferation and stimulates differentiation. *Biochem Biophys Res Commun* 1987; 142: 775–82.

38. Brasitus TA, Dudeja PK, Dahiya R, Halline A. Dexamethasone induced alterations in lipid composition and fluidity of rat proximal-small-intestinal brush-border membranes. *Biochem J* 1987; 248: 455–61.

39. Neutra MR, Forstner JF. Gastrointestinal mucus: synthesis, secretion, and function. In: Johnson LR, ed. *Physiology of the gastrointestinal tract*, 2nd ed. New York: Raven Press, 1987: 975–1009.

40. Marsh MN, Trier JS. Morphology and cell proliferation of subepithelial fibroblasts in adult mouse jejunum. II. Radioautographic studies. *Gastroenterology* 1974; 67: 636–45.
41. Kedinger M, Simon-Assmann P, Bouziges F, Haffen K. Epithelial-mesenchymal interactions in intestinal epithelial differentiation. *Scand J Gastroenterol* 1988; 23 (suppl 151): 62–9.
42. Parker FG, Barnes EN, Kaye GI. The pericryptal fibroblast sheath. IV. Replication, migration, and differentiation of the subepithelial fibroblasts of the crypt and villus of the rabbit jejunum. *Gastroenterology* 1974; 67: 607–21.
43. Simon-Assmann P, Bouziges F, Arnold C, Haffen K, Kedinger M. Epithelial-mesenchymal interactions in the production of basement membrane components in the gut. *Development* 1988; 102: 339–47.
44. Quaroni A, Isselbacher KJ. Study of intestinal cell differentiation with monoclonal antibodies to intestinal cell surface components. *Dev Biol* 1985; 111: 267–79.
45. Potten CS, Morris RJ. Epithelial stem cells *in vivo*. *J Cell Sci Suppl* 1988; 10: 45–62.
46. Gordon JI, Hermiston ML. Differentiation and self-renewal in the mouse gastrointestinal epithelium. *Curr Opin Cell Biol* 1994; 6: 795–803.
47. Gordon JI, Schmidt GH, Roth KA. Studies of intestinal stem cells using normal, chimeric, and transgenic mice. *FASEB J* 1992; 6: 3039–50.
48. Picciano MF. Human milk: nutritional aspects of a dynamic food. *Biol Neonate* 1998; 74: 84–93.
49. Xanthou M, Bines J, Walker WA. Human milk and intestinal host defense in newborns: an update. *Adv Pediatr* 1995; 42: 171–208.
50. Koldovsky O, Thornburg W. Hormones in milk. *J Pediatr Gastroenterol Nutr* 1987; 6: 172–96.
51. Britton JR, Koldovsky O. Corticosteroid increases gastrointestinal luminal proteolysis in suckling rats. *Biol Neonate* 1988; 54: 330–8.
52. Koldovsky O. Hormonal and dietary factors in the development of digestion and absorption. In: Winick M, ed. *Nutrition and development*. New York: John Wiley & Sons, 1972: 135–200.
53. Yeh K-Y, Yeh M, Holt PR. Hormonal regulation of adaptive intestinal growth in artificially reared pups. *Am J Physiol* 1987; 253: G802–8.
54. Diamond JM. Hard-wired local triggering of intestinal enzyme expression. *Nature* 1986; 324: 408.
55. Reddy BS, Wostmann BS. Intestinal disacchridases activities in growing germ-free and conventional rats. *Arch Biochem Biophys* 1966; 113: 609–16.
56. Bry L, Falk PG, Midtvedt T, Gordon JI. A model of host-microbial interactions in an open mammalian ecosystem. *Science* 1996; 273: 1380–3.
57. Chu SW, Walker WA. Developmental changes in the activities of sialyl- and fucosyltransferases in rat small intestine. *Biochim Biophys Acta* 1986; 883: 496–500.
58. Moog F. The functional differentiation of the small intestine. III. Influence of the pituitary-adrenal system on the differentiation of phosphatase in the duodenum of the suckling mouse. *J Exp Zool* 1953; 124: 329–46.
59. Doell RG, Kretchmer N. Intestinal invertase: precocious development of activity after injection of hydrocortisone. *Science* 1964; 143: 42–4.
60. Galand G. Brush border membrane sucrase-isomaltase, maltase-glucoamylase and trehalase in mammals. Comparative development, effects of glucocorticoids, molecular mechanisms, and phylogenetic implications. *Comp Biochem Physiol* 1989; 94B: 1–11.
61. Buddington RK, Diamond JM. Ontogenetic development of intestinal nutrient transporters. *Annu Rev Physiol* 1989; 51: 601–19.
62. Henning SJ. Plasma concentrations of total and free corticosterone during development in the rat. *Am J Physiol* 1978; 235: E451–6.
63. Martin GR, Henning SJ. Enzymic development of the small intestine: are glucocorticoids necessary? *Am J Physiol* 1984; 246: G695–9.
64. Yeh K-Y, Moog F. Influence of the thyroid and adrenal glands on the growth of the intestine of the suckling rat, and on the development of intestinal alkaline phosphatase and disaccharidase activities. *J Exp Zool* 1977; 200: 337–48.
65. Galand G. Effect of antiglucocorticoid (RU-38486) on hydrocortisone induction of maltase-glucoamylase, sucrase-isomaltase and trehalase in brush border membranes of suckling rats. *Experentia* 1988; 44: 516–18.
66. Henning SJ, Helman TA, Kretchmer N. Studies on normal and precocious appearance of jejunal sucrase in suckling rats. *Biol Neonate* 1975; 26: 249–62.
67. Herbst JJ, Koldovsky O. Cell migration and cortisone induction of sucrase activity in jejunum and ileum. *Biochem J* 1972; 126: 471–6.

68. Nanthakumar NN, Henning SJ. Ontogeny of sucrase-isomaltase gene expression in rat intestine: responsiveness to glucocorticoids. *Am J Physiol* 1993; 264: G306–11.
69. Koldovsky O, Sunshine P, Kretchmer N. Cellular migration of intestinal epithelia in suckling and weaned rats. *Nature* 1966; 212: 1389–90.
70. Yeh K-Y. Cell kinetics in the small intestine of suckling rats. I. Influence of hypophysectomy. *Anat Rec* 1977; 188: 69–76.
71. Walters JR, Howard A, Rumble HE, *et al.* Differences in expression of homeobox transcription factors in proximal and distal human small intestine. *Gastroenterology* 1997; 113: 472–7.
72. Kawabata M, Imamura T, Miyazono K. Signal transduction by bone morphogenetic proteins (BMP). *Cytokine Growth Factor Rev* 1998; 9: 49–61.
73. Riggins GJ, Kinzler KW, Vogelstein B, Thiagalingam S. Frequency of Smad gene mutations in human cancers. *Cancer Res* 1997; 57: 2578–80.
74. Kedinger M, Lefebvre O, Duluc I, Freund JN, Simon-Assmann P. Cellular and molecular partners involved in gut morphogenesis and differentiation. *Phil Trans R Soc Lond B Biol Sci* 1998; 353: 847–56.
75. Yeh K-Y, Holt PR. Ontogenic timing mechanism initiates the expression of rat intestinal sucrase activity. *Gastroenterology* 1986; 90: 520–6.
76. Quaroni, A. Development of fetal rat intestine in organ and monolayer culture. *J Cell Biol* 1985; 100: 1611–22.
77. Menard D, Corriveau L, Arsenault P. Differential effects of epidermal growth factor and hydrocortisone in human fetal colon. *J Pediatr Gastroenterol Nutr* 1990; 10: 13–20.
78. Menard D, Arsenault P, Pothier P. Biologic effects of epidermal growth factor in human fetal jejunum. *Gastroenterology* 1988; 94: 656–63.
79. Perr H, Oh P, Johnson D. Developmental regulation of transforming growth factor β–mediated collagen synthesis in human intestinal muscle cells. *Gastroenterology* 1996; 110: 92–101.
80. Foltzer-Jourdainne C, Raul F. Effect of epidermal growth factor on the expression of digestive hydrolases in the jejunum and colon of newborn rats. *Endocrinology* 1990; 127: 1763–9.
81. Haffen K, Kedinger M, Simon-Assmann P. Mesenchyme-dependent differentiation of epithelial progenitor cells in the gut. *J Pediatr Gastroenterol Nutr* 1987; 6: 14–23.
82. Le Douarin N. Etude experimentale de l'organogenese du tube digestif et du foie chez l'embryon de poulet. *Bull Biol Fr Belg* 1964; 98: 543–676.
83. Kedinger M, Simon-Assmann PM, Lacroix B, *et al.* Fetal gut mesenchyme induces differentiation of cultured intestinal endodermal and crypt cells. *Dev Biol* 1986; 113: 474–83.
84. Kedinger M, Simon-Assmann P, Bouziges F, *et al.* Smooth muscle actin expression during rat gut development and induction in fetal skin fibroblastic cells associated with intestinal embryonic epithelium. *Differentiation* 1990; 43: 87–97.
85. Del Buono R, Fleming KA, Morey AL, Hall PA, Wright NA. A nude mouse xenograft model of fetal intestine development and differentiation. *Development* 1992; 114: 67–73.
86. Lacroix B, Kedinger M, Simon-Assmann PM, Haffen K. Enzymatic response to glucocorticoids of the chick intestinal endoderm associated with various mesenchymal cell types. *Biol Cell* 1985; 54: 235–40.
87. Kedinger M, Simon-Assmann P, Alexandre E, Haffen K. Importance of a fibroblastic support for *in vitro* differentiation of intestinal endodermal cells and for their response to glucocorticoids. *Cell Differ* 1987; 20: 171–82.
88. Apelqvist A, Ahlgren U, Edlund H. Sonic hedgehog directs specialised mesoderm differentiation in the intestine and pancreas. *Curr Biol* 1997; 7: 801–4.
89. Roberts DJ, Smith DM, Goff DJ, Tabin C. Epithelial-mesenchymal signaling during the regionalization of the chick gut. *Development* 1998; 125: 2791–801.
90. Beaulieu JF. Extracellular matrix components and integrins in relationship to human intestinal epithelial cell differentiation. *Prog Histochem Cytochem* 1997; 31: 1–78.
91. Simon-Assmann P, Bouziges F, Freund JN, Perrin-Schmitt F, Kedinger M. Type IV collagen mRNA accumulates in the mesenchymal compartment at early stages of murine developing intestine. *J Cell Biol* 1990; 110: 849–57.
92. Simon-Assmann P, Kedinger M, De Arcangelis A, Rousseau V, Simo P. Extracellular matrix components in intestinal development. *Experientia* 1995; 51: 883–900.
93. Desloges N, Simoneau A, Jutras S, Beaulieu JF. Tenascin may not be required for intestinal villus development. *Int J Dev Biol* 1994; 38: 737–9.

94. Beaulieu JF, Vachon PH, Chartrand S. Immunolocalization of extracellular matrix components during organogenesis in the human small intestine. *Anat Embryol (Berl)* 1991; 183: 363–9.

95. Ferguson A, Gerskowitch VP, Russell RI. Pre- and post-weaning disaccharidase patterns in isografts of fetal mouse intestine. *Gastroenterology* 1973; 64: 292–7.

96. Smith BT, Sabry K. Glucocorticoid-thyroid synergism in lung maturation: a mechanism involving epithelial-mesenchymal interaction. *Proc Natl Acad Sci USA* 1983; 80: 1951–4.

97. Dow K, Sabry EK, Smith BT. Evidence for epithelial-mesenchymal interactions mediating glucocorticoid effects in developing chick liver. *Cell Tissue Res* 1983; 231: 83–91.

98. Staehling-Hampton K, Hoffmann FM, Baylies MK, Rushton E, Bate M. dpp Induces mesodermal gene expression in *Drosophila*. *Nature* 1994; 372: 783–6.

99. Sekimoto T, Yoshinobu K, Yoshida M, *et al.* Region-specific expression of murine *Hox* genes implies the *Hox* code-mediated patterning of the digestive tract. *Genes Cells* 1998; 3: 51–64.

100. Zhang Y, Musci T, Derynck R. The tumor suppressor *Smad*4/DPC 4 as a central mediator of *Smad* function. *Curr Biol* 1997; 7: 270–6.

101. Spencer J, MacDonald T. Ontogeny of human mucosal immunity. In: MacDonald T, ed. *Ontogeny of the immune system of the gut.* Boca Raton: CRC Press, 1990: 23–41.

102. Trier JS. Structure and function of intestinal M cells. *Gastroenterol Clin North Am* 1991; 20: 531–47.

103. Simon TC, Gordon JI. Intestinal epithelial cell differentiation: new insights from mice, flies and nematodes. *Curr Opin Genet Dev* 1995; 5: 577–86.

DISCUSSION

Dr. Zoppi: Two lactases are found in the human intestinal tract. One is a specific β-galactosidase and the second is a nonspecific esterase. Were you talking about the first or the second?

Dr. Nanthakumar: The first. We use a specific inhibitor that will inhibit lysosomal lactase and we can then assay for the specific activity of the β-galactosidase.

Dr. Büller: In looking at the grafted intestine for 10 to 12 months, what happened to the lactase? It should have come down if it is hardwired. You have a lovely experiment to show that.

Dr. Nanthakumar: In human intestine, however, it takes 2 to 3 years for lactase to come down.

Dr. Büller: If the experiment is done with rat intestine, what would happen?

Dr. Nanthakumar: The lactase will come down. When fetal rat or mouse tissue is grafted in the gut, it first expresses lactase but then when the sucrase comes up, the lactase goes down.

Dr. Naim: Did you look at the biosynthesis and structural features of lactase in these human xenografts, as compared with the normal situation?

Dr. Nanthakumar: We are getting started on this, but mice are small, so only a very small amount of tissue is in the graft. At the moment, our success rate is approximately 50% to 70%. We are putting all our efforts in maximizing the success rate so we can do better experiments. We are also trying to use immunocompromised rats, which can accommodate much larger amounts of tissue and which withstand the surgery better. At the moment, we are concentrating on the method, although your question is one of the things we would eventually like to explore.

Dr. Naim: Only small explants are needed for these experiments—not very much material.

Dr. Ménard: Have you had the opportunity to look at the response of the human xenograft to glucocorticoids or growth factors?

Dr. Nanthakumar: We are doing these experiments at the moment. We are not yet in a position to report on this, but it looks as though glucocorticoids may have a primary effect on lactase expression.

Dr. Lentze: In xenografts, you have a model where the pieces of gut are completely deprived of luminal factors. So you have a model with zero luminal influence, but the clock of development is still ticking. Did you try to manipulate the mice in any way, such as fasting or overfeeding, to trigger other events in these xenografts?

Dr. Nanthakumar: We are at the moment trying to see if specific bacterial toxins or nutrients placed in the xenograft lumen have an effect on any of the markers we have been following. We are certainly thinking along the lines you suggest.

Dr. Marini: In the human preterm baby, a difference is seen if glucocorticoids are given before birth or a few days after birth. Before birth, a clear reduction is seen in enterocolitis; after birth, there may be risk of harm. It is clear that even in normal mice or rats, steroid use accelerates maturation. Is the effect the same if they are given before birth or after birth? Have you any experience with this in your model?

Dr. Nanthakumar: Our data suggest that if they are given at a time corresponding to prenatal administration, they will accelerate gut maturation, but we are only looking at a very limited number of markers. We need to look at a number of different transporters, immune functions, and other factors before making any statement about what is likely to be happening in the human gut.

Dr. Marini: Another problem is one of nutrition. These animals are fed with natural milk, which contains many factors that can affect the gut, not only nutrients but stimulating factors.

Dr. Nanthakumar: Indeed, growth factors found in milk have been implicated in the maturation of the gut. We are in the process of analyzing some of these at present.

Dr. N. Wright: You told us that 5′-bromodeoxyuridine (BrdU) inhibited the precocious action of glucocorticoids but stimulated normal development. What is the mechanism of that? Is it related to the mutagenic action of BrdU?

Dr. Nanthakumar: Developmental change in organs such as liver or pancreas is superimposed on differentiation in the small intestine. For example, pancreatic amylase is turned on in the differentiated cell itself, whereas in the small intestine, even in the suckling animal, the epithelial differentiation program results in the suckling animal turning on lactase and not sucrase. As the development progresses, however, the differentiation program itself is switched on and it now expresses high sucrase and low lactase. When glucocorticoids are given, it takes 24 hours to see an effect, because the hormone seems to act somewhere in the proliferated cells (1,2). However, other studies (3–5) have clearly shown that the hormone effect requires both mesenchyme and epithelium. And, depending on which species and which region of the gut and mesenchyme are being examined, essential primary signals come from the epithelium, but secondary signals, which are also important, come from the mesenchyme. As to the molecular details, we have no idea as yet.

Dr. N. Wright: But why does BrdU inhibit the precocious stabilization of glucocorticoids. What is the mechanism of that?

Dr. Nanthakumar: During pancreatic development, or hematopoietic development, myogenesis, and so on, if when the nucleosome opens up repressor protein is bound in those regions, incorporation of BrdU affects the rate of dissociation and association of transcription factors at those developmental sites. It was shown long ago that only one gene nick is required for myogenesis (6–9).

Dr. Milla: CDX2 and other similar transcription factors seem to be the key to how the epithelium starts to differentiate. Have you any insight into what the downstream targets of CDX2 might be?

Dr. Nanthakumar: The situation is very complicated. Two CDX forms, CDX1 and CDX2, are expressed in different compartments. CDX forms are expressed from the time of the first pre-endodermal cell from the initial state of endodermal development. However, it has clearly been shown that CDX is important in activating marker genes such as sucrase or carbonic anhydrase in the colon. However, CDXs are expressed way ahead, whereas sucrase is expressed at the right time during the postnatal development. This suggests that the elements that CDX bind are usually repressed or inaccessible to CDX during development. At the proper developmental time, however, they open up and CDX can bind and then they activate the transcription factor. However, we have no idea what the mechanism is and how it happens.

Dr. Lé: Can you tell us about the different processes that are triggered by CDX?

Dr. Nanthakumar: At the moment we know that CDX2 knockout mice do not develop, because CDX2 is necessary for preimplantation extra-embryonic endoderm. So, the fetus never implants and does not develop. Stage-specific induction of CDX2 is being developed in Trabers' laboratory to show whether CDX2 is required for gut development, and if so at what point.

Dr. Mäki: Could CDX2 be involved in TGF-β function? We have shown that TGF-β is very necessary in epithelial cell differentiation.

Dr. Nanthakumar: Drusilla Roberts has shown, using the chick gut development model, that a member of the TGF-β family called ''BMP4'' protein is clearly important in epithelium-mesenchyme communication and it is likely that this is the mechanism whereby the TGF-β family is important for development and maintenance. TGF-β and several other factors are extremely important in the way in which epithelium and lymphocytes in the mesenchyme respond during specific inflammatory processes.

Dr. Delvin: I have a question about CDX and the homeobox genes. I thought that homeobox genes were active very early on during embryogenesis. So, in a model such as yours, do you think you can fully appreciate the role of those genes? Has most of the cell programming not already been established in your model, so the cells are already dedicated to a particular role, even though the clock has not yet been started?

Dr. Nanthakumar: In the fly, the homeotic genes have a much simpler developmental program than in mammals. In the mouse are found four families of *Hox* genes that regulate anterior-posterior development, whereas in *Drosophila* only one family is seen. In the mammal, functional redundancy is clearly shown and these genes talk to each other. A gradient of expression of the *Hox* genes is necessary for proper development. However, in certain tissues such as CDX and PDX2, different homeotic genes called ''nonclustered homeotic genes'' are found, which are important in specific functions of specific tissues. When those genes are inactivated, they affect only certain parts of the program. To answer your question: various homeotic genes exist in epithelia and various homeotic genes in the mesenchyme, and when a proper combination of these is achieved, normal developmental progression occurs at the right time.

Dr. Ghoos: What is the physiologic meaning of having sucrase activity in the colon?

Dr. Nanthakumar: During the second trimester in the human fetus, the epithelium from the small intestine and from the colon look almost exactly the same and the colon functions like the small intestine. During the third trimester, colonic mucosa loses the villi and assumes the normal colonic appearance. Thus, at 20 weeks, the colon expresses intestine-specific markers, because it looks and functions like the small intestine. A hypothesis related to colon cancer is that the colon regresses in development and if cells are immortalized at this stage, they may express intestine-specific markers.

REFERENCES

1. Herbst JJ, Koldovsky O. Cell migration and cortisone induction of sucrase activity in jejunum and ileum. *Biochem J* 1972; 126: 471–6.
2. Koldovsky O, Sunshine P, Kretchmer N. Cellular migration of intestinal epithelia in suckling and weaned rats. *Nature* 1966; 212: 1389–90.
3. Haffen K, Kedinger M, Simon-Assmann P. Mesenchyme-dependent differentiation of epithelial progenitor cells in the gut. *J Pediatr Gastroenterol Nutr* 1987; 6: 14–23.
4. Kedinger M, Simon-Assmann P, Lacroix B, *et al*. Fetal gut mesenchyme induces differentiation of cultured intestinal endodermal and crypt cells. *Dev Biol* 1986; 113: 474–83.
5. Kedinger M, Simon-Assmann P, Alexandre E, Haffen K. Importance of a fibroblastic support for *in vitro* differentiation of intestinal endodermal cells and for their response to glucocorticoids. *Cell Growth Differ* 1987; 20: 171–82.
6. Tapscott SJ, Lassar AB, Davis RL, Weintraub H. 5-Bromo-2′-deoxyuridine blocks myogenesis by extinguishing expression of MyoD1. *Science* 1989; 245: 532–6.
7. Davis RL, Weintraub H, Lassar AB. Expression of a single transfected cDNA converts fibroblasts to myoblasts. *Cell* 1987; 51: 987–1000.
8. O'Neil MC, Stockdale FE. 5-Bromodeoxyuridine inhibition of differentiation. Kinetics of inhibition and reversal in myoblasts. *Dev Biol* 1974; 37: 117–32.
9. Pinney DF, Pearson-White SH, Konieczny SF, Latham KE, Emerson CP Jr. Myogenic lineage determination and differentiation: evidence for a regulatory gene pathway. *Cell* 1988; 53: 781–93.

Gastrointestinal Functions, edited by Edgard E. Delvin and Michael J. Lentze. Nestlé Nutrition Workshop Series, Pediatric Program, Vol. 46, Nestec Ltd., Vevey/Lippincott Williams & Wilkins, Philadelphia © 2001.

Role of Extracellular Matrix Proteins on Human Intestinal Cell Function: Laminin–Epithelial Cell Interactions

Jean-François Beaulieu

Department of Anatomy and Cell Biology, University of Sherbrooke, Faculty of Medicine, Sherbrooke, Québec, Canada

The intestinal epithelium is a very dynamic tissue, which depends on a variety of factors for the regulation of its growth as well as for the expression of digestive functions during development and in the adult (1,2). Over the last 10 years, it has become increasingly evident that among these factors are extracellular matrix molecules, a series of large and mostly insoluble bioactive glycoproteins. As in many other organs in the intestine, the epithelium lies on a thin and continuous sheet of specialized extracellular matrix, the basement membrane, which separates epithelial cells from the interstitial connective tissue or stroma. It is now recognized that basement membrane composition defines the necessary microenvironment required for multiple cellular functions during development and at maturity: proliferation, migration, tissue-specific gene expression, and, ultimately, apoptosis (3). These functions are themselves mediated by various cell membrane receptors, many of which are members of the integrin superfamily (4).

The intact intestine, and particularly the small intestine, represents an attractive system where cell–matrix interactions can be analyzed in relationship to growth and differentiation. First, during development, the process of endodermal differentiation into a functional epithelium is closely related to intestinal morphogenesis; indeed, the ontogenic appearance of the main epithelial cell types takes place precisely at the time that short villi begin to form, while a gradual confinement of the proliferative cell population occurs with crypt formation. Second, the epithelium is in constant and rapid renewal in the mature intestine. Its functional unit, the crypt–villus axis, consists of spatially separated proliferative and differentiated cell populations located in the crypt and on the villus, respectively.

After a brief summary of the development and functional aspects of the crypt–villus unit in the human small intestine, current knowledge will be summarized about basement membrane composition and the expression of integrins in relationship to the cell state in human intestinal cells, which has been comprehensively reviewed (5,6). Then, to address the potential role of extracellular matrix molecules on intes-

59

tinal functions, focus turns to cell–laminin interactions. First, it will be shown that analysis of the spatial and temporal distribution of these functional molecules in a well-organized structure (e.g., the intact intestinal epithelium) represents a powerful approach to evaluating the potential implication of individual components in a normal environment. Second, with the availability of *in vitro* models that can recapitulate the crypt–villus axis, evidence will be provided showing that it also becomes possible to investigate these cell–matrix interactions more directly in order to define cause and effect relations on intestinal cell differentiation.

DEVELOPMENT AND CHARACTERISTICS OF THE CRYPT–VILLUS UNIT IN THE HUMAN SMALL INTESTINE

Ontogeny

In contrast with most laboratory animals, the crypt–villus unit develops relatively early during human ontogeny, being essentially established by mid-pregnancy (7). At 8 weeks, the intestinal wall consists simply of stratified endoderm surrounded by concentric mesenchymal cell layers. Between 9 and 10 weeks, villus formation begins by mesenchymal infiltration of the stratified epithelium, so that by 12 weeks the entire small intestine is covered by short villi lined with a simple columnar epithelium. In parallel with this morphologic development, many of the digestive enzymes associated with absorptive cells are expressed on the villi. Crypts begin to develop around 16 weeks. By 20 weeks, the fetal small intestinal mucosa already morphologically resembles the adult with well-developed crypts and villi and many of the same digestive capacities.

Properties

The crypt–villus functional unit can be defined by typical morphologic and functional properties displayed by the mature villus enterocytes that distinguish them from crypt cells. The villi are mainly lined by functional absorptive and goblet cells, whereas the crypts contain stem cells and proliferative and poorly differentiated cells, as well as a subset of differentiated secretory cells, namely Paneth's, goblet, and enteroendocrine cells. The differentiation of each cell type (8) takes place as the cells move either upward toward the villus (adsorptive, mucus, and endocrine cells) or downward to concentrate at the bottom of the crypt (Paneth's cells). The compartmentalization of distinct cell populations according to their functional state is a well-documented phenomenon that can be exemplified by the analysis of the localization of various markers along the crypt–villus axis. It is noteworthy that in all species studied, the crypt–villus junction represents a physical limit from which enterocytes acquire their final functional characteristics. For instance, immunostaining to detect maltase-glucoamylase, a marker of the functional enterocyte, is restricted to villus cells, whereas MIM-1/39, a specific marker for secretory granules, is expressed only by crypt cells. However, in several instances, it appears that in the human, in contrast with the situation observed in laboratory animals, some of the classical enterocytic markers can be expressed by immature cells located below this border. For instance, aminopeptidase N and dipeptidylpeptidase IV have been found constitutively expressed by both proliferative and differentiated intestinal cells. These differences have to be considered when choosing markers to study human intestinal cell differentiation both *in situ* and *in vitro*. More importantly, they show that the regulation of gene expression along the crypt–villus axis differs fundamentally between human and animal models (7).

EPITHELIAL BASEMENT MEMBRANE COMPOSITION

The epithelial basement membrane of the human small intestine has been found to contain all the major components specific to most basement membranes, as well as some nonexclusive macromolecules also found in the interstitial extracellular matrix (Fig. 1). Basement membrane–associated components (e.g., tenascin and fibronectin) have been well characterized for their differential and complementary expression along the crypt–villus axis in both the adult and developing small intestine

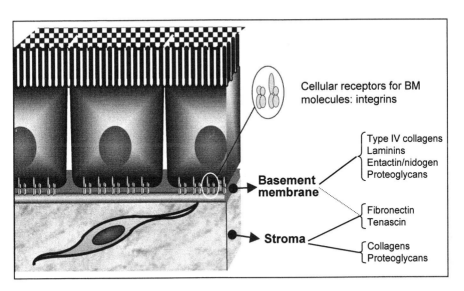

FIG. 1. Organization of the epithelial–stromal interface in the human intestine. The basement membrane, which is localized at the interface between the two tissues, contains basement membrane-specific macromolecules (e.g., type IV collagens and laminins) as well as associated basement membrane components (e.g., tenascin and fibronectin). Cellular receptors for basement membrane molecules (e.g., integrins) are involved in the mediation of cell adhesion, migration, and gene expression regulating cell proliferation and differentiation. (Adapted from Beaulieu J-F. Extracellular matrix components and integrins in relationship to human intestinal epithelial cell differentiation. *Prog Histochem Cytochem* 1997;31:1–78.)

TABLE 1. *Extracellular matrix molecules and integrins identified in association with human intestinal epithelial cells*

Basement membrane molecules	Basement membrane–associated molecules	Integrins
Type IV collagen α_1/α_2 chains	Fibronectin HI	$\alpha_1\beta_1$ I
Type IV collagen α_5/α_6 chains H	Tenascin HI	$\alpha_2\beta_1$ HI
Laminin-1 HI	SPARC/BM40/osteonectin H	$\alpha_3\beta_1$ HI
Laminin-2 HI	Osteopontin H	$\alpha_5\beta_1$ HI
Laminin-5 I	Decorin HI	$\alpha_6\beta_1$
Entactin/nidogen		$\alpha_7\beta_1$ HI
Heparan sulfate proteoglycans		$\alpha_9\beta_1$ H
		$\alpha_6\beta_4$ I

H, differently expressed during development; I, differently expressed along the crypt-villus axis.
Adapted from Beaulieu J-F. Extracellular matrix components and integrins in relationship to human intestinal epithelial cell differentiation. *Prog Histochem Cytochem* 1997;31:1–78; Beaulieu J-F. Integrins and human intestinal cell functions. *Front Biosci* 1999;4:310–21.

(Table 1) (5,9,10). Specific basement membrane components (e.g., the classical type IV collagen, heterotrimeric laminin, and various proteoglycans) were initially reported to be expressed at the base of all epithelial cells, whereas some of their integrin receptors were found to be expressed under distinctive crypt–villus gradients (Table 1). However, with the considerable progress in the characterization of basement membrane macromolecules over the past few years, it has become evident that type IV collagen, laminin, and heparan sulfate proteoglycans are large protein families, with isoforms subject to differential spatial and temporal patterns of expression in the small intestine.

Type IV Collagens

The classical form of type IV collagen is composed of α_1(IV) and α_2(IV) collagen chains, which assemble as an $[\alpha_1(IV)]_2\alpha_2(IV)$ complex. This major basement membrane component forms an intricate framework from which other basement membrane molecules associate (3). Study of the type IV collagen α_1(IV) to α_6(IV) chains in the adult human small intestine at protein and transcript levels confirmed the constitutive expression of the α_1 and α_2 chains in the epithelial basement membrane (11). Although the α_3(IV) and α_4(IV) chains were not detected, the α_5(IV) and α_6(IV) were also identified (11,12). Interestingly, in contrast to the α_1(IV) and α_2(IV) chains, which originate from the mesenchymal compartment, the α_5(IV) and α_6(IV) chains were found to be produced by both epithelial and mesenchymal cells *in situ* and *in vitro* (12,13). Another particularity of these newly identified type IV collagen chains is their distinct expression throughout intestinal development, the α_6(IV) chain being expressed constitutively at all stages, whereas the α_5(IV) chain is subject to a downregulation from the fetus to the adult (11,12). The significance of α_6(IV) chain expression in the adult epithelial basement membrane without its presumed

α_5(IV) partner remains to be determined at a functional level but represents a good example of basement membrane compositional change throughout development.

Proteoglycans

Proteoglycans were historically identified according to their associated glycosaminoglycan chains. However, this class of complex glycoproteins has been completely redefined over recent years by the characterization of the transcripts encoding their protein cores. Although some of the basement membrane proteoglycans have been identified, such as perlecan, which seems to be ubiquitously expressed in the epithelial basement membrane of the intestine, the identity of other identified heparan sulfate proteoglycans still needs to be better documented (5,9). Evidence also indicates that some chondroitin sulfate proteoglycans may be epithelial basement membrane components in the gut (5,9). Thus, as illustrated by recent studies (14), further analysis of proteoglycans in the small intestinal mucosa should allow for a better appreciation of their potential involvement.

Laminins

As with the other basement membrane molecules, laminin also was initially thought to be a single $\alpha\beta\gamma$ heterotrimeric molecule, but has been redefined as a multigene family of related proteins (15). Indeed, five α, three β, and two γ chains have been identified, which can associate to form 11 distinct laminins. Quantitatively, laminins are important basement membrane molecules. Functionally, in addition to their contribution to basement membrane network organization (3), they

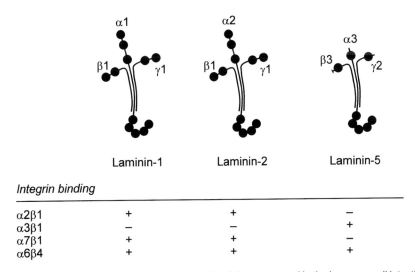

Integrin binding

	Laminin-1	Laminin-2	Laminin-5
$\alpha2\beta1$	+	+	−
$\alpha3\beta1$	−	−	+
$\alpha7\beta1$	+	+	−
$\alpha6\beta4$	+	+	+

FIG. 2. Schematic representation of the three laminins expressed in the human small intestine and identification of their corresponding binding integrins.

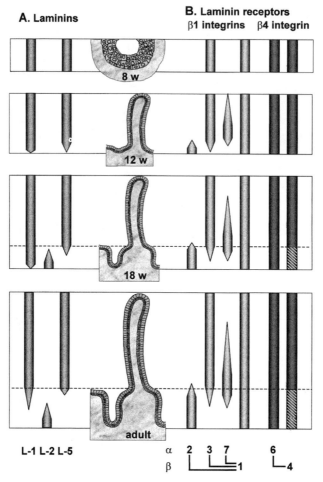

FIG. 3. Developmental expression and distribution of laminins and laminin-binding integrins along the crypt–villus unit in the human small intestine. **A.** Laminin-1 (L-1) and laminin-5 (L-5) are present very early during development, whereas laminin-2 appears only at the time crypts develop. In the adult, laminin-1 and laminin-2 show complementary distribution, whereas laminin-5 is restricted to the villus. **B.** Among the laminin-binding integrins, $\alpha_2\beta_1$ is only detected after 10 weeks in the intervillous area and remains confined to the crypts after 16 weeks, whereas the expression and distribution of $\alpha_3\beta_1$ coincides with laminin-5, its ligand. In contrast, the laminin-1 binding integrin $\alpha_7\beta_1$ is primarily expressed in the upper crypt and lower part of the villus. The integrin $\alpha_6\beta_4$ is found ubiquitously in both the developing and adult intestinal epithelium but its crypt form is inactive. (Adapted from Beaulieu J-F. Extracellular matrix components and integrins in relationship to human intestinal epithelial cell differentiation. *Prog Histochem Cytochem* 1997; 31:1–78; and Beaulieu J-F. Integrins and human intestinal cell functions. *Front Biosci* 1999; 4: 310–21.)

have been shown to regulate several cellular activities including the promotion of adhesion, growth, polarization, and differentiation, depending on the cell type studied. Furthermore, the variability in their spatial and temporal expression in particular tissues and organs suggests that different laminins could perform distinct functions (3,15).

The expression of laminins in the small intestinal basement membrane has received much attention since the reciprocal expression of laminin-1 ($\alpha_1\beta_1\gamma_1$; Fig. 2) and laminin-2 ($\alpha_2\beta_1\gamma_1$) along the crypt–villus axis was reported (16–18). The occurrence of laminin-1 as an upper crypt–villus form and laminin-2 as a lower crypt form (Fig. 3A) indeed suggested for the first time a possible relationship between laminin expression and functional intestinal cell differentiation. Laminin-5 ($\alpha_3\beta_3\gamma_2$; Fig. 2) is the only other laminin yet identified in the human intestine (19,20). These observations are of interest as this laminin has previously been reported only in basement membranes of stratified epithelia, in association with anchoring filaments of hemidesmosomes. It is noteworthy that true hemidesmosomes are not present in the human small intestinal epithelium, consistent with the fact that type VII collagen and some of the major hemidesmosomal proteins are lacking (19). However, its localization—essentially restricted to the villus in the human small intestine (Fig. 3A)—coincides well with that of HD1/plectin, another important hemidesmosomal component (20).

LAMININ RECEPTORS IN THE HUMAN SMALL INTESTINE

Because of the differential expression of laminin variants along its crypt–villus unit, the human small intestinal epithelium has emerged as one of the most promising systems to study laminins in relationship to the cell state. Furthermore, their corresponding cell receptors have also been found to be differentially expressed throughout development as well as along the crypt–villus axis in the adult. Among these receptors, it is mainly (although not exclusively; 21) integrins that mediate cell interactions with laminins. Integrins are a family of transmembrane $\alpha\beta$ heterodimer glycoproteins that bind selectively to various extracellular matrix molecules and trigger intracellular cascades of signaling events leading to the modulation of gene expression (Fig. 4).

Expression of integrins has been determined in the human intestinal epithelium (5,6) on the basis that this may provide important information on their potential involvement in cell–laminin interactions *in situ*. As summarized in Fig. 2, the principal integrins present in intestinal epithelial cells that can bind to laminins are $\alpha_2\beta_1$, $\alpha_3\beta_1$, $\alpha_7\beta_1$, and $\alpha_6\beta_4$. Analysis of the laminin-binding integrins in the developing crypt–villus functional unit of the human small intestine revealed interesting features. The $\alpha_2\beta_1$ and $\alpha_3\beta_1$ integrins were found at the basal domain of intestinal cells according to strict complementary staining patterns (18,19,22), $\alpha_2\beta_1$ being predominant in the crypts (in the intervillous area before 16 weeks) and $\alpha_3\beta_1$ on the villus (Fig. 3B). The expression of the $\alpha_7\beta_1$ integrin has also been analyzed (23). The presence of the α_7B subunit was closely paralleled with the acquisition

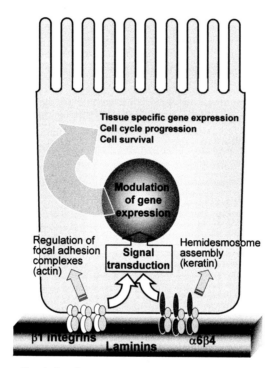

FIG. 4. Integrin-mediated signaling events in epithelial cells. Adhesion of cells to basement membrane molecules such as laminins triggers integrin clustering and activation of various molecules regulating the assembly of focal adhesion complexes (β_1 integrins) or hemidesmosomes $\alpha_6\beta_4$, as well as various signaling pathways involved in the modulation of gene expression governing cell survival, cell cycle progression, and tissue-specific gene expression. (Adapted from Beaulieu J-F. Integrins and human intestinal cell functions. *Front Biosci* 1999; 4: 310–21.)

of differentiation characteristics during development and along the crypt–villus axis in the adult, being restricted to the upper part of the crypt and the lower villus region (Fig. 3B). On the other hand, $\alpha_6\beta_4$ was found to be uniformly distributed at the base of epithelial cells from the bottom of the crypt to the tip of the villus (16,17,19). However, difficulties in interpreting the widespread distribution of this integrin arose from the existence of variants, referred to as α_6A, α_6B, and β_4A to E (24). Recent studies from our laboratory indicate that the intestinal form of this integrin appears to be $\alpha_6\beta_4$A but that the β_4A subunit is distinct immunologically between crypts and villi (25; Fig. 3B).

CELL–LAMININ INTERACTIONS IN THE REGULATION OF INTESTINAL FUNCTIONS

Observations showing the expression of several primary laminin-binding integrins in the intestinal epithelium and their differential localization along the crypt–villus axis, in concert with compositional changes in laminin-1, -2, and -5 (Fig. 3), reveal the potential complexity of the organization of epithelial cell–laminin interactions involved in the maintenance of a relatively simple system such as the human intestinal epithelium. The analysis of the distribution of these functional molecules in a spatially well-organized structure represents a powerful way of estimating the potential implication of individual components in a normal environment. Nevertheless, to recapitulate the mechanisms involved, several questions relating to the basic organization of laminin and integrin subunits—such as the exact forms and variants expressed, their relative quantitative importance, the specificity of their interactions and, more importantly, their precise involvement in the regulation of specific cell functions—also need to be addressed by means of more direct approaches.

Intestinal Cell Models

The roles of cell–laminin interactions have been investigated in various intestinal experimental models, principally human intestinal cell lines. Although mostly of colon adenocarcinoma origin, these cell lines (e.g., Caco-2) have been used advantageously to study the role of laminins on intestinal cell functions, namely cell differentiation (26). The development in recent years of normal human intestinal epithelial cell lines (e.g., the HIEC cell line) that are comparable with the undifferentiated cells of the crypt (27) has begun contributing to a better understanding of laminin–cell interactions in the intestinal model.

Laminins in Intestinal Cell Differentiation

The identification of laminin-1 at the base of villus cells and laminin-2 in crypt cells in the intact intestine prompted our laboratory to investigate this relationship further in the Caco-2 enterocytic model. A close relationship between laminin-1 deposition and sucrase–isomaltase expression was demonstrated at the cell level. For instance, subclones of the Caco-2/15 cell line in which laminin-1 deposition was impaired were found to express considerably less sucrase–isomaltase at their apical pole (26). Furthermore, growth of Caco-2/15 cells on purified human laminin-1 and laminin-2 showed that both substrates can promote intestinal cell marker expression but that only laminin-1 has the ability to precociously induce functional differentiation markers such as sucrase-isomaltase and lactase-phlorizin hydrolase (26). The data thus provided suggest that intestinal differentiation-related gene expression is specifically promoted by laminins and is susceptible to differential modulation by variant forms of this family (26). Additional evidence that laminin-1 plays an important role in regulating cell differentiation was obtained by transfecting Caco-2 cells with an antisense laminin (α1-chain complementary DNA [cDNA] fragment) (28). On the other hand, laminin-1 failed to induce expression of differentiation markers in the cryptlike cell line HIEC (Perreault N, et al., unpublished data, 1998), although it stimulates cell adhesion and spreading (25).

Laminin-Binding Integrins in the Regulation of Intestinal Functions

In the light of observations showing that laminin-1 can regulate intestinal cell differentiation *in vitro* and that laminin-binding integrins (e.g., $\alpha_2\alpha_1$, $\alpha_3\beta_1$, $\alpha_7\beta_1$, and $\alpha_6\beta_4$) are detected in the intact human intestinal epithelium under particular patterns of distribution along the crypt–villus axis, the expression of these laminin-binding integrins has been analyzed in HIEC and Caco-2 cells. These studies provided evidence that the $\alpha_7\beta_1$ and $\alpha_6\beta_4$ integrins may play a role in laminin-1 mediated intestinal differentiation, whereas $\alpha_2\beta_1$ and $\alpha_3\beta_1$ are less likely to be involved.

$\alpha_2\beta_1$

Considered to be a laminin-1 and collagen receptor, the $\alpha_2\beta_1$ integrin was found to be expressed at a relatively high level in HIEC and undifferentiated Caco-2 cells (23), as with most other intestinal cell lines including those derived from colon adenocarcinomas (6,29). Although good evidence indicates that $\alpha_2\beta_1$ may act in cooperation with $\alpha_6\beta_4$ for attachment to laminin-1 in some of these cells (29), it has also been shown to mediate glandular formation in collagen gels (30). This latter observation is reminiscent of what is observed during gland formation in the developing fetal small intestine (18). In the adult, $\alpha_2\beta_1$ is predominantly associated with the proliferative crypt cells lying on a basement membrane that contains type IV collagens (22) but which lacks laminin-1 (16). Together, these observations would suggest that in the intestinal epithelium the $\alpha_2\beta_1$ integrin acts primarily as a collagen receptor involved in gland morphogenesis and maintenance, rather than as a laminin receptor mediating differentiation.

$\alpha_3\beta_1$

The $\alpha_3\beta_1$ heterodimer has been shown to act as a specific laminin-5 receptor (6,29). Surprisingly, considering the *in situ* situation where both laminin-5 and $\alpha_3\beta_1$ are present predominantly at the base of the differentiated villus cells (Fig. 3), Caco-2 cells appear to express extremely low levels of both of these molecules, even under the differentiated state (Basora N, et al., unpublished data, 1998). These observations suggest that the laminin-5-$\alpha_3\beta_1$ interaction may not be essential for intestinal differentiation, a possibility that would fit well with the recent demonstration, in the epidermis, that the function of $\alpha_3\beta_1$ appears to be in cell attachment and basement membrane organization (31).

$\alpha_7\beta_1$

The $\alpha_7\beta_1$ integrin has been well characterized as a laminin-1 and laminin-2 receptor, mediating laminin functions during myogenic differentiation (32). The particular distribution of its $\alpha_7\beta_1$ form in the differentiating compartment of the intact intestine (Fig. 3B) suggests a role for this integrin in the differentiation process. *In vitro*, a relation between $\alpha_7\beta_1$ expression and the acquisition of enterocytic functions was established in Caco-2 cells, while the integrin was found absent from all undifferentiated intestinal cell lines tested, including HIEC (23). These observations clearly suggest that $\alpha_7\beta_1$ can act as a laminin-1 receptor mediating intestinal cell differentiation.

$\alpha_6\beta_4$

The integrin $\alpha_6\beta_4$ has been extensively studied in the skin where it contributes to hemidesmosomes (33). In intestinal cells, it has been shown to act as a high-affinity receptor for laminin-1 and laminin-5 (25,34). One interesting feature pertaining to the β_4 subunit is its particularly long cytoplasmic domain involved in the activation of various signaling pathways, namely Ras/MAP kinases and phosphatidylinositol 3-OH kinase, as well as in the modulation of the cyclin-dependent kinase inhibitors p21/WAF/Cip1 and p27/Kip (4,33). The $\alpha_6\beta_4$ integrin was thought to be ubiquitously expressed by intestinal epithelial cells *in situ* and *in vitro*, suggesting a poor relationship with cell differentiation. However, distinct forms of the integrin were recently identified in the human intestinal epithelium (25). *In vitro*, it was shown that Caco-2 cells express a full-length β_4A subunit, whereas the undifferentiated HIEC cells express a novel β_4A subunit that lacks the C terminal segment of the cytoplasmic domain (β_4Actd-). Interestingly, the $\alpha_6\beta_4Actd-$ integrin expressed by the undifferentiated cells of the crypts was found to be nonfunctional for adhesion to laminin,

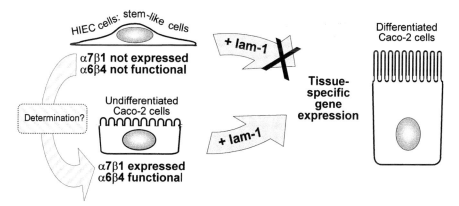

FIG. 5. A working model for laminin-1 mediated intestinal cell differentiation. In this model, $\alpha_7\beta_1$ and $\alpha_6\beta_4$ would act as the main modulators of tissue-specific gene expression. Caco-2 cells spontaneously express laminin-1 and its deposition at the substratum gradually occurs after confluence. Plating undifferentiated Caco-2 cells on laminin-1 accelerates the process, whereas laminin-2 has no specific effect. Furthermore, plating the cryptlike HIEC cells on the same substrates has no significant effect as these undifferentiated cells do not express $\alpha_7\beta_1$ and their $\alpha_6\beta_4$ is not functional.

indicating that the expression of a functional form of $\alpha_6\beta_4$ is related to intestinal differentiation (25).

Together, these data provide a good indication of which integrins are most able to mediate the effects of laminin-1 on intestinal cell differentiation. As depicted in Fig. 5, our working model now includes $\alpha_7B\beta_1$ and $\alpha_6\beta_4$ as the main modulators of tissue-specific gene expression.

CONCLUSIONS AND PERSPECTIVES

The regulation of intestinal epithelial cell proliferation, migration, and differentiation remains incompletely understood, but obviously involves cell–matrix interactions. Summarized in this chapter is the current knowledge concerning epithelial basement membrane composition in the human small intestine, with an outline of the potential role of these bioactive basement membrane molecules in regard to laminins. Evidence has been presented that spatial and temporal compositional changes in the expression of laminins, as well as in their specific cell receptors, occur in the human small intestine in relationship to the cell state. Further investigation of these observations with adequate *in vitro* models has confirmed the existence of a direct relationship between basement membrane molecules and the modulation of gene expression, as illustrated by the effects of laminin-1 on intestinal differentiation-related marker expression. It has also allowed significant progress in the identification of the surface receptors most likely to be involved in the mediation of these effects.

The challenges for the next years will be to extend these studies further in both normal and pathologic states. Better documentation of cell–matrix interactions occurring in the developing and adult intestine is required. First, the intestinal epithelial basement membrane composition still needs to be further defined. For example, it is likely that the role of proteoglycans has been underestimated; similarly, potential basement membrane–associated molecules other than tenascin and fibronectin have received little attention in the human intestine until now. Second, substantial progress has been made concerning the biology of extracellular matrix–binding molecules such as integrins and their expression by intestinal epithelial cells. However, the direct cause and effect relationships between the activation of particular receptors and the expression of specific cell functions remains, in several instances, to be demonstrated. One example is the integrin $\alpha_9\beta_1$, a tenascin receptor, which has been found to be associated with proliferative intestinal cells (35,36). The question whether this receptor can directly trigger the genes responsible for the activation of proliferation in normal intestinal cells remains open. On the other hand, our knowledge of the direct involvement of these molecules in gastrointestinal pathology other than cancers is practically nonexistent. However, in a context where extracellular matrix proteins have been proposed to be part of an integrated communication system in the normal and diseased intestinal mucosa (37), it is likely that progress in the basic knowledge of intestinal cell–matrix interactions will lead to significant developments in the next few years.

ACKNOWLEDGMENTS

The original work and preparation of this review was supported by grants from the Medical Research Council of Canada (MT-11289 and GR-15186) and from the ''Fonds pour la Formation de Chercheurs et l'Aide à la Recherche.''

REFERENCES

1. Podolsky DK, Babyatsky MW. Growth and development of the gastrointestinal tract. In: Yamada T, ed. *Textbook of gastroenterology*, 2nd ed. Philadelphia: Lippincott, 1995: 546–77.
2. Montgomery RK, Mulberg AE, Grand RJ. Development of the human gastrointestinal tract. Twenty years of progress. *Gastroenterology* 1999; 116: 702–31.
3. Timpl R, Brown JC. Supramolecular assembly of basement membranes. *Bioessays* 1996; 18: 123–32.
4. Giancotti FG. Integrin signaling: specificity and control of cell survival and cell cycle progression. *Curr Opin Cell Biol* 1997; 9: 691–700.
5. Beaulieu J-F. Extracellular matrix components and integrins in relationship to human intestinal epithelial cell differentiation. *Prog Histochem Cytochem* 1997; 31: 1–78.
6. Beaulieu J-F. Integrins and human intestinal cell functions. *Front Biosci* 1999; 4: 310–21.
7. Ménard D, Beaulieu J-F. Human intestinal brush border membrane hydrolases. In: Bkaily G, ed. *Membrane physiopathology*. Norwell: Kluwer, 1994: 319–41.
8. Leblond CP. The life history of cells in renewing systems. *Am J Anat* 1981; 160: 114–59.
9. Simon-Assmann P, Kedinger M, De Archangelis A, Rousseau V, Simo P. Extracellular matrix components in intestinal development. *Experientia* 1995; 51: 883–900.
10. Bélanger I, Beaulieu J-F. Tenascin in the developing and adult human intestine. *Histol Histopathol* 2000; 15: 577–85.
11. Beaulieu JF, Vachon PH, Herring-Gillam E, *et al.* Expression of the α_5(IV) collagen chain in the fetal human small intestine. *Gastroenterology* 1994; 107: 957–67.
12. Simoneau A, Herring-Gillam FE, Vachon PH, *et al.* Identification, distribution, and tissular origin of the α_5(IV) and α_6(IV) collagen chains in the developing human intestine. *Dev Dyn* 1998; 212: 437–47.
13. Vachon PH, Durand J, Beaulieu J-F. Basement membrane formation and re-distribution of β_1 integrins in a human intestinal co-culture system. *Anat Rec* 1993; 236: 567–76.
14. Li M, Choo B, Wong ZM, Filmus J, Buick RN. Expression of OCI-5/glypican 3 during intestinal morphogenesis: regulation by cell shape in intestinal epithelial cells. *Exp Cell Res* 1997; 235: 3–12.
15. Engvall E, Wewer UM. Domains of laminin. *J Cell Biochem* 1996; 61: 493–501.
16. Beaulieu J-F, Vachon PH. Reciprocal expression of laminin A-chain isoforms along the crypt–villus axis in the human small intestine. *Gastroenterology* 1994; 106: 829–39.
17. Simon-Assmann P, Duclos B, Orian-Rousseau V, *et al.* Differential expression of laminin isoforms and α_6-β_4 integrins subunits in the developing human and mouse intestine. *Dev Dyn* 1994; 201: 71–85.
18. Perreault N, Vachon PH, Beaulieu JF. Appearance and distribution of laminin A chain isoforms and integrin α_2, α_3, α_6, β_1, and β_4 subunits in the developing human small intestinal mucosa. *Anat Rec* 1995; 242: 242–50.
19. Leivo I, Tani T, Laitinen L, *et al.* Anchoring complex components laminin-5 and type VII collagen in the intestine: association with migration and differentiating enterocytes. *J Histochem Cytochem* 1996; 44: 1267–77.
20. Orian-Rousseau V, Aberdam D, Fontano L, *et al.* Developmental expression of laminin-5 and HD1 in the intestine—epithelial to mesenchymal shift for the laminin γ_2 chain subunit deposition. *Dev Dyn* 1996; 206: 12–23.
21. Weiser MM, Sykes DE, Piscatelli JJ, Rao M. The role of the non-integrin 67 kDa laminin receptor in enterocyte proliferation, adhesion and motility. In: Halter F, Winton D, Wright NA, eds. *The gut as a model in cell and molecular biology*. Dordrecht: Kluwer, 1997: 149–64.

22. Beaulieu J-F. Differential expression of the VLA family of integrins along the crypt-villus axis in the human small intestine. *J Cell Sci* 1992; 102: 427–36.
23. Basora N, Vachon PH, Herring-Gillam FE, Perreault N, Beaulieu JF. Relation between integrin $\alpha_7 B\beta_1$ expression in human intestinal cells and enterocytic differentiation. *Gastroenterology* 1997; 113: 1510–21.
24. de Melker AA, Sonnenberg A. Integrins: alternative splicing as a mechanism to regulate ligand binding and integrin signaling events. *Bioessays* 1999; 21: 499–509.
25. Basora N, Boudreau F, Perreault N, *et al.* Expression of functionally distinct integrin beta4A subunit variants in relation to the differentiation state in human intestinal cells. *J Biol Chem* 1999; 274: 29819–25.
26. Vachon PH, Beaulieu J-F. Extracellular heterotrimeric laminin promotes differentiation in human enterocytes. *Am J Physiol* 1995; 268: G857–67.
27. Perreault N, Beaulieu J-F. Use of the dissociating enzyme thermolysin to generate viable human normal intestinal epithelial cell cultures. *Exp Cell Res* 1996; 224: 354–64.
28. De Archangelis A, Neuville P, Boukamel R, Lefebvre O, Kedinger M, Simon-Assmann P. Inhibition of laminin α_1-chain expression leads to alteration of basement membrane assembly and cell differentiation. *J Cell Biol* 1996; 133: 417–30.
29. Mercurio AM. Laminin receptors: achieving specificity through cooperation. *Trends Cell Biol* 1995; 5: 419–23.
30. Liu D, Gagliardi G, Nasim MM, *et al.* TGF-α can act as a morphogen and/or mitogen in a colon-cancer cell line. *Int J Cancer* 1994; 56: 603–8.
31. DiPersio CM, Hodivala-Dilke KM, Jaenisch R, Kreidberg JA, Hynes RO. $\alpha_3\beta_1$ integrin is required for normal development of the epidermal basement membrane. *J Cell Biol* 1997; 137: 729–42.
32. Vachon PH, Xu H, Liu L, *et al.* Integrins ($\alpha_7\beta_1$) in muscle function and survival; disrupted expression in merosin-deficient congenital muscular dystrophy. *J Clin Invest* 1997; 100: 1870–81.
33. Nievers MG, Schaapveld RQJ, Sonnenberg A. Biology and function of hemidesmosomes. *Matrix Biol* 1999; 18: 5–17.
34. Lee EC, Lotz MM, Steel GD, Mercurio AM. The integrin $\alpha_6\beta_4$ is a laminin receptor. *J Cell Biol* 1992; 117: 671–8.
35. Basora N, Desloges N, Chang Q, *et al.* Expression of the $\alpha_9\beta_1$ integrin in human colonic epithelial cells: resurgence of the fetal phenotype in a subset of colon cancers and adenocarcinoma cell lines. *Int J Cancer* 1998; 75: 738–43.
36. Desloges N, Basora N, Perreault N, Bouatrouss Y, Sheppard D, Beaulieu J-F. Regulated expression of the integrin $\alpha_9\beta_1$ in the epithelium of the developing human gut and in intestinal cell lines: relation with cell proliferation. *J Cell Biochem* 1998; 71: 536–45.
37. Fiocchi C. Intestinal inflammation: a complex interplay of immune and nonimmune cell interactions. *Am J Physiol* 1997; 273: G769–75.

DISCUSSION

Dr. Goulet: At least two intestinal diseases with a very early neonatal onset exist—"tufting" disease and epithelial dysplasia. As such children have diseases restricted to the gastrointestinal tract, including the colon and the small bowel, can you tell us about the specificity of the laminin–integrin system you described with respect to other epithelia, such as the renal tubular epithelium?

Dr. Beaulieu: The specificity depends on the molecule expressed. Extracellular matrix molecules have their own peculiarities and receptors. We do not know yet, exactly, what pathways are linked to these receptors. Depending on the circumstance, they can activate cell proliferation or tissue-specific gene expression leading to cell differentiation, or just mediate migration or adhesion. At this point, we can only say that this laminin–integrin system is involved in basic processes such as cell proliferation and differentiation.

Dr. Goulet: But the diseases I am referring to are certainly innate genetic diseases according to their population distribution and the number of cases in a family, so a primary defect probably exists. In one of these specific diseases, we described a defect in one type of integrin, but that is not the only defect we have seen. Specifically, have you any experimental model involving knockout mice in which you can suppress the integrin or laminin isoforms?

Dr. Beaulieu: In the mouse, targeted integrin mutations have mostly been found to be embryonic or perinatally lethal, which in most cases precludes the direct evaluation of cell functions pertaining to specific organs. With respect to the $\alpha_7\beta_1$ integrin, mutation of this gene generates a form of muscular dystrophy but does not seem to cause any impairment to differentiation of the gut (i.e., for the mouse). It may be different for the human because expression of integrins and laminins differs between the two species. For example, laminin-1 does not seem to be expressed in the same compartments in the mouse and human intestine. Furthermore, the $\alpha_7\beta_1$ integrin is not found in mouse intestinal epithelium. Therefore, better documentation is needed for the expression of these molecules in the human gut before further exploring their cell functions. Likely of functional importance is the fact that in various diseases, such as those you referred to as well as in Crohn's disease, these molecules are redistributed. Once we have identified the molecules susceptible to play a role *in vivo*, we will be able to better investigate their functions using *in vitro* systems.

Dr. Zoppi: What happens to laminin protein in a situation such as a chronic, nonspecific diarrhea where the function of intestinal alkaline phosphatase has been shown to be altered?

Dr. Beaulieu: Not much is known about the expression and involvement of laminins in this pathology. To my knowledge, no specific extracellular matrix molecule is known to specifically modulate an enzyme such as alkaline phosphatase.

Dr. Lévy: Given your findings in inflammatory bowel disease, especially Crohn's disease, do you think that inflammatory cytokines can influence the expression of laminin?

Dr. Beaulieu: Yes, this is one of our working hypotheses. Cytokines are likely to influence epithelial cells and their underlying myofibroblasts to upregulate the expression of laminin-1 and 5. They could also be involved in the disappearance of laminin-2 from the pericryptal region by a mechanism involving extracellular proteases, which have been found to be induced by proinflammatory cytokines.

Dr. Lévy: You have incubated Caco-2 cells with laminin and you have demonstrated an induction of the differentiation process. What are the mechanisms involved?

Dr. Beaulieu: We think that laminin-1 is specifically recognized by integrins such as $\alpha_7\beta_1$ and $\alpha_6\beta_4$, which in combination with growth factors, generate signals to the nucleus to activate genes involved in the regulation of cell differentiation.

Dr. Alpers: It was not clear to me in your model whether laminin is being made only by cells in the lamina propria or by epithelial cells as well, taking into account that epithelial cells also make fibronectin, for instance. Which cells do you think are involved? And depending on which they are, does that help you decide whether this is a primary event or whether it is merely a secondary event as the cell differentiates and makes the various integrins?

Dr. Beaulieu: We have studied the origin of these molecules in the human fetal intestine and have confirmed that type IV collagen originates from mesenchymal cells, as in the mouse. Laminins seem to originate from both the epithelial and mesenchymal compartments, although laminin-2 seems to be produced predominantly by the epithelium. Tenascin originates exclusively from the mesenchyme, *whereas 95% of the fibronectin* is from the mesenchyme as well. The mesenchyme, therefore, is important in the production of basement membrane molecules, which would support the hypothesis of a primary event.

Dr. Brandtzaeg: For integrins to be involved in signal transduction, some sort of conformational change needs to occur. Do you have any method to distinguish between integrins that are in their native form or in their activated form in the system?

Dr. Beaulieu: One way is to look at focal adhesion kinase phosphorylation. This gives some idea of whether a β_1 integrin has been activated. Another important aspect relative to signal transduction is the generation of clusters of integrins, which depends on ligand recognition. Cell adhesion to ligands in a specific integrin-dependent manner is, thus, another indication. The next step in activation is a complex cascade involving various elements, which depends on integrins and other elements such as growth factors present in the (adhesion) complex.

Dr. Nanthakumar: I was under the impression that knockout mice have been generated for integrin $\alpha_6\beta_4$, and they are born alive but die later. If they are born with absence of $\alpha_6\beta_4$ and the crypt–villus structure is properly formed at the time of birth, what is the contribution of $\alpha_6\beta_4$?

Dr. Beaulieu: In these mice, the epithelia detach from the underlying mesenchyme, so adhesion appears to be greatly impaired in the gut. Functional alterations have also been reported. This is a good example of cooperation between multiple laminin integrins. Knockout does not seem to completely impair intestinal development, which suggests rescue mechanisms by other integrins. For instance, $\alpha_3\beta_1$ has been shown to compensate for the nonfunctional $\alpha_6\beta_4$. This suggests strong cooperation between different integrins.

Dr. Lentze: You showed that sucrase-isomaltase depends on laminin-1 in Caco-2 cells. What adaptive changes occur in the intestine, for instance in short bowel, where either morphology and function is enhanced because of luminal or hormonal factors? Are laminins and integrins dependent on luminal or hormonal factors for enhancement, for example in adaptive changes in short bowel?

Dr. Beaulieu: We believe that laminin and integrin expression is regulated by growth factors and cytokines. For instance, well-known targets of tumor growth factor-beta (TGF-β) are integrins and extracellular matrix molecules. Integrin expression is mostly dependent on TGF-β, but many molecules such as laminins and tenascins also depend on the status of TGF-β, and that is just one example. This field still needs to be better documented.

Dr. Gall: Is there direct evidence that activating the integrin leads to gene expression, or could it be just an effect on the cytoskeleton and altering membrane trafficking?

Dr. Beaulieu: Some of the best evidence is from the experiments I presented on the differential effect of laminin-1 and laminin-2 on sucrase-isomaltase expression. These laminins are similar because they share two of the three chains, and the third is homologous. The specific induction of sucrase-isomaltase at the transcript level with one laminin but not the other is a good indication of activation of gene expression. Also, plating Caco-2 cells on laminin-1 results in the activation of various kinases (e.g., focal adhesion kinase), supporting the idea that laminin activates integrin signaling in these cells. The specific pathways leading to gene expression, however, remains to be identified.

Dr. N. Wright: In looking at the epidermis, Jones and Watt (1) showed that, although all cells in the epidermis show $\beta1$ integrin, certain cells in the rete peg were integrin bright cells. One integrin bright cell per rete peg was seen, and it turns out that these were the stem cells—they had the highest clonogenic capacity when they were sorted. Looking at your $\alpha_2\beta_1$ staining pattern, did you find any difference in integrin expression within the stem cell zone?

The idea is that these integrin bright cells are held very tightly on the basal lamina, so that is the way the cell divisions are polarized. Is there an equivalence in intestinal crypt? Do you find variation in β1 integrin expression within the crypt?

Dr. Beaulieu: Although we looked for this kind of feature in the intestinal crypt, we never found an integrin or an extracellular matrix molecule to be concentrated in a very small region. Some of these molecules tend to be limited to the bottom of the crypts, but none of them were found to be restricted to the stem cell zone. My feeling is that either we have not yet looked for the right integrin subunit or variant, or another mechanism anchors stem cells in the intestinal crypt.

REFERENCE

1. Jones PH, Watt FM. Separation of human epidermal cells from transit amplifying cells on the basis of differences in integrin function and expression. *Cell* 1993; 21: 713–24.

Gastrointestinal Functions, edited by Edgard E. Delvin and
Michael J. Lentze. Nestlé Nutrition Workshop Series, Pediatric
Program, Vol. 46, Nestec Ltd., Vevey/Lippincott Williams &
Wilkins, Philadelphia © 2001.

Human Intestinal Nutrient Transporters

Ernest M. Wright

Department of Physiology, UCLA School of Medicine, Los Angeles, California, USA

Over the past decade, advances in molecular biology have revolutionized studies
on intestinal nutrient absorption in humans. Before the advent of molecular biology,
the study of nutrient absorption was largely limited to *in vivo* and *in vitro* animal
model systems. This did result in the classification of the different transport systems
involved, and in the development of models for nutrient transport across enterocytes
(1).

Nutrients are either absorbed passively or actively. Passive transport across the
epithelium occurs down the nutrient's concentration gradient by simple or facilitated
diffusion. The efficiency of simple diffusion depends on the lipid solubility of the
nutrient in the plasma membranes—the higher the molecule's partition coefficient,
the higher the rate of diffusion. Facilitated diffusion depends on the presence of
simple carriers (uniporters) in the plasma membranes, and the kinetic properties of
these uniporters. The rate of facilitated diffusion depends on the density, turnover
number, and affinity of the uniporters in the brush border and basolateral membranes.
The "active" transport of nutrients simply means that energy is provided to transport
molecules across the gut against their concentration gradient. It is now well recognized that active nutrient transport is brought about by Na^+ or H^+ cotransporters
(symporters) that harness the energy stored in ion gradients to drive the uphill transport of a solute. The rate of active transport of a nutrient depends on the density
and kinetics of these cotransporters.

The models for passive and active nutrient absorption across the intestinal mucosa
have evolved from those derived for sugar absorption (Fig. 1). Fructose is passively
absorbed across the intestine by two different uniporters in the brush border and
basolateral membranes of enterocytes (2), *GLUT5* in the brush border and *GLUT2*
in the basolateral membrane (Table 1) (5–26). In humans, the amount of fructose
absorption is limited by the number of brush border *GLUT5* transporters, and this
accounts for the fact that 80% of the population shows malabsorption symptoms
after ingesting 50 g of the sugar (27). Other nutrients (e.g., organic ions) are also
passively absorbed across the gut by having two uniporters expressed in series in
the brush border and basolateral membranes.

Glucose and galactose are actively absorbed by a cotransporter and a uniporter
expressed in series. These sugars are accumulated within the cell across the brush

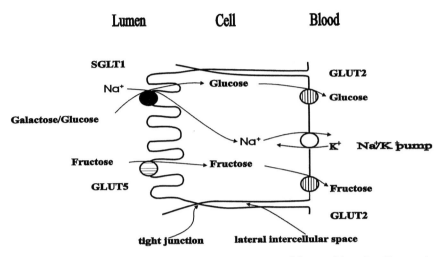

FIG. 1. A model for nutrient absorption across enterocytes of the small intestine. The passive transport of fructose across the brush border and basolateral membranes of the epithelium is accomplished by two uniporters, *GLUT5* and *GLUT2*. The active transport of glucose and galactose across the epithelium occurs in two stages: the first is the accumulation of the sugar within the epithelium by the brush border Na$^+$/glucose cotransporter, *SGLT1*; the second stage is the transport of sugar out of the cell across the basolateral membrane by the uniporter, *GLUT2*. Similar models account for the passive and active absorption of other nutrients across the intestine.

border membrane by an Na$^+$/glucose cotransporter (*SGLT1*), and then leave the cell across the basolateral membrane into the blood by facilitated diffusion through *GLUT2* (28). Similar models have been proposed to explain the active absorption of vitamins, bile salts, phosphate, dicarboxylates, amino acids, peptides, and trace ions. In some cases, it is the pH gradient across the brush border membrane rather than the Na$^+$ gradient that drives uptake, for example the *PEPT1* and *NRAMP* cotransporters (Table 1).

The actual identification of the transport proteins proved to be elusive, owing to the inherent problems in working with rare integral membrane proteins. For example, the brush border Na$^+$/glucose cotransporter only accounts for 0.1% of the total protein in the brush border, and it was very difficult to purify and assay by conventional biochemical techniques. In fact, it took almost 25 years to identify the transporter protein (29).

The rapid advances of the past decade have come through the power of molecular biology and the development of heterologous expression systems for transport proteins. Nevertheless, it took the development of a novel cloning strategy by Coady, Hediger, and Ikeda in my laboratory—expression cloning (30,31)—to remove the major bottleneck to cloning membrane transporters. Rather than screening complementary DNA (cDNA) libraries with oligonucleotide probes or antibodies, which required the purification of rare membrane proteins, a functional screening approach

TABLE 1. *Human intestinal nutrient transporters*

Gene	Substrate	Location	Reference
I. Na$^+$ cotransporters			
IA. Na$^+$/glucose family			
1. *SGLT1* (SLC5A1)	Glucose, galactose	BBM	3
2. *SMVT1* (SLC5A6)	Biotin, pantothenate, lipoate	BBM	4
3. *NIS* (SLC5A5)	Iodide	BBM	5
4. *SMIT* (SLC5A3)	Myoinositol	BBM	6
IB. Na$^+$/ascorbate			
1. *SVCT2* (SLC23A1)	Ascorbate	BBM	7
IC. Na$^+$/bile salt			
1. *ASBT* (SLC10A2)	Cholate, taurocholate	BBM	8
ID. Na$^+$/phosphate			
1. *NaPi-IIB* (SLC34A3)	Phosphate	BBM	9
IE. Na$^+$/dicarboxylate			
1. *NaDC1* (SLC13A2)	Citrate, succinate	BBM	10
2. *ratNaDC2* (SLC13A3)	Citrate, succinate	BLM	11
IF. Na$^+$/nucleoside			
1. *SPNT1/CNT2* (SLC28A2)	Inosine, uridine	BBM	12
2. *CNT2* (SLC28AZ)	Inosine, uridine	BBM	13
IG. Na$^+$/carnitine			
1. *OCTN2* (SLC22A5)	Carnitine	BBM	14, 15
IH. Na$^+$/H$^+$/K$^+$/glutamate			
1. *EAAT3/EAAC1* (SLC1A1)	Glutamate, aspartate	BBM	16
II. H$^+$/peptide			
1. *PEPT1* (SLC15A1)	Di- and tripeptides	BBM	17
IIB. H$^+$/divalent cations			
1. *DCT1/NRAMP2* (SLC11A2)	Zn, Fe, Cd, Mn, Co, Ni	BBM	18
III. Uniporters			
IIIA. Multiple facilitator family (MFS)			
1. *GLUT2* (SLC2A2)	Glucose, galactose, fructose	BBM	19
2. *GLUT5* (SLC2A5)	Fructose	BBM	20
IIIB. Organic cation			
1. *OCT1* (SLC22A2)	TEA, choline	BLM	21
2. *OCT2* (SLC22A)	TEA, choline	BLM	21
IIIC. Folate			
1. *RFC1/FOLT1* (SLC19A1)	Reduced folate	BBM?	22
IIID. Nucleoside			
1. *ENT1* (SLC29A1)	Purine and pyrimidine nucleosides		23
2. *ENT2* (SLC29A2)	Purine and pyrimidine nucleosides		24, 25
IIIE. Neutral amino acids			
1. *LAT2* (SLC7A6)			
2. *4F2hc* (SLC3A2)	Tyrosine, phenylalanine	BLM	26

BBM, brush border membrane; BLM, basolateral membranes; TEA, tetraethyl ammonium.
Transporters cloned from human intestinal cDNA libraries, or cloned from other human libraries and known to be expressed in the small intestine. The human gene nomenclature used in the table (www.gene.ucl.ac.uk/nomenclature/) is that employed by the database Online Mendelian Inheritance in Man (OMIM) for human genetic disorders (www.ncbi.nlm.nih.gov/Omim).

was used. This rested on the finding that *Xenopus laevis* oocytes have the remarkable ability to efficiently translate foreign complementary RNA (cRNA) from virtually any source and, in the case of membrane proteins, correctly target the functional protein to the plasma membrane. The rate of sodium-dependent sugar uptake into native oocytes is extraordinarily small (< 0.25 pmol/h for 50 μM αMDG), but this increases by more than an order of magnitude after injecting 50 ng of intestinal polyA$^+$ RNA into the oocytes (30). Then, this radioactive tracer assay was used to isolate a clone from a rabbit intestinal cDNA that coded for the Na$^+$/glucose cotransporter. Injection of cRNA from the plasmid pMJC 429 into oocytes increased sodium-dependent uptake more than 1,000 times above background (31), and the characteristics of this cloned transport were very similar to those of the native brush border transporter (28,32). The human transporter was cloned soon after using the rabbit cDNA to screen a human intestinal cDNA library (3).

Expression cloning is now the method of choice to identify genes coding for membrane transporters. Of the 23 human nutrient transporter clones listed in Table 1, more than half were directly or indirectly isolated by expression cloning and their function characterized by expression in oocytes. Generally, the transporter clones were first isolated from animal cDNA libraries by expression cloning and then from human cDNA libraries by homology screening. In some instances, the cDNA clones were isolated from nonintestinal libraries (e.g., renal or liver libraries) and these genes were subsequently shown to be expressed in the human intestine by Northern blot or reverse transcriptase polymerase chain reaction (RT-PCR) analysis. The functional characteristics of these cloned transporters closely match the properties of the transporters in intestinal brush border and basolateral membranes.

HUMAN INTESTINAL TRANSPORTERS

Thus far, some 23 transporters belonging to 15 gene families have been shown to be expressed in the human intestine (Table 1). Given the pace of research and the advances of the human genome project, this number is expected to grow rapidly. Ion and water channels, pumps, and ion exchangers expressed in the intestine are not included in Table 1. The list is divided into the secondary active transporters expressed in the brush border, and the uniporters expressed in the basolateral membrane. Interestingly, some gene families (the Na$^+$/dicarboxylate and *GLUT* families) contain members that are expressed either in the brush border or in the basolateral membrane. In yet another family, the organic ion family, the protein can behave as a uniporter and a cotransporter (see below). This is just one example of a single gene product with multiple functions.

All but one of the transporters listed in Table 1 are monomeric (or homomultimeric) proteins (i.e., the expression of each gene in cells produces the fully functional protein). The exception is the large neutral amino acid–facilitated transporter (system L), where two gene products, *LAT2* and *4F2*, are required for activity (26). Each of the transporter gene families codes for a polytopic membrane proteins of 40–80 kd with a secondary structure profile that is unique in terms of the number

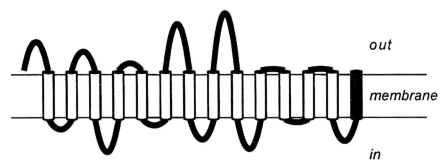

FIG. 2. The secondary structure model for the *SGLT1* family of membrane proteins. The model shows that the protein is formed by 14 transmembane α helices linked by external and internal hydrophilic loops of various lengths. Both the N- and C-termini are shown to be on the extracellular face of the membrane. In the case of some family members (e.g., *NIS* and the bacterial proline transporter, *putP*, the 14th helix is missing and the C-terminus of the protein lies in the intracellular compartment. (From Turk E, Wright EM. Membrane topology motifs in the SGLT cotransporter family. *J Membr Biol* 1997; 159: 1–20; figure kindly provided by Dr. E. Turk.)

of transmembrane helices and the position of large hydrophilic loops between helices (Fig. 2). In the case of the Na^+/glucose cotransporter family, a core is found of 13 transmembrane helices and a large cytoplasmic domain following helix 13 (33). The *SGLT1* family of sodium cotransporters now includes some 55 proteins found in bacteria, yeast, and animal cells. They include transporters for sugars, amino acids, vitamins, and iodide (Table 1). Both the bacterial and animal sugar transporters have 14 transmembrane helices (Fig. 2) with a large intracellular loop between helices 13 and 14. The 14th helix is missing in the thyroid Na^+/iodide and the *Escherichia coli* Na^+/proline transporters. Most of the other human nutrient transporters listed in Table 1 are predicted to have 12 transmembrane helices, but others are thought to have 8 to 11 helices.

The overexpression of the cloned transporters in oocytes and cultured cells has permitted detailed studies of transport kinetics and substrate specificity. In the case of the *SGLT1* family of proteins, the high level of expression in *Xenopus* oocytes ($> 10^{11}$ copies/cell) gives such a high signal-to-noise ratio that it has been possible to unravel details about the transport cycle that were previously unknown. We have pioneered the use of novel biophysical methods to examine the kinetics of the glucose, iodide, myoinositol, and peptide cotransporters, and others have used similar methods to study the ascorbate, phosphate, citrate, and glutamate cotransporters. The cotransporters work by very similar mechanisms. Our model for Na^+/glucose cotransport is shown in Fig. 3.

Transport occurs by an ordered, six-state kinetics scheme, where two sodium ions first bind to the external surface of the protein and this produces a conformation change that permits sugar to bind (32). Once the external ligands are bound, the protein undergoes a conformation change that exposes the ligands to the cytoplasmic surface, where the sugar and Na^+ dissociate and the empty carrier then ''reorientates'' to the original state. The catalytic cycle results in the transport of two sodium

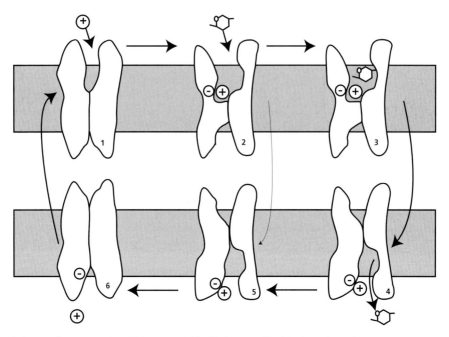

FIG. 3. Six-state ordered kinetic model for Na$^+$-sugar, Na$^+$ leak, and passive water transport. The model assumes that (*a*) the transporter has a valency of -2 (for simplicity depicted by $-$); (*b*) in the external membrane surface (with states C1, 2, 3), two sodium ions (depicted by $+$) bind to the transporter before the sugar molecule; (*c*) sugar is transported simultaneously with Na$^+$ via the conformational change C3 = C4; (*d*) in the internal membrane surface (with states C4, 5, 6), the sugar molecule dissociates from the transporter before the sodium ions; and (*e*) membrane voltage affects the conformational change of the empty transporter C1 = C6, and Na$^+$ binding to the transporter C1 = C2. The protein behaves as an Na$^+$-sugar cotransporter (cycle C1, 2, 3, 4, 5, 6) in the presence of sugar. In the absence of sugar, the protein behaves as an Na$^+$ uniporter (Na$^+$ leak, cycle C1, 2, 5, 6).

ions and one sugar molecule into the cell. The rate and direction of Na$^+$/sugar transport is determined by the concentration of ligands on each side of the membrane and the membrane potential. Voltage is predicted to influence both the rate of sodium binding to the external surface and the distribution of the unloaded protein between the outward and inward facing conformations. In the absence of sugar, the protein behaves as a sodium uniporter with similar kinetics to Na+/glucose cotransport. The turnover number for the uniport mode is only about 10% of that for the cotransport mode.

In addition to their role as uniporters and cotransporters, these proteins also behave as water transporters, low conductance water channels, and water cotransporters (34–36). The human Na$^+$/glucose cotransporter transports about 225 water molecules during each turnover of the Na$^+$/glucose catalytic cycle. The stoichiometry of cotransport, 2 Na$^+$/1 glucose/225 water molecules, is independent of the sodium and glucose concentrations, voltage, temperature, and osmotic gradient. Water cotransport even occurs against an osmotic gradient. We estimate that Na$^+$/glucose/

water cotransport accounts for approximately 4 L of intestinal water absorption a day (i.e., a major fraction of the total water absorption). The cotransport of water by *SGLT1* provides a molecular explanation for the link between intestinal glucose, salt, and water absorption, and for oral rehydration therapy. Water cotransport has also been described for other cotransporters (e.g., *NIS* and *NaDC1*), but the number of water molecules cotransported per turnover ranges from 50 to 500.

GENETIC DISORDERS OF NUTRIENT ABSORPTION

The most well-known disorder of nutrient absorption is glucose-galactose malabsorption (GGM). This is characterized by the neonatal onset of severe watery diarrhea, which results in death unless the child's fluid and electrolyte balance is restored (37,38). The diarrhea rapidly ceases with fasting or removing the offending sugars (lactose, glucose, and galactose) from the diet, but promptly resumes with oral feeding of foods containing these sugars. Fructose absorption (Fig. 1) is unaffected, and this forms the basis for the successful management of the children on special formulas. The most reliable diagnostic test for GGM is the hydrogen breath test, where oral administration of glucose or galactose greatly increases breath hydrogen in patients with GGM but not in controls. We are aware of about 200 cases worldwide.

With the cloning and mapping of the human *SGLT1* gene, we set out to search for the mutations causing GGM (39–42). Mutations that account for the disorder were identified in 33 of 34 GGM patients examined. In 17 kindreds, the patients bore homozygous mutations; in another 10 kindreds, the mutations were heterozygous. The mutations in the *SGLT1* gene included 23 missense, 4 splice-site, and 3 nonsense mutations. The splice-site and nonsense mutations result in the production of severely truncated, nonfunctional proteins. Of the missense mutations, 22 result in the production of the full-length cotransporter where the primary defect in sugar transport is caused by mistrafficking of the protein in the cell (i.e., the transporter is not inserted into the plasma membrane). In the 23rd case, the full-length protein is inserted into the brush border membrane of the patient's enterocytes but it is unable to transport glucose and galactose into the cell. All the partial reactions of the transporter are normal (Fig. 3), except for the translocation of the bound sugar through the membrane. This mutation provided important clues about the site of sugar translocation through the cotransporter (43).

Although GGM is a rare autosomal recessive disorder, the large number of mutations in the *SGLT1* gene does raise a question about the carriers of these mutations: Is there any reduction in capacity of the heterozygotes to absorb sugar? This is pertinent in view of the fact that a positive hydrogen breath test occurs in approximately 10% of the normal adult population (27).

Another disorder caused by mutations in a gene coding for an intestinal transporter is primary bile acid malabsorption (44). This is an idiopathic intestinal disorder associated with congenital diarrhea, steatorrhea, a reduction in plasma cholesterol, and a reduced circulation of bile acids in the body. So far, two missense mutations in the bile acid transporter (*ASBT*), *Leu243Pro* and *Thr262Met*, were identified that abolish bile salt transport. Unlike most of the missense GGM mutations, these mutations in the bile salt transporter do not cause trafficking or missorting defects in transfected *COS* cells. Finally, mutations in the Na^+/carnitine transporter have recently been shown to cause primary systemic carnitine deficiency, SCD (15). Four mutations have been found in three SCD pedigrees, and all result in defects in protein production.

It is to be expected that mutations in the other intestinal nutrient transporters will be uncovered that produce defects in absorption. These disorders may be autosomal recessive or dominant, depending on the oligomeric structure of the transporter proteins.

ACKNOWLEDGMENTS

Our studies of intestinal nutrient transporters are supported by grants from the National Institutes of Health (DK44582, DK19567 and DK44602). I thank my past and current colleagues for their invaluable contributions to these studies.

REFERENCES

1. Johnson LR, Alpers DH, Christensen J, Jacobson ED, Walsh JH, eds. *Physiology of the gastrointestinal tract*, 3rd ed. New York: Raven Press, 1994.
2. Corpe CP, Burant CF, Hoekstra JH. Intestinal fructose absorption: clinical and molecular aspects. *J Pediatr Gastroenterol Nutr* 1999; 28: 364–74.
3. Hediger MA, Turk E, Wright EM. Homology of the human intestinal Na^+/glucose and *E. coli* Na^+/proline cotransporters. *Proc Natl Acad Sci USA* 1989; 86: 5748–52.
4. Prasad PD, Wang HP, Huang W, *et al.* Molecular and functional characterization of the intestinal Na^+-dependent multivitamin transporter. *Arch Biochem Biophys* 1999; 366: 95–106.
5. Smanik PA, Liu Q, Furminger TL, *et al.* Cloning of the human sodium iodide symporter. *Biochem Biophys Res Commun* 1996; 226: 339–45.
6. Berry GT, Mallee JJ, Kwon HM, *et al.* The human osmoregulatory Na^+/*myo*-inositol cotransporter gene (SLC5A3): molecular cloning and localization to chromosome 21. *Genomics* 1995; 25: 507–13.
7. Tsukaguchi H, Toku T, Mackenzie B, *et al.* A family of mammalian Na^+-dependent L-ascorbic acid transporters. *Nature* 1999; 399: 70–5.
8. Wong MH, Oelkers P, Dawson PA. Identification of a mutation in the ileal sodium-dependent bile acid transporter gene that abolishes transport activity. *J Biol Chem* 1995; 270: 27228–34.
9. Field JA, Zhang L, Brun KA, Brooks DP, Edwards RM. Cloning and functional characterization of a sodium-dependent phosphate transporter expressed in human lung and small intestine. *Biochem Biophysical Res Commun* 1999; 258: 578–82.
10. Pajor AM. Molecular cloning and functional expression of a sodium-dicarboxylate cotransporter from rabbit kidney. *Am J Physiol (Renal Fluid Electrolyte Physiol)* 1996; 270: F642–8.
11. Chen XM, Tsukaguchi H, Chen XZ, Berger UV, Hediger MA. Molecular and functional analysis of SDCT2, a novel rat sodium-dependent dicarboxylate transporter. *J Clin Invest* 1999; 103: 1159–68.
12. Wang J, Su SF, Dresser MJ, Schaner ME, Washington CB, Giacomini KM. Na^+-dependent purine nucleoside transporter from human kidney: cloning and functional characterization. *Am J Physiol (Renal Fluid Electrolyte Physiol)* 1997; 273: F1058–65.
13. Ritzel MW, Yao SY, Huang MY, Elliott JF, Cass CE, Young JD. Molecular cloning and functional expression of cDNAs encoding a human Na^+-nucleoside cotransporter (HCNT1). *Am J Physiol* 1997; 272: C707–14.
14. Tamai I, Ohashi R, Nezu J, *et al.* Molecular and functional identification of sodium ion–dependent, high affinity human carnitine transporter OCTN2. *J Biol Chem* 1998; 273: 20378–82.
15. Nezu J, Tamai I, Oku A, *et al.* Primary systemic carnitine deficiency is caused by mutations in a gene encoding sodium ion–dependent carnitine transporter. *Nat Genet* 1999; 21: 91–4.

16. Arriza JL, Fairman WA, Wadiche JI, Murdoch GH, Kavanaugh MP, Amara SG. Functional comparisons of three glutamate transporter subtypes cloned from human motor cortex. *J Neurosci* 1994; 14: 5559–69.

17. Liang R, Fei YJ, Prasad PD, *et al.* Human intestinal H$^+$ peptide cotransporter: cloning, functional expression, and chromosomal localization. *J Biol Chem* 1995; 270: 6456–83.

18. Gunshin H, Mackenzie B, Berger UV, *et al.* Cloning and characterization of a mammalian proton-coupled metal-ion transporter. *Nature* 1997; 388: 482–8.

19. Fukumoto H, Seino S, Imura H, *et al.* Sequence, tissue distribution, and chromosomal localization of mRNA encoding a human glucose transporter-like protein. *Proc Natl Acad Sci USA* 1981; 85: 5435–8.

20. Kayano T, Burant CF, Fukumoto H, *et al.* Human facilitative glucose transporters. Isolation, functional characterization, and gene localization of cDNAs encoding an isoform (GLUT5) expressed in small intestine, kidney, muscle, and adipose tissue and an unusual glucose transporter pseudogene-like sequence (GLUT6). *J Biol Chem* 1990; 265: 13276–82.

21. Gorboulev V, Ulzheimer JC, Akhoundova A, *et al.* Cloning and characterization of two human polyspecific organic cation transporters. *DNA Cell Biol* 1997; 7: 871–81.

22. Nguyen TT, Dyer DL, Dunning DD, Rubin SA, Grant KE, Said HM. Human intestinal folate transport: cloning, expression, and distribution of complementary RNA, *Gastroenterol* 1997; 112: 783–91.

23. Griffiths M, Beaumont N, Yao SY, *et al.* Cloning of a human nucleoside transporter implicated in the cellular uptake of adenosine and chemotherapeutic drugs. *Nat Med* 1997; 1: 89–93.

24. Griffiths M, Yao SY, Abidi F, *et al.* Molecular cloning and characterization of a nitrobenzylthioinosine-insensitive (ei) equilibrative nucleoside transporter from human placenta. *Biochem J* 1997; 328: 739–43.

25. Crawford CR, Patel DH, Naeve C, Belt JA. Cloning of the human equilibrative, nitrobenzylmercaptopurine riboside (NBMPR)-insensitive nucleoside transporter ei by functional expression in a transport-deficient cell line. *J Biol Chem* 1998; 9: 5288–93.

26. Pineda M, Fernández E, Torrents D, *et al.* Identification of a membrane protein, LAT-2, that co-expresses with 4F2 heavy chain, an L-type amino acid transport activity with broad specificity for small and large zwitterionic amino acids. *J Biol Chem* 1999; 274: 19738–44.

27. Montes RG, Gottal RG, Bayless TM, Hendrix TR, Perman JA. Breath hydrogen testing as a physiology laboratory exercise for medical students. *Am J Physiol* 1992; 262: S25–8.

28. Wright EM, Hirayama BA, Loo DDF, Turk E, Hager K. Intestinal sugar transport. In: Johnson LR, Alpers DH, Christensen J, Jacobson ED, Walsh JH, eds. *Physiology of the gastrointestinal tract*, Vol 2, 3rd ed. New York: Raven Press, 1994; 1751–75.

29. Peerce BE, Wright EM. Conformational changes in the intestinal brush border Na$^+$-glucose cotransporter labeled with fluorescein isothiocyanate. *Proc Natl Acad Sci USA* 1984; 81: 2223–6.

30. Hediger MA, Ikeda T, Coady M, Gundersen CB, Wright EM. Expression of size selected mRNA encoding the intestinal Na$^+$/glucose cotransporter in *Xenopus laevis* oocytes. *Proc Natl Acad Sci USA* 1987; 84: 2634–7.

31. Hediger MA, Coady MJ, Ikeda K, Wright EM. Expression cloning and cDNA sequencing of the Na$^+$/glucose cotransporter. *Nature* 1987; 350: 354–6.

32. Wright EM, Loo DDF, Panayotova-Heiermann M, *et al.* Structure and function of the Na$^+$/glucose cotransporter. *Acta Physiol Scand* 1998; 163: 257–64.

33. Turk E, Wright EM. Membrane topology motifs in the SGLT cotransporter family. *J Membr Biol* 1997; 159: 1–20.

34. Loo DDF, Zeuthen T, Chandy G, Wright EM. Cotransport of water by the Na$^+$/glucose cotransporter. *Proc Natl Acad Sci USA* 1996; 93: 13367–70.

35. Loo DDF, Hirayama BA, Meinild AK, Chandy G, Zeuthen T, Wright EM. Passive water and ion transport by cotransporters. *J Physiol (Lond)* 1999; 518: 195–202.

36. Meinild AK, Klaerke DA, Loo DDF, Wright EM, Zeuthen T. The human Na$^+$-glucose cotransporter is a molecular water pump. *J Physiol (Lond)* 1998; 508: 15–21.

37. Wright EM. Glucose galactose malabsorption. *Am J Physiol* (*Gastrointest Liver Physiol*) 1998; 98: G879–82.

38. Wright EM, Martín GM, Turk E. Familial glucose-galactose malabsorption and hereditary renal glycosuria. In: Scriver CR, Beaudet AL, Sly WS, Valle D, eds. *Metabolic basis of inherited disease*, 8th ed. New York: MacGraw Hill, 2000.

39. Turk E, Zabel B, Mundlos S, Dyer J, Wright EM. Glucose/galactose malabsorption caused by a defect in the Na$^+$/glucose cotransporter. *Nature* 1991; 350: 354–6.

40. Martín GM, Turk E, Lostao MP, Kerner C, Wright EM. Defects in Na^+/glucose cotransporter (SGLT1) trafficking and function cause glucose-galactose malabsorption. *Nat Genet* 1996; 12: 216–20.
41. Martín MG, Lostao MP, Turk E, Lam J, Kreman M, Wright EM. Compound missense mutations in the sodium/D-glucose cotransporter result in trafficking defects. *Gastroenterology* 1997; 112: 1206–12.
42. Lam JT, Martín MG, Turk E, *et al.* Missense mutations in SGLT1 cause glucose-galactose malabsorption by trafficking defects. *Biochim Biophys Acta* 1999; 1453: 297–303.
43. Loo DDF, Hirayama B, Gallardo EM, Lam J, Turk E, Wright EM. Conformational changes couple Na^+ and glucose transport. *Proc Natl Acad Sci USA* 1998; 95: 7789–94.
44. Oelkers P, Kirby LC, Heubi JE, Dawson PA. Primary bile acid malabsorption caused by mutations in the ileal sodium-dependent bile acid transporter gene (SLC10A2). *J Clin Invest* 1997; 8: 1880–7.

DISCUSSION

Dr. Black: You hinted at the polymorphism issue. Are there are thoughts about whether the different expressions of the proteins permit different rate constants? And what drives expression of the gene? Do different polymorphisms result in different levels of expression of the genes and active transport across membranes?

Dr. E. Wright: These heterologous expression systems provide an answer to your first question. You can express protein at different levels and look at the kinetic properties, and the only thing that varies with the level of expression is V_{max}—the total amount of transport. But, if a polymorphism in a gene can produce any kind of defect, it can produce a defect in transcription, translation, RNA stability, trafficking, or function in the membrane, which is a real challenge to sort out. I have just entered into a consortium with a group in San Francisco who are going to look for polymorphisms in 50 genes in 450 individuals to determine whether they are present and what are their consequence. Our preliminary results are that polymorphisms are few and far between.

Dr. Zoppi: What happens to D-xylose in glucose/galactose malabsorption?

Dr. E. Wright: A misconception about D-xylose exists. It is assumed to be passively absorbed, but in fact it is absorbed by the sodium-glucose transporter with a very low affinity. The affinity for glucose is probably about 0.1 to 0.2 mmol/L, the affinity for D-xylose is about 50 mmol/L. So xylose is not a good reference point as a passively absorbed sugar, as it is definitely transported by the sodium-glucose transporter (1).

Dr. Memon: Where are these transporters for cations expressed in the gastrointestinal mucosa?

Dr. E. Wright: The 23 genes discussed all are present in the small intestine in the enterocyte. Most of the sodium-dependent and proton-dependent ones are in the brush border membrane of the enterocyte; most of the facilitated transporters are in the basolateral membrane of the enterocyte.

Dr. Memon: I was referring to the cation transporters that are meant for zinc and other minerals.

Dr. E. Wright: The immunocytochemistry of this has not been published, but it is thought that they are present in the brush border membrane. For divalent cations such as copper, adenosine triphosphatase (ATPase) is also present. Copper ATPase is a close relative of the sodium pump family, and is the protein responsible for Menke's disease, in which copper is accumulated in the cell but cannot be pumped out across the basolateral surface.

Dr. Memon: Are these proteins affected in any way by a deficiency of micronutrients?

Dr. E. Wright: We do not know that yet. A great explosion has occurred in molecular biology, but very little on the function of these proteins. A good heterologous expression system is needed to be able to study this. No one, to my knowledge, is investigating function, but at least we have the tools—DNA probes and appropriate antibodies—to start asking those kinds of questions.

Dr. Goulet: What types of transporter are involved in the very rare syndrome of congenital sodium chloride malabsorption?

Dr. E. Wright: Only nutrient absorption has been discussed. Other proteins such as the sodium-proton exchanger or the congenital chloridorrhea chloride transports were not included in this discussion. A candidate gene for chloride deficiency has been identified by a Finnish group (2). The calcium transporter for the brush border membrane has eventually been cloned, and there appears to be a calcium channel, very much like the sodium channel I_{Na}.

Dr. Bjarnason: I take it that you are not a fan of the Pappenheimer model of glucose absorption? (3–5).

Dr. E. Wright: I do not agree with it at all. I respect Pappenheimer's studies; some problems exist, however, and other people have been unable to show a paracellular pathway for water or sugar.

Dr. Bjarnason: I totally agree with your reservations. It just reminds me of how many papers of ours have been rejected because of those papers!

Dr. Ghoos: What happens to the hydrogen breath test if only 25 g of glucose is given? Fifty grams is a heavy load.

Dr. E. Wright: This was in adults, and 50 g was the standard test (6).

Dr. Ghoos: Fructose is the main cause of diarrhea in children at 5 to 6 years of age. At what age does fructose absorption become optimal?

Dr. E. Wright: Toddler's diarrhea is mostly brought about by mothers giving children fruit juice and high fructose levels prematurely. What has happened in those children is that the fructose transporter, *GLUT5*, is not maximally expressed. The level increases with age, but I do not know when fructose absorption is optimal in children.

Dr. Ghoos: Could there be "facilitated transport" of glucose? You have shown that a proportion of normal adults are unable to absorb a 50-g dose of glucose, but what happens if the same dose is given in a meal with fat and amino acids?

Dr. E. Wright: I have no idea. Many variables are seen in nutrition, such as gastrointestinal motility, gastric emptying time, transit times, and so on. These variables can all be altered by meal composition. Obviously, gastric emptying can be influenced dramatically by whether glucose, amino acids, or fat are present in the meal, which has to be taken into account.

Dr. Ghoos: Coming back to that dose of glucose, could the effect simply depend on gastric emptying and osmotic load?

Dr. E. Wright: Possibly, but I think not.

Dr. Alpers: One natural example of heterogeneity is *SGLT2*. What is the stoichiometry of that? Why is it there? Does it provide a clue for what might be found in the intestine?

Dr. E. Wright: *SGLT2* is present in the kidney. It is the primary mechanism for the reabsorption of glucose from the glomerular filtrate. In the kidney, *SGLT2* is in the third segment of the proximal tubule to absorb the dregs of the glucose. But *SGLT2* is not in the human intestine. Otherwise, with these patients with glucose-galactose malabsorption, a sodium-dependent glucose absorption would be found at some level through *SGLT2*. So, evidence thus far indicates that *SGLT2* is a kidney isoform, and it is not in the intestine.

Dr. Alpers: I was asking a different question. Is there anything known about the stoichiometry or the function of *SGLT2* that might provide a clue to the kinds of changes that might be found when the heterogeneity of *SGLT1* is identified in the intestine?

Dr. E. Wright: The dogma is that the Na^+ Hill coefficient for *SGLT2* is 1 (i.e., one sodium and one glucose are transported). The confusion is: *SGLT1* has two sodiums and one glucose.

Dr. Endres: If 70% of healthy volunteers have fructose malabsorption, that should also be true for patients with hereditary fructose intolerance. From our study of 56 patients with this disease of intermediary metabolism, no evidence indicated that the amount of fructose absorbed varies from patient to patient. It was calculated in a US dental journal that fructose tolerance in the adult fructose-intolerant patient is approximately 15 to 20 mg/kg/d, which is much less than a single dose of 50 g of fructose. Would you agree with the fact that no difference is seen in these patients is because the probands were only malabsorbers, and that a very small amount of fructose in the patients leads to the same clinical symptoms?

Dr. E. Wright: The fructose intolerance that you have studied and described is obviously a disorder of fructose metabolism. A group in Chicago has looked intensively for *GLUT5* mutations in children who are malabsorbing fructose, and they found none (2). I think absorption is normal, but it is the effects of the lesion in the fructose metabolic pathway that is a problem in fructose intolerance.

Dr. Lentze: Reports are seen of children who cannot tolerate any fructose at all; they get diarrhea immediately. Do they have no expression of the *GLUT5* transporter, or what is the mechanism of their complete intolerance?

Dr. E. Wright: I do not know. A group in Chicago looked for mutations in *GLUT5* in such patients and could not find any.

Dr. Hamilton: I was very interested and quite puzzled by your comments on water transport associated with glucose absorption. Do you have any further comments on that, particularly in relationship to the function of the intestinal tract?

Dr. E. Wright: Just to reiterate, what we have shown is that with a variety of cotransport proteins a stoichiometric relationship exists between the transport of ligand and the transport of water. That transport of water is fixed for any given protein. For some proteins (e.g., the hydrogen/amino acid cotransporter), however, it can be as low as 50 water molecules per turnover and for a KCl cotransporter it can be 500 water molecules per turnover, so this is something related to the properties of the protein. This tight relationship between sodium, glucose, and water explains the role of glucose in water absorption in the normal intestine and oral rehydration therapy. Glucose is needed for water absorption. People always thought that glucose was required for metabolism to turn on the sodium pump, which turned on sodium transport, which turned on water transport. The linkage is much more direct—it is a linkage between water, sodium, and glucose going through the protein.

Dr. Delvin: But, other transporters are involved in water transport, for example aquaporin, which is found in the kidney. Is it also found in the membranes of the intestine, and what are its relationships, in terms of lineage, with these other transporters?

Dr. E. Wright: Aquaporin-1 is the major water channel of the proximal tubule and that accounts for a lot of the water absorption. However, animals with aquaporin knockout are still able to reabsorb water from the proximal tubule, although their passive water permeability goes down. In the intestine, no concrete evidence is found for functional expression of aquaporins in the intestinal mucosa.

Dr. Gall: Two comments: first, we cannot show active water transport in the presence of glucose in intestinal tissue, either brush border membranes or in Ussing chambers; second, we have unreported evidence that aquaporin-3 is expressed in the basolateral membrane, and aquaporin-8 in the brush border. And we can block water transport in the system.

Dr. E. Wright: The aquaporins will only explain water transport if an osmotic gradient exists. If no osmotic gradient exists, no net water transport will occur. What the *SGLT1* will do is transport water against an osmotic gradient.

Dr. Gall: Yes, but we cannot show that in Ussing chambers or in brush border membrane vesicles. When we add glucose, we cannot show transport of water.

Dr. E. Wright: In experiments that I did 30 years ago as a doctoral student, this was something that could shown quite clearly—glucose stimulated water transport across the rat small intestine, by an order of magnitude.

Dr. Lévy: What is the role of glycosylation? Did you find any defects in glycosylation, which is a very important process in the intracellular trafficking of proteins?

Dr. E. Wright: Glycosylation is not required on this particular protein, *SGLT1*, for either trafficking or function. We have mutated out the N-linked glycosylation site, no glycosylation occurs and, in those mutants with the N-linked glycosylation site removed, absolutely no effect is seen. The protein traffics normally, and it is functional. Thus, in this particular case, glycosylation does not appear to be of any significance.

REFERENCES

1. Hager K, Hazama A, Kwon HM, *et al.* Kinetics and specificity of the renal Na$^+$/*myo*-inositol cotransporter expressed in xenopus oocytes. *J Membr Biol* 1995, 143: 103–13.
2. Wasserman D, Hoekstra JH, Tolia V, *et al.* Molecular analysis of the fructose transporter gene (*GLUT5*) in isolated fructose malabsorption. *J Clin Invest* 1996; 98: 2398–402.
3. Pappenheimer JR, Reiss KZ. Contribution of solvent drag through intercellular junctions to absorption of nutrients by the small intestine of the rat. *J Membr Biol* 1987; 100: 123–36.
4. Pappenheimer JR. Paracellular intestinal absorption of glucose, creatinine, and mannitol in normal animals: relation to body size. *Am J Physiol* 1990; 254: G290–9.
5. Madara JL, Pappenheimer JR. Structural basis for physiological regulation of paracellular pathways in intestinal epithelia. *J Membr Biol* 1987; 100: 149–64.
6. Montes RG, Gottal RG, Bayless TM, Hendrix TR, Perman JA. Breath hydrogen testing as a physiology laboratory exercise for medial students. *Am J Physiol* 1992; 262: S25–8.

Gastrointestinal Functions, edited by Edgard E. Delvin and
Michael J. Lentze. Nestlé Nutrition Workshop Series, Pediatric
Program, Vol. 46, Nestec Ltd., Vevey/Lippincott Williams &
Wilkins, Philadelphia © 2001.

Development, Regulation, and Function of Secretory Immunity

Per Brandtzaeg

*Institute of Pathology, Medical Faculty, University of Oslo; Laboratory for
Immunohistochemistry and Immunopathology (LIIPAT), Department of Pathology, The National
Hospital, Rikshospitalet, Oslo, Norway*

The surface area covered by mucosal epithelia probably amounts to more than 200 times that of the skin, thus comprising almost 400 m^2 in an adult individual. This extensive and generally vulnerable monolayered epithelial barrier is protected by numerous innate chemical and physical mechanisms that cooperate intimately with adaptive, specific mucosal immunity. The main humoral mediators of the local specific immune system are secretory IgA (SIgA) and IgM (SIgM); the former class of antibodies constitutes the largest noninflammatory defense system of the body (1–3). Although the secretory antibody system is mainly directed against colonization of pathogens and penetration of ''dangerous'' antigens, it is also involved in immune exclusion of innocuous, soluble proteins present in food (Fig. 1). However, the latter types of antigen as well as components of indigenous bacteria generally induce poorly understood suppressive mechanisms collectively called ''oral tolerance'' when induced through the gut (4,5). This complex phenomenon of mucosally induced tolerance apparently explains why most individuals show no adverse immune reactions to persistent contact with food proteins and the normal microbial flora.

Successful interaction between local innate and specific immunity is a prerequisite for health because the various mucosae are favored as portals of entry by most infectious agents, allergens, and carcinogens. The neonatal period is particularly critical in this respect, as the newborn is immediately exposed to numerous microorganisms, foreign proteins, and chemicals. This chapter contains a summary of how secretory immunity develops, and a discussion of the mechanisms involved in the regulation and function of this adaptive first-line defense system. Its contribution to immune exclusion is virtually lacking during a variable period after birth; breastfeeding, therefore, is important, not only as a natural immunologic ''substitution therapy'' but most likely also because immune-modulating factors in breast milk may enhance the development of the infant's mucosal immune system (6).

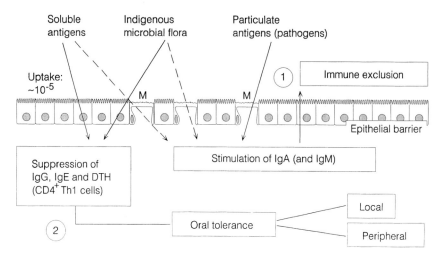

FIG. 1. Schematic depiction of two major adaptive immune mechanisms induced in the gut. (1) Immune exclusion limits epithelial colonization of pathogens and inhibits penetration of harmful foreign material. This first line of defense is principally mediated by secretory antibodies of the IgA (and IgM) class in cooperation with various nonspecific, innate protective factors (not shown). Secretory immunity is preferentially stimulated by particulate antigens and pathogenic infectious agents taken up through M cells (M) as indicated (see Fig. 2). (2) Penetrating, soluble dietary antigens (magnitude of uptake indicated) and the normal microbial flora are less stimulatory for secretory immunity (*broken arrows*) but induce, instead, suppression of proinflammatory humoral immune responses (IgG and IgE antibodies) as well as delayed-type hypersensitivity (DTH) mediated by activated T helper cells (CD4+) of the γ interferon-producing Th1 subset. This complex and poorly defined phenomenon is called "oral tolerance"; it may exert downregulatory effects both locally and in the periphery.

IMMUNE EXCLUSION AND MUCOSAL HOMEOSTASIS

Induction and Dissemination of Local Specific Immunity

After the first period of passive humoral immunity, survival depends on the infant's specific immune responses. In this respect, the SIgA system is the best defined part of adaptive mucosal immunity (7,8). The relative resistance of SIgA against many microbial and endogenous gastrointestinal proteases makes it well suited for surface protection (3,9). In addition, SIgM may have a protective effect, particularly in early infancy and in selective IgA deficiency, but antibodies of this isotype are more easily degraded in the gut lumen than SIgA (10,11).

Primary B-cell responses that give rise to secretory antibodies seem to be elicited mainly in specialized lymphoepithelial structures where antigens are sampled from the mucosal surface (1,8,11–13). Such organized gut-associated lymphoid tissue (GALT) includes aggregated (Peyer's patches) and scattered secondary B-cell follicles (Fig. 2). In the human, Peyer's patches are mainly found in the distal ileum, whereas most of the solitary lymphoid follicles occur in the appendix and distal large bowel. All these components of GALT appear functionally similar; they contain a characteristic follicle-associated epithelium (FAE) with "membrane" (M) cells

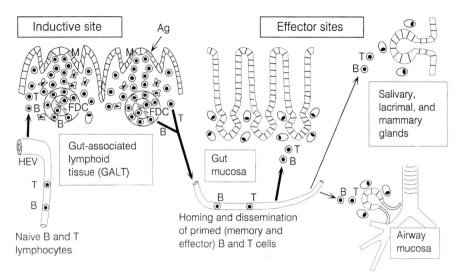

FIG. 2. Schematic depiction of homing in the integrated or so-called "common" human mucosal immune system. Naive B and T lymphocytes are recruited to organized gut-associated lymphoid tissue (GALT) through high endothelial venules (HEV) in the parafollicular T-cell zone. Such lymphoepithelial inductive sites contain activated B-cell follicles with follicular dendritic cells (FDC) and the domes are covered with a specialized epithelium where "membrane" (M) cells transport luminal antigens (Ag) inward. Antigen-primed B and T lymphocytes migrate through lymph and reach peripheral blood for subsequent homing to mucosal effector sites. Their extravasation is particularly efficient in the gut lamina propria (*heavy arrow*) but dissemination also takes place from GALT to more distant effector sites in an integrated manner as indicated (*thin arrows*).

capable of transporting live and dead antigens into the underlying lymphoid tissue (11–13).

Although GALT constitutes the major part of mucosa-associated lymphoid tissue (MALT), induction of mucosal immune responses can probably also take place in the palatine tonsils and other lymphoepithelial structures of the Waldeyer pharyngeal ring, including nasal-associated lymphoid tissue (NALT) such as the adenoids (14). Accumulating evidence suggests that a certain regionalization exists in the mucosal immune system, especially a dichotomy between the gut and the upper aerodigestive tract with regard to homing properties and terminal differentiation of B cells (11,12). This disparity may be explained by microenvironmental differences in the antigenic repertoire as well as in the lymphoid and vascular adhesion molecules involved in local leukocyte extravasation (13). It appears that primed immune cells preferentially home to effector sites corresponding to the inductive sites where they initially responded to an antigen. Because bronchus-associated lymphoid tissue (BALT) is lacking in normal lungs of newborns and adults (15), the Waldeyer ring with the palatine tonsils and adenoids probably represents a significant component of MALT in humans, providing primed B cells for secretory effector sites of the upper aerodigestive tract (11,12,14).

Critical Role of Secretory Immunity in Infancy

The appearance of secretory antibodies in breast milk, directed against both intestinal and respiratory infectious agents, is a reflection of the MALT–mammary gland axis of B-cell migration (3,6,12), and the protective value of breastfeeding is highlighted in relationship to infections in the newborn period, particularly in developing countries. Mucosal pathogens are now a major killer of children below the age of 5 years, being responsible for more than 14 million deaths annually. Diarrheal disease alone claims a toll of 5 million children a year, or approximately 500 deaths every hour. These figures document the need for mucosal vaccines to enhance surface defense against common infectious agents, in addition to advocating breastfeeding. Convincing epidemiologic documentation suggests that the risk of dying from diarrhea is reduced 14 to 24 times in breastfed children (16,17). Indeed, exclusively breastfed infants are better protected against a variety of infections (16,18), atopic allergy (19), and celiac disease (20). Moreover, recent experiments in neonatal rabbits strongly suggest that SIgA is a crucial protective component of breast milk (21). The role of secretory antibodies for mucosal homeostasis is furthermore supported by the fact that knockout mice lacking SIgA and SIgM show increased mucosal leakiness (22).

Efficiency of Receptor-Mediated Secretory Antibody Transport

The remarkable magnitude of GALT as an inductive site for B cells is documented by the fact that at least 80% of all immunoglobulin (Ig)-producing blasts and plasma cells (collectively called immunocytes) in an adult are located in the intestinal lamina propria (11). Some 90% of these terminally differentiated mucosal B cells normally produce mainly dimers or larger polymers of IgA, collectively called "pIgA" (7,8). Such polymers (as well as pentameric IgM) are efficiently transported externally as SIgA and SIgM antibodies by a transmembrane epithelial glycoprotein of approximately 100 kd called "secretory component" (SC), or the polymeric Ig receptor (pIgR), which is constitutively expressed basolaterally on intestinal crypt cells and other serous types of glandular cell (7,11). After transcytosis to the apical surface, SIgA and SIgM are released to the lumen by cleavage of the pIgR, and only the C terminal smaller receptor domain remains for degradation in the epithelial cell; the 80-kd extracellular part is incorporated into the SIg molecules as bound SC, thereby conferring protection against proteolytic degradation—particularly to SIgA in which SC becomes covalently linked (Fig. 3). In adult humans, more pIgA (40 mg/kg body weight) is translocated to the intestinal secretions by this receptor-mediated mechanism every day than the total daily IgG production (~30 mg/kg) (23). Therefore, the gut is quantitatively the most important effector organ of adaptive humoral immunity.

Excess of unoccupied pIgR is released apically to the lumen by proteolytic cleavage in the same manner as SIgA and SIgM to form the so-called free SC (Fig. 3). This 80-kd fragment (identical to bound SC) occurs in most secretions and, by equilibrium with the bound component, it exerts a stabilizing effect on the quaternary

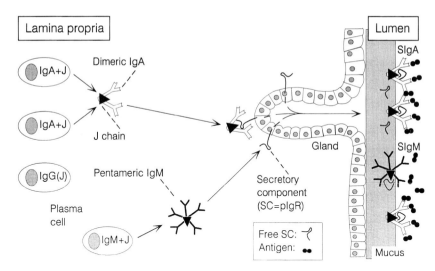

FIG. 3. Model for external transport of J-chain-containing dimeric IgA and pentameric IgM by the transmembrane secretory component (SC) or polymeric Ig receptor (pIgR) expressed basolaterally on glandular epithelial cells. The polymeric Ig molecules are produced with incorporated J chain (IgA + J and IgM + J) by mucosal plasma cells. The resulting secretory Ig molecules (SIgA and SIgM) act in a first line of defense by performing immune exclusion of antigens in the mucus layer on the epithelial surface (to the right). Although J chain is often produced by mucosal IgG plasma cells, it does not combine with this Ig class but is degraded intracellularly (J). Locally produced (and serum-derived) IgG, therefore, is not subjected to active external transport. Free SC (depicted in the mucus) is generated when unoccupied pIgR (at the top) is cleaved at the apical face of the epithelial cell.

structure of SIgM, in which SC remains noncovalently linked (7,8). In various ways, free SC may also contribute to innate mucosal defense (see below).

Constitutive and Cytokine-Induced Regulation of the pIg Receptor

As first proposed by our laboratory in the early 1970s, the receptor-mediated epithelial transport mechanism is shared by pIgA and pentameric IgM because they contain a common 15-kd polypeptide called J (joining) chain produced by the mucosal immunocytes (7,11,24). The J chain constitutes an essential part of the pIgR binding site in the Ig polymers (25). The pIgR belongs to the Ig superfamily (8) and binds the two ligands noncovalently in a somewhat different manner through the first of its five extracellular Ig-like domains (26). Although the receptor expression is constitutively regulated, it can be upregulated synergistically by the immunoregulatory cytokines γ interferon (IFN-γ) and interleukin 4 (IL-4) (8,26,27). Also, the proinflammatory cytokines tumor necrosis factor-α (TNF-α) and IL-1 can enhance pIgR expression in the human HT-29 adenocarcinoma cell line (26,27).

Our recent molecular experiments with the same cell line have shown that IFN-γ, IL-4, and TNF-α enhance pIgR expression by transcriptional activation (28), and,

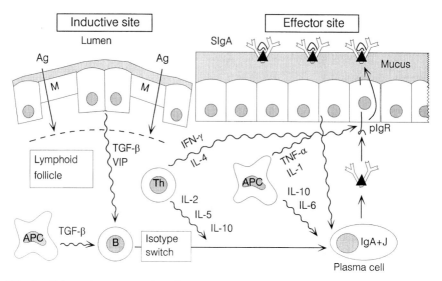

FIG. 4. Schematic representation of regulatory aspects of secretory immunity that take place in inductive compartment (on the left) and at mucosal effector site (on the right). Various cytokines are apparently involved in isotype switching and terminal differentiation of mucosal B cells to promote the striking generation of plasma cells that produce dimeric IgA with J chain (IgA + J) at secretory effector sites. Some of these cytokines may be derived from antigen-presenting cells (APC), T helper cells (Th), or the epithelium, as indicated. In the gut, both transforming growth factor β (TGF-β) and vasoactive intestinal peptide (VIP) may act as IgA switch factors. Certain Th- and APC-derived cytokines also upregulate epithelial expression of the transmembrane secretory component or polymeric Ig receptor (pIgR), thereby providing a regulatory link between the immunologic activity at the effector site and the magnitude of local external transport of secretory IgA (SIgA).

thus, they can provide an immunoregulatory link between the level of a local immune response and the antibody transport function of the receptor (Fig. 4). We and others have cloned and characterized the promoter region of the receptor gene; DNA elements that bind transcription factors belonging to the basic helix-loop-helix leucine zipper family and the interferon regulatory factor family seem to be most important for the constitutive and IFN-γ-enhanced pIgR transcription, respectively (26).

Immunohistochemical observations on celiac disease, chronic gastritis, and Sjögren's syndrome all show an immune response–associated enhancement of secretory immunity; signs of upregulated pIgR expression and increased uptake of IgA are seen in glandular epithelia in all these immunologically active lesions (27). Nevertheless, the pIgR-mediated epithelial transport capacity may be insufficient in certain patients with an unusual intestinal IgA cell expansion, resulting in excessive amounts of pIgA in serum (29).

Regulation of the pIg Receptor by Other Mediators

In addition to cytokines, other soluble factors can modulate the expression of pIgR both *in vitro* and *in vivo*. Butyrate, which is an abundant fermentation product in the colon, can enhance the stimulatory effect of IL-1 and TNF-α in HT-29 cells, particularly in the presence of IFN-γ, but decreases the stimulatory effect of IL-4, even in the presence of IFN-γ (30). It is currently not known whether this reflects the *in vivo* response of the large bowel epithelium. Furthermore, both constitutive and cytokine-enhanced pIgR expression appear to depend on adequate presence of vitamin A (retinoic acid) and the nutritional state of the subject (31,32). In the rat kidney, pIgR mRNA levels were found to be upregulated by a vasopressin-coupled pathway in response to variations in water intake (33). Moreover, parasympathetic and sympathetic autonomic nerve stimulation of rat submandibular glands increased the output SIgA significantly (2.6 and 6 times, respectively); this might reflect an effect of neurotransmitters on the secretory epithelial cells, although an influence of nerves on the local immunocytes could be a contributing factor (34).

Protective Function of SIgA Antibodies and Free Secretory Component

The main purpose of the secretory antibody system is, in cooperation with innate mucosal defense mechanisms, to perform immune exclusion (Fig. 1). Most importantly, SIgA inhibits colonization and invasion by pathogens, and pIgR transported pIgA and pentameric IgM antibodies may even inactivate viruses (e.g., rotavirus and influenza virus) inside secretory epithelial cells and carry the pathogens and their products back to the lumen (35–39), thus avoiding any cytolytic damage to the epithelium (Fig. 5). Both the agglutinating and virus-neutralizing antibody effects of pIgA are superior to those of monomeric antibodies (1), and SIgA antibodies may block microbial invasion efficiently (40). Thus, individuals negative for human immunodeficiency virus (HIV) who live with HIV-positive partners for several years often appear to be protected by specific SIgA antibodies in their genital tract (41). A potentially important additional anti-infectious defense function is the ability of IgA antibodies to induce loss of bacterial plasmids that code for adherence-associated molecules and resistance to antibiotics (42).

Induction of SIgA responses has also been shown to interfere significantly with mucosal uptake of soluble macromolecules in experimental animals (1). Collectively, therefore, the functions of locally produced pIgA would be to inhibit mucosal colonization of microorganisms as well as the penetration of antigens, and this effect is most probably enhanced by the relatively high levels of polyreactive SIgA antibodies (43,44). In the gut, interaction of SIgA with the intestinal superantigen protein Fv (Fv fragment binding protein) may, moreover, build an immune fortress by forming large complexes of intact or degraded antibodies with different specificities (45), thereby probably reinforcing immune exclusion.

It has been claimed that SIgA is capable of antibody-dependent, cell-mediated cytotoxicity and can promote phagocytosis through FcαRI (CD89) present on macrophages and granulocytes, enhance sticking of certain bacteria to mucus, interfere with growth factors (e.g., iron) and enzymes necessary for pathogenic bacteria and parasites, and exert positive influences on the inductive phase of mucosal immunity by promoting antigen uptake in GALT (1,3). The latter possibility adds to the importance of breastfeeding in providing a supply of relevant SIgA antibodies to the infant's gut.

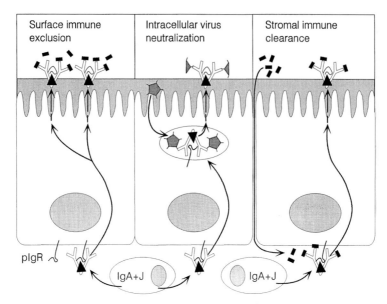

FIG. 5. Schematic representation of three levels at which dimeric IgA or secretory IgA (SIgA) may provide immune protection after being produced with J chain (IgA + J) by plasma cells in the lamina propria. **Left**: Dimeric IgA is transported by the transmembrane secretory component or polymeric Ig receptor (pIgR) across epithelial cells and released into the lumen as SIgA antibodies that perform immune exclusion by interaction with luminal antigens (■). **Middle**: Dimeric IgA antibodies interact with viral antigens within epithelial cells during pIgR-mediated transport, thereby performing intracellular virus neutralization and removal of viral products. **Right**: Dimeric IgA antibodies interact with antigens in the mucosal lamina propria and shuttle them back to the lumen by pIgR-mediated transport.

Interestingly, potentially tissue-damaging eosinophils possess not only FcαRI but apparently also a receptor for free or bound SC (46). This probably explains why SIgA has particularly strong eosinophil-degranulating properties (47,48) and, in this respect, appears to be more potent than cross-linked IgE antibodies, which instead may be more involved in the recruitment and priming of these cells (49). Also, SIgA has been shown to induce degranulation of IL-3 primed basophils (50). Thus, by interacting with eosinophils and basophils (and perhaps also mast cells), SIgA provides a proinflammatory potential for the secretory immune system when immune exclusion fails, such as in parasitic mucosal infestations.

However, currently, it is difficult to know how the balance between SIgA and free SC can influence eosinophil activation, because free SC in solution (but presumably not on a surface) may be blocking in this respect (46,48). Free SC, moreover, may block epithelial adhesion of *Escherichia coli* (51), and a pneumococcal surface protein (SpsA) has recently been shown to interact with both free and bound SC (52). Such observations suggest that, phylogenetically, SC has originated from the innate defense system.

Noninflammatory Mucosal Clearance of Antigens

Intact antigens have been shown to cross the normal gut barrier and enter the blood stream, even in adults, particularly after food intake, although the actual level of uptake remains uncertain (1). Work performed in experimental animals with mucosal application of ^{125}I-labeled albumin has been difficult to interpret because of marker instability; both degradation of the carrier molecule and release of the label can result in considerable overestimation of protein penetrability as determined by scintillation counting compared with data based on immunologic quantification (53).

Several routes can be visualized for the penetration of intact soluble antigen through the normal intestinal epithelium: passive paracellular diffusion or uptake through epithelial discontinuities (e.g., the cell extrusion zones of the villus tips); translocation through enterocytes by endocytosis and subsequent exocytosis; or transport by M cells in GALT. The relative importance of these different mechanisms remains unknown; and the consequences in terms of sensitization or induction of oral tolerance probably depend on the route of uptake as well as on the nature of the antigen (soluble, lectinlike, or particulate). These possibilities have been reviewed in detail elsewhere (1,4,54).

Quantitative studies performed on peripheral blood have provided some information about the absorption of intact dietary antigens in healthy human adults. Paganelli and Levinsky (55) found up to 3 ng/ml of β-lactoglobulin in peripheral blood after an intake of 1.2 L of bovine milk. Kilshaw and Cant (56) often detected both β-lactoglobulin and ovalbumin in peripheral blood as well as in breast milk of lactating women, the levels ranging from 110 pg/ml to 6.4 ng/ml in the latter fluid. Husby et al. (57) reported a serum level up to 10 ng/ml of ovalbumin, which corresponds to approximately 10^{-5} of the amount consumed. Most of the antigen appeared in the circulation after 2 to 5 hours and it was present partly in immune complexes.

Receptor-mediated clearance of immune complexes from the gut lamina propria to the lumen may take place because pIgR expressing epithelial monolayers have been shown to translocate undegraded antigens bound to pIgA antibodies from the basolateral side to the apical culture medium (58). Interestingly, monomeric IgA or IgG antibodies, when cross linked through antigen to pIgA of the same specificity, also contributed to this pIgR-mediated epithelial transport of immune complexes. Secretory epithelia, thus, may participate in noninflammatory removal from the mucosa of locally trapped antigens (Fig. 5).

Additional IgA-Mediated Putative Homeostatic Mechanisms

Experimental evidence also suggests that IgA in gut mucosa may influence local homeostasis by its binding to FcαRI on mucosal leukocytes. First, monomeric IgA—and particularly pIgA or IgA containing immune complexes—is able to suppress the attraction of neutrophils, eosinophils, and monocytes, thereby reducing the availability of the numerous potent inflammatory mediators that may be released from these cells (1). Second, IgA can downregulate the secretion of proinflammatory cytokines such as TNF-α from activated monocytes (59), and perhaps also from mucosal macrophages. Third, activation of neutrophils and monocytes that results in generation of reactive oxygen intermediates (respiratory burst) may also be inhibited by IgA (60). On the other hand, pIgA or aggregated monomeric IgA can trigger resting monocytes to show increased activity such as TNF-α secretion (61) and can also cause eosinophil degranulation (see above). This proinflammatory potential of IgA probably reflects the need for additional local antigen elimination mechanisms when mucosal immune exclusion fails, such as in intestinal parasitic infestations. Altogether, these divergent, experimental *in vitro* results emphasize that the contribution of IgA to normal mucosal homeostasis must be remarkably fine-tuned.

Advantage of IgA Over IgM in the Secretory Immune System

In normal adults, external secretions contain much more SIgA than SIgM, which is mainly explained by the striking predominance of local pIgA-producing cells (11). However, in well-controlled, quantitative studies of jejunal fluid and parotid saliva, the concentration ratio of IgA to IgM is found to be 2.4 to 4.9 times greater than the corresponding local immunocyte class production ratio (62–65). This estimate is based on the observation of a fairly similar synthetic rate in IgA- and IgM-producing cells (66). Notably, mucosal IgA plasma cells release a variable amount of monomeric IgA in addition to pIgA (7), whereas IgM-producing cells are virtually restricted to polymer secretion (67). On a molar basis, therefore, these calculations mean that the external transfer of pIgA is favored at least 6 to 12 times over that of pentameric IgM, suggesting the existence of significant biological variables of secretory immunity other than the local immunocyte distribution. Such variables could reflect differences in diffusion properties across the stromal matrix and basement membrane, in the affinity of the Ig polymers for pIgR, or in the efficiency of the pIgR-mediated epithelial transcytosis of the two ligands.

In a recent *in vitro* study, we examined the impact of these variables on the epithelial transport of pIgA and pentameric IgM (68). *In vivo* observations suggest that monomeric IgA, as is the case with IgG, diffuses more easily across basement membranes than pentameric IgM; the latter is mainly found intravascularly (78%), whereas most of the former (60%) is abundantly distributed in interstitial tissue fluid. In addition, some SIgA (2%) present in intestinal juice appears to be derived from serum pIgA, whereas much less (<1%) SIgM originates from serum IgM (69). Therefore, we compared the diffusion properties of pIgA and pentameric IgM as well as their binding to, and translocation by, polarized Madin–Darby canine kidney (MDCK) cells transfected to express the human pIgR. Not unexpectedly, pIgA diffused more readily than pentameric IgM through various filters used to support the MDCK monolayers. This result was supported by *in situ* immunofluorescence staining of the intestinal mucosa that showed preferential retention of pentameric IgM, both in lamina propria vessel walls and in epithelial basement membrane zones (68). The jejunal basement membrane is composed of a fine collagen network, with an estimated pore size of 13.5 nm (70). Radiographic analyses of the Fc region of pentameric IgM, combined with computerized molecular modeling (71), and electron microscopical analysis (72), suggest a molecular diameter in the range of 30 to 40 nm. Thus, the size of pentameric IgM most probably imposes severe restriction on its diffusion across basement membranes *in vivo* and, hence, its access to the pIgR. Also, it is possible that some of the retained pentameric IgM is broken down along with the proteolytic turnover of basement membranes, although this ligand was transcytosed as efficiently as pIgA by the human pIgR (68).

Altogether, the pIgA molecule appears to be particularly well designed for efficient protection of mucosal surfaces by possessing molecular characteristics that make it well-suited, both for efficient external transfer and for survival in exocrine secretions. Also, pIgA serves to maintain local immunologic homeostasis, both by performing immune exclusion as SIgA antibodies and by its anti-inflammatory action within the mucosa. These properties of pIgA may collectively have represented an evolutionary advantage over IgM in selecting SIgA as the dominant secretory antibody class in humans. Therefore, pIgA appears to be a ''smaller and smarter'' antibody than pentameric IgM in terms of mucosal defense.

POSTNATAL DEVELOPMENT OF SECRETORY IMMUNITY

Mucosal B-Cell System

Peyer's patches and other GALT structures are well-developed at birth, discrete T- and B-cell areas being apparent as early as 19 weeks of gestation (73). However, secondary follicles with germinal centers signifying B-cell activation do not occur until some weeks after birth; this reflects their dependency on exogenous environmental stimulation. The germinal center B cells of murine Peyer's patches express small amounts of surface IgA along with less IgM or IgG (74). Such isotype skewing reflects B-cell switching in the course of clonal differentiation to precursors for IgA-producing immunocytes, the preferential induction of which is the hallmark of GALT (13).

The fact that the postnatal immune activation of GALT is retarded parallels the temporary immaturity of systemic immunocompetence observed in the newborn period (5,75,76). Thus, very few B cells with IgA-producing capacity (presumably GALT derived) are present in the peripheral blood of newborns ($< 8/10^6$ mononuclear cells); after 1 month, however, this number is remarkably increased ($\sim 500/10^6$ mononuclear cells), reflecting the progressive environmental stimulation of GALT (77). An initial early increase in positive cells can be seen in preterm infants, especially in those with intrauterine infections, although IgM production predominates in these cases. In agreement with these observations in peripheral blood, only occasional IgM- and IgG-producing intestinal immunocytes are present at birth, and local IgA immunocytes are either absent or extremely rare even until after 10 days of age (10). The numbers of mucosal IgM- and IgA-producing cells increase rapidly after 2 to 4 weeks, the latter class becoming predominant at 1 to 2 months and usually peaking at about 12 months.

An early SIgM antibody response is probably of protective value, but it is known that specific immunity to certain bacterial capsular polysaccharides is poor or lacking before 2 years of age. This creates a window of susceptibility at the time of disappearance of protective maternal IgG antibodies together with weaning and deprivation of passively acquired SIgA from breast milk. The basis for the impaired immune response to polysaccharides is unclear, but reduced levels of complement receptor 2 (CR2, CD21) expression on B cells and follicular dendritic cells, together with low complement activity in newborns, may result in lack of CR2/B-cell receptor synergy, thereby contributing to defective B-cell activation (78). Compelling evidence indicates that the interaction of the complement split product C3d with CR2 is an extremely important link between innate immunity and specific B-cell responses (79).

Individual Variations in the Development of Mucosal Homeostasis

It should be noted that the postnatal mucosal B-cell development shows large individual variation (10). To some extent this variability might be genetically determined and could exert an important impact on children's health when their SIgA-mediated immune exclusion and other noninflammatory mucosal antigen-handling mechanisms are transiently inefficient.

On the basis of IgA measurements in serum, it has been suggested that infants and children at hereditary risk of atopy have a retarded postnatal development of their IgA system (80,81). Perhaps their SIgA-mediated immune exclusion and other noninflammatory mucosal antigen-handling mechanisms are transiently deficient. This notion was later supported by quantitation of jejunal immunocytes; a significantly reduced IgA response to luminal antigens, without any IgM compensation, was found in the mucosa of atopic children (82). Another study showed an inverse relationship between the serum IgE concentration and the number of IgA-producing cells in jejunal mucosa of children with food allergy (83). More recently, it was reported that infants born to atopic parents have a significantly higher prevalence of salivary IgA deficiency than age-matched control infants (84). Interestingly, Kilian et al. (85) found that the throats of infants aged 18 months with presumably IgE-mediated clinical problems contained significantly higher proportions of IgA1 protease-producing bacteria than age-matched healthy controls.

Therefore, a combination of reduced SIgA-dependent epithelial barrier function and hereditary increased IgE responses might often underlie the pathogenesis of mucosal hypersensitivity, at least in many of the atopic children. This notion accords with the increased frequency of infections, atopic allergies, and gluten-dependent enteropathy (celiac disease) seen in subjects with permanent selective IgA deficiency, although compensatory overproduction of SIgM, to some extent, may counteract the adverse consequences of their absent mucosal IgA responses (10,86).

Role of Antigen Exposure in the Development of IgA-Producing Cells

The antigenic and mitogenic load on the mucosa appears to be a decisive factor for the postnatal development of the secretory immune system. Antigenic constituents of food clearly exert a stimulatory effect, as suggested by fewer lamina propria IgA-producing cells in mice fed on hydrolyzed milk proteins (87) as well as in parenterally fed babies (88). However, the indigenous microbial flora is of utmost importance, as indicated by the fact that the intestinal IgA system of germ-free or specific pathogen-free mice is normalized after approximately 4 weeks of conventionalization (89,90). Bacteroides and *E. coli* strains seem to be particularly stimulatory for the development of intestinal IgA immunocytes (91,92). Interestingly, early colonization of infants with a nonenteropathogenic strain of *E. coli* has recently been reported to have a long-term beneficial effect in reducing both infections and allergies (93).

Decreased amounts of both dietary and microbial antigens, thus, can explain why the numbers of colonic IgA- and IgM-producing immunocytes were found to be decreased by approximately 50% after 2 to 11 months in children who had been subjected to defunctioning colostomies (94). Postnatal and prolonged observations on defunctioned ileal segments in lambs have even more strikingly revealed a scarcity of immunocytes in the lamina propria; this result was explained by reduced local accumulation of B-cell blasts and might involve both hampered migration from GALT to the mucosa and, subsequently, decreased local proliferation and differentiation (95). It follows that the postnatal development of the mucosal IgA system is usually much faster in developing countries than in the industrialized parts of the world (10). This difference apparently holds true even in malnourished children (96), which reflects the fact that mucosal immunity is highly adaptable to the antigenic load of the environment.

In the light of these findings, a reduced SIgA-dependent barrier function could contribute to the increased frequency of certain diseases in industrialized countries, particularly allergies and other inflammatory disorders. The possible beneficial effect of probiotic preparations, therefore, has been evaluated in several experimental and clinical studies. Interestingly, especially viable preparations containing *Lactobacillus* spp. and *Bifidobacterium* spp. have been reported to enhance the IgA system, both in humans and in experimental animals (97–101), apparently in a T-cell–dependent manner (102).

Nutrition and Intestinal Immunity

An early immunohistochemical study of children with low protein-energy intake reported selective reduction of intestinal IgA-producing immunocytes (103). This was supported by experiments in rodents with prolonged and severe malnutrition (104); hampered homing of IgA-expressing B cells from GALT might be involved (105). Severe vitamin A deficiency appears to have a particularly marked adverse effect on mucosal IgA antibody responses (106), but with no consistent downregulation of epithelial IgA transport (107), although cytokine-mediated upregulation of pIgR *in vitro* appears to depend on this vitamin (31). Interestingly, although energy deficiency reduces intestinal pIgA expression in weanling mice (32), it has been reported that undernourished children respond to bacterial overgrowth in the gut with enhanced synthesis as well as upregulated external transfer of IgA (108). It is of great clinical importance that the detrimental effects of severe malnutrition on the SIgA system can be reversed by nutritional rehabilitation (109).

CONCLUSIONS

Secretory immunity depends on an intimate cooperation between mucosal B cells and the pIgR/SC-expressing epithelia. The obvious biological significance of the striking J-chain expression shown by disseminated MALT-derived immunocytes is that IgA and IgM polymers with high affinity for pIgR/SC can be produced at secretory effector sites and become readily available for active external transport.

Considerable evidence supports the notion that intestinal immunocytes are largely derived from B cells initially induced in GALT, but insufficient knowledge exists concerning intestinal uptake, processing, and presentation of luminal antigens as a basis for the extensive and continuous priming and expansion of mucosal B cells. Also, it is not clear how the germinal-center reaction in GALT, compared with other parts of MALT (e.g., tonsils), so strikingly promotes preferential isotype switching to IgA and a high level of J-chain expression.

Although the B-cell migration from GALT to the intestinal lamina propria is guided by rather well-characterized adhesion molecules, the chemotactic stimuli involved in extravasation and microcompartmental distribution of various B-cell subsets remain elusive. Importantly, the homing mechanisms of mucosal B cells appear to be remarkably regionalized. Retention and accumulation of the extravasated B cells at secretory effector sites are influenced by antigen-driven local proliferation and differentiation. However, little is known about the necessary stimulatory signals for this process.

The mucosal barrier normally allows some penetration of intact soluble antigens so a need probably always exists for immune elimination in the lamina propria. If immune exclusion is impaired (e.g., in IgA deficiency) or too large an antigen load is found on the epithelial barrier (e.g., in chronic infection), activated nonspecific amplification mechanisms involved in immune elimination may cause hypersensitivity which is observed clinically as mucosal disease. Although the immunopathogenic mechanisms are rather well understood in some of intestinal disorders (e.g., atopic food allergy and celiac disease), the cause of their initiation, possibly involving abrogation of oral tolerance, generally remains unexplained.

Clinical observations in humans, as well as studies of pIgR/SC knockout mice, suggest that secretory immunity is not the only important part of intestinal mucosal defense; thus, it is becoming increasingly evident that innate local immunity is crucial and much more complex than previously believed. The cooperation between innate and adaptive mucosal immunity needs exploration to better understand how homeostasis of mucous membranes normally is maintained.

The relationship between induction of intestinal IgA responses and oral tolerance remains somewhat of an enigma (4). Experiments in CD8 knockout mice have suggested that this phenotype of T lymphocytes (the predominant intraepithelial lymphocyte subset) is crucial for downregulation of the mucosal B-cell system (110). The hyporesponsiveness of the intestinal immune system appears to be robust, because even a strong immunogen such as cholera toxin (CT) is unable to abrogate it, although oral tolerance cannot be induced in the presence of CT (110). On the other hand, transforming growth factor β has also been shown to be important in promoting IgA switching (Fig. 4) in mice immunized with CT (111), and this cytokine is believed to be one of the major mediators of oral tolerance in murine test systems (112). It is not yet possible to extrapolate such apparently contradictory information to the human mucosal immune system.

It is well established in the human gut that the mucosal immune system responds to infection with local IgA and IgM production (113), and it appears that the level of this secretory antibody response may determine whether clinical symptoms will or will not occur (114). In experimental animals, antibody-dependent immune exclusion has been shown to operate even for small molecules such as chemical carcinogens (115,116). However, further studies are needed because a rational basis for manipulation of local immunity by vaccines is still not satisfactorily established.

ACKNOWLEDGMENTS

Studies in my laboratory are supported by the Norwegian Cancer Society, the Research Council of Norway, Anders Jahre's foundation, and Rakel and Otto Kr. Bruun's Legacy. I thank Ms. Marit Henningsen and Mr. Erik K. Hagen for excellent secretarial assistance.

REFERENCES

1. Brandtzaeg P, Baklien K, Bjerke K, Rognum TO, Scott H, Valnes K. Nature and properties of the human gastrointestinal immune system. In: Miller K, Nicklin S, eds. *Immunology of the gastrointestinal tract*, Vol 1. Boca Raton: CRC Press, 1987: 1–85.
2. Russell MW, Reinholdt J, Kilian M. Anti-inflammatory activity of human IgA antibodies and their Fabα fragments: inhibition of IgG-mediated complement activation. *Eur J Immunol* 1989; 19: 2243–9.
3. Goldblum RM, Hanson LÅ, Brandtzaeg P. The mucosal defense system. In: Stiehm ER, ed. *Immunologic disorders in infants & children*, 4th ed. Philadelphia: WB Saunders, 1996: 159–99.
4. Brandtzaeg P. History of oral tolerance and mucosal immunity. *Ann NY Acad Sci* 1996; 778: 1–27.
5. Brandtzaeg P. Development and basic mechanisms of human gut immunity. *Nutr Rev* 1998; 56: S5–18.
6. Brandtzaeg P. Development of the mucosal immune system in humans. In: Bindels JG, Goedhart AC, Visser HKA, eds. *Recent developments in infant nutrition*. London: Kluwer Academic Publishers, 1996: 349–76.
7. Brandtzaeg P. Role of J chain and secretory component in receptor-mediated glandular and hepatic transport of immunoglobulins in man. *Scand J Immunol* 1985; 22: 111–46.
8. Brandtzaeg P. Molecular and cellular aspects of the secretory immunoglobulin system. *APMIS* 1995; 103: 1–19.
9. Kilian M, Reinholdt J, Lomholt H, Poulsen K, Frandsen EV. Biological significance of IgA1 proteases in bacterial colonization and pathogenesis: critical evaluation of experimental evidence. *APMIS* 1996; 104: 321–38.
10. Brandtzaeg P, Nilssen DE, Rognum TO, Thrane PS. Ontogeny of the mucosal immune system and IgA deficiency. *Gastroenterol Clin North Am* 1991; 20: 397–439.
11. Brandtzaeg P, Farstad IN, Johansen F-E, Morton HC, Norderhaug IN, Yamanaka T. The B-cell system of human mucosae and exocrine glands. *Immunol Rev* 1999; 171: 45 -87.
12. Brandtzaeg P, Baekkevold ES, Farstad IN, *et al.* Regional specialization in the mucosal immune system: what happens in the microcompartments? *Immunol Today* 1999; 20: 141–51.
13. Brandtzaeg P, Farstad IN, Haraldsen G. Regional specialization in the mucosal immune system: primed cells do not always home along the same track. *Immunol Today* 1999; 20: 267–77.

14. Brandtzaeg P. Regionalized immune function of tonsils and adenoids. *Immunol Today* 1999; 20: 383–4.
15. Tschernig T, Kleemann WJ, Pabst R. Bronchus-associated lymphoid tissue (BALT) in the lungs of children who had died from sudden infant death syndrome and other causes. *Thorax* 1995; 50: 658–60.
16. Hanson LÅ, Ashraf R, Carlsson B, *et al.* Save the children. In: Hanson LÅ, Köhler L, eds. *Peace, health and development.* Göteburg, Sweden. NHV Report, 1993; 4: 31–8.
17. Anonymous. A warm chain for breastfeeding [Editorial]. *Lancet* 1994; 344: 1239–41.
18. Wright AL, Bauer M, Naylor A, Sutcliffe E, Clark L. Increasing breastfeeding rates to reduce infant illness at the community level. *Pediatrics* 1998; 101: 837–44.
19. Saarinen UM, Kajosaari M. Breastfeeding as prophylaxis against atopic disease: prospective follow-up study until 17 years old. *Lancet* 1995; 346: 1065–9.
20. Brandtzaeg P. Development of the intestinal immune system and its relation to coeliac disease. In: Mäki M, Collin P, Visakorpi JK, eds. *Coeliac disease.* Proceedings of the Seventh International Symposium on Coeliac Disease. Coeliac Disease Study Group, Tampere, 1997: 221–44.
21. Dickinson EC, Gorga JC, Garrett M, *et al.* Immunoglobulin A supplementation abrogates bacterial translocation and preserves the architecture of the intestinal epithelium. *Surgery* 1998; 124: 284–90.
22. Johansen F-E, Pekna M, Norderhaug IN, *et al.* Absence of epithelial immunoglobulin A transport, with increased mucosal leakiness, in polymeric immunoglobulin receptor/secretory component-deficient mice. *J Exp Med* 1999; 190: 915–21.
23. Conley ME, Delacroix DL. Intravascular and mucosal immunoglobulin A: two separate but related systems of immune defense? *Ann Intern Med* 1987; 106: 892–9.
24. Brandtzaeg P. Presence of J chain in human immunocytes containing various immunoglobulin classes. *Nature* 1974; 252: 418–20.
25. Brandtzaeg P, Prydz H. Direct evidence for an integrated function of J chain and secretory component in epithelial transport of immunoglobulins. *Nature* 1984; 311: 71–3.
26. Norderhaug IN, Johansen F-E, Schjerven H, Brandtzaeg P. Regulation of the formation and external transport of secretory immunoglobulins. *Crit Rev Immunol* 1999; 19: 481–508.
27. Brandtzaeg P, Halstensen TS, Huitfeldt HS, *et al.* Epithelial expression of HLA, secretory component (poly-Ig receptor), and adhesion molecules in the human alimentary tract. *Ann NY Acad Sci* 1992; 664: 157–79.
28. Nilsen EM, Johansen F-E, Kvale D, Krajci P, Brandtzaeg P. Different regulatory pathways employed in cytokine-enhanced expression of secretory component and epithelial HLA class I genes. *Eur J Immunol* 1999; 29: 168–79.
29. Brandtzaeg P, Baklien K. Characterization of the IgA-immunocyte population and its product in a patient with excessive intestinal formation of IgA. *Clin Exp Immunol* 1977; 30: 77–88.
30. Kvale D, Brandtzaeg P. Constitutive and cytokine induced expression of HLA molecules, secretory component, and intercellular adhesion molecule-1 is modulated by butyrate in the colonic epithelial cell line HT-29. *Gut* 1995; 36: 737–42.
31. Sarkar J, Gangopadhyay NN, Moldoveanu Z, Mestecky J, Stephensen CB. Vitamin A is required for regulation of polymeric immunoglobulin receptor (pIgR) expression by interleukin-4 and interferon-gamma in a human intestinal epithelial cell line. *J Nutr* 1998; 128: 1063–9.
32. Ha CL, Woodward B. Depression in the quantity of intestinal secretory IgA and in the expression of the polymeric immunoglobulin receptor in caloric deficiency of the weanling mouse. *Lab Invest* 1998; 78: 1255–66.
33. Rice JC, Spence JS, Megyesi J, Safirstein RL, Goldblum RM. Regulation of the polymeric immuno-globulin receptor by water intake and vasopressin in the rat kidney. *Am J Physiol* 1998; 274: F966–77.
34. Carpenter GH, Garrett JR, Hartley RH, Proctor GB. The influence of nerves on the secretion of immunoglobulin A into submandibular saliva in rats. *J Physiol (Lond)* 1998; 512: 567–73.
35. Mazanec MB, Kaetzel CS, Lamm ME, Fletcher D, Nedrud JG. Intracellular neutralization of virus by immunoglobulin A antibodies. *Proc Natl Acad Sci USA* 1992; 89: 6901–5.
36. Mazanec MB, Coudret CI, Fletcher D. Intracellular neutralization of influenza virus by immunoglob-ulin A anti-hemagglutinin monoclonal antibodies. *J Virol* 1995; 69: 1339–43.
37. Bomsel M, Heyman M, Hocini H, *et al.* Intracellular neutralization of HIV transcytosis across tight epithelial barriers by anti-HIV envelope protein dIgA or IgM. *Immunity* 1998; 9: 277–87.
38. Burns JW, Siadat-Pajouh M, Krishnaney AA, Greenberg HB. Protective effect of rotavirus VP6-specific IgA monoclonal antibodies that lack neutralizing activity. *Science* 1996; 272: 104–7.

39. Fujioka H, Emancipator SN, Aikawa M, *et al.* Immunocytochemical colocalization of specific immunoglobulin A with sendai virus protein in infected polarized epithelium. *J Exp Med* 1998; 188: 1223–9.

40. Hocini H, Bélec L, Iscaki S, *et al.* High-level ability of secretory IgA to block HIV type 1 transcytosis: contrasting secretory IgA and IgG responses to glycoprotein 160. *AIDS Res Hum Retrovirus* 1997; 13: 1179–85.

41. Mazzoli S, Trabattoni D, Lo Caputo S, *et al.* HIV-specific mucosal and cellular immunity in HIV-seronegative partners of HIV-seropositive individuals. *Nat Med* 1997; 3: 1250–7.

42. Porter P, Linggood MA. Novel mucosal anti-microbial functions interfering with the plasmid-mediated virulence determinants of adherence and drug resistance. *Ann NY Acad Sci* 1983; 409: 564–78.

43. Quan CP, Berneman A, Pires R, Avrameas S, Bouvet JP. Natural polyreactive secretory immunoglobulin A autoantibodies as a possible barrier to infection in humans. *Infect Immun* 1997; 65: 3997–4004.

44. Bouvet JP, Dighiero G. From natural polyreactive autoantibodies to a la carte monoreactive antibodies to infectious agents: is it a small world after all? *Infect Immun* 1998; 66: 1–4.

45. Bouvet J-P, Piràs R, Quan CP. Protein Fv (Fv fragment binding protein): a mucosal human superantigen reacting with normal immunoglobulins. In: Zouali M, ed. *Human B cell superantigens*. Austin, Texas: RG Landes, 1996: 179–87.

46. Lamkhioued B, Gounni AS, Gruart V, Pierce A, Capron A, Capron M. Human eosinophils express a receptor for secretory component. Role in secretory IgA-dependent activation. *Eur J Immunol* 1995; 25: 117–25.

47. Abu-Ghazaleh RI, Fujisawa T, Mestecky J, Kyle RA, Gleich GJ. IgA-induced eosinophil degranulation. *J Immunol* 1989; 142: 2393–400.

48. Motegi Y, Kita H. Interaction with secretory component stimulates effector functions of human eosinophils but not of neutrophils. *J Immunol* 1998; 161: 4340–6.

49. Peebles RS, Liu MC, Adkinson NF, Lichtenstein LM, Hamilton RG. Ragweed-specific antibodies in bronchoalveolar lavage fluids and serum before and after segmental lung challenge: IgE and IgA associated with eosinophil degranulation. *J Allergy Clin Immunol* 1998; 101: 265–73.

50. Iikura M, Yamaguchi M, Fujisawa T, *et al.* Secretory IgA induces degranulation of IL-3-primed basophils. *J Immunol* 1998; 161: 1510–15.

51. Giugliano LG, Ribeiro STG, Vainstein MH, Ulhoa CJ. Free secretory component and lactoferrin of human milk inhibit the adhesion of enterotoxigenic *Escherichia coli*. *J Med Microbiol* 1995; 42: 3–9.

52. Hammerschmidt S, Talay SR, Brandtzaeg P, Chhatwal GS. SpsA, a novel pneumococcal surface protein with specific binding to secretory immunoglobulin A and secretory component. *Mol Microbiol* 1997; 25: 1113–24.

53. Brandtzaeg P, Tolo K. Mucosal penetrability enhanced by serum-derived antibodies. *Nature* 1977; 266: 262–3.

54. Sanderson IR, Walker WA. Uptake and transport of macromolecules by the intestine: possible role in clinical disorders (an update). *Gastroenterology* 1993; 104: 622–39.

55. Paganelli R, Levinsky RJ. Solid phase radioimmunoassay for detection of circulating food protein antigens in human serum. *J Immunol Methods* 1980; 37: 333–41.

56. Kilshaw PJ, Cant AJ. The passage of maternal dietary proteins into human breast milk. *Int Arch Allergy Appl Immunol* 1984; 75: 8–15.

57. Husby S, Jensenius JC, Svehag S-E. Passage of undegraded dietary antigen into the blood of healthy adults. Quantification, estimation of size distribution, and relation of uptake to levels of specific antibodies. *Scand J Immunol* 1985; 22: 83–92.

58. Kaetzel CS, Robinson JK, Chintalacharuvu KR, Vaerman JP, Lamm ME. The polymeric immunoglobulin receptor (secretory component) mediates transport of immune complexes across epithelial cells: a local defense function for IgA. *Proc Natl Acad Sci USA* 1991; 88: 8796–800.

59. Wolf HM, Fischer MB, Pühringer H, Samstag A, Vogel E, Eibl MM. Human serum IgA downregulates the release of inflammatory cytokines (tumor necrosis factor-α, interleukin-6) in human monocytes. *Blood* 1994; 83: 1278–88.

60. Wolf HM, Vogel E, Fischer MB, Rengs H, Schwarz H-P, Eibl MM. Inhibition of receptor-dependent and receptor-independent generation of the respiratory burst in human neutrophils and monocytes by human serum IgA. *Pediatr Res* 1994; 36: 235–43.

61. Devière J, Vaerman J-P, Content J, et al. IgA triggers tumor necrosis factor α secretion by mono-cytes: a study in normal subjects and patients with alcoholic cirrhosis. Hepatology 1991; 13: 670–5.

62. Brandtzaeg P, Fjellanger I, Gjeruldsen ST. Human secretory immunoglobulins. I. Salivary secretions from individuals with normal or low levels of serum immunoglobulins. Scandinavian Journal of Haematology 1970; Suppl. No. 12: 1–83.

63. Müller F, Frøland S, Hvatum M, Radl J, Brandtzaeg P. Both IgA subclasses are reduced in parotid saliva from patients with AIDS. Clin Exp Immunol 1991; 83: 203–9.

64. Feltelius N, Hvatum M, Brandtzaeg P, Knutson L, Hällgren R. Increased jejunal secretory IgA and IgM in ankylosing spondylitis: normalization after treatment with sulphasalazine. J Rheumatol 1994; 21: 2076–81.

65. Prigent-Delecourt L, Coffin B, Colombel JF, Dehennin JP, Vaerman JP, Rambaud JC. Secretion of immunoglobulins and plasma proteins from the colonic mucosa: an in vivo study in man. Clin Exp Immunol 1995; 99: 221–5.

66. Gitlin D, Sasaki T. Immunoglobulins G, A, and M determined in single cells from human tonsil. Science 1969; 164: 1532–4.

67. Alberini CM, Bet P, Milstein C, Sitia R. Secretion of immunoglobulin M assembly intermediates in the presence of reducing agents. Nature 1990; 347: 485–7.

68. Natvig IB, Johansen F-E, Nordeng TW, Haraldsen G, Brandtzaeg P. Mechanism for enhanced external transfer of dimeric IgA over pentameric IgM. Studies of diffusion, binding to the human polymeric Ig receptor, and epithelial transcytosis. J Immunol 1997; 159: 4330–40.

69. Jonard PP, Rambaud JC, Dive C, Vaerman JP, Galian A, Delacroix DL. Secretion of immunoglobu-lins and plasma proteins from the jejunal mucosa. Transport rate and origin of polymeric immuno-globulin A. J Clin Invest 1984; 74: 525–35.

70. Inoue S. Basic structure of basement membranes is a fine network of ''cords,'' irregular anastomos-ing strands. Microsc Res Technol 1994; 28: 29–47.

71. Perkins SJ, Nealis AS, Sutton BJ, Feinstein A. Solution structure of human and mouse immunoglobu-lin M by synchrotron x-ray scattering and molecular graphics modelling. A possible mechanism for complement activation. J Mol Biol 1991; 221: 1345–66.

72. Davis AC, Roux KH, Pursey J, Shulman MJ. Intermolecular disulfide bonding in IgM: effects of replacing cysteine residues in the mu heavy chain. EMBO J 1989; 8: 2519–26.

73. Spencer J, MacDonald TT. Ontogeny of human mucosal immunity. In: MacDonald TT, ed. Ontogeny of the immune system of the gut. Boca Raton: CRC Press, 1990: 23–50.

74. Butcher EC, Rouse RV, Coffman RL, Nottenburg CN, Hardy RR, Weissman IL. Surface phenotype of Peyer's patch germinal center cells: implications for the role of germinal centers in B cell differentiation. J Immunol 1982; 129: 2698–707.

75. Holt PG. Postnatal maturation of immune competence during infancy and childhood. Pediatr Allergy Immunol 1995; 6: 59–70.

76. MacDonald TT, Spencer J. Development of gastrointestinal immune function and its relationship to intestinal disease. Curr Opin Gastroenterol 1993; 9: 946–52.

77. Stoll BJ, Lee FK, Hale E, et al. Immunoglobulin secretion by the normal and the infected newborn infant. J Pediatr 1993; 122: 780–6.

78. Griffioen AW, Franklin SW, Zegers BJ, Rijkers GT. Expression and functional characteristics of the complement receptor type 2 on adult and neonatal B lymphocytes. Clin Immunol Immunopathol 1993; 69: 1–8.

79. Dempsey PW, Allison ME, Akkaraju S, Goodnow CC, Fearon DT. C3d of complement as a molecu-lar adjuvant: bridging innate and acquired immunity. Science 1996; 271: 348–50.

80. Taylor B, Norman AP, Orgel HA, Stokes CR, Turner MW, Soothill JF. Transient IgA deficiency and pathogenesis of infantile atopy. Lancet 1973; ii: 111–13.

81. Soothill JF. Some intrinsic and extrinsic factors predisposing to allergy. Proc R Soc Med 1976; 69: 439–42.

82. Sloper KS, Brook CG, Kingston D, Pearson JR, Shiner M. Eczema and atopy in early childhood: low IgA plasma cell counts in the jejunal mucosa. Arch Dis Child 1981; 56: 939–42.

83. Perkkiö M. Immunohistochemical study of intestinal biopsies from children with atopic eczema due to food allergy. Allergy 1980; 35: 573–80.

84. van Asperen PP, Gleeson M, Kemp AS, et al. The relationship between atopy and salivary IgA deficiency in infancy. Clin Exp Immunol 1985; 62: 753–7.

85. Kilian M, Husby S, Host A, Halken S. Increased proportions of bacteria capable of cleaving IgA1 in the pharynx of infants with atopic disease. Pediatr Res 1995; 38: 182–6.

86. Brandtzaeg P, Nilssen DE. Mucosal aspects of primary B-cell deficiency and gastrointestinal infections. *Curr Opin Gastroenterol* 1995; 11: 532–40.
87. Sagie E, Tarabulus J, Maeir DM, Freier S. Diet and development of intestinal IgA in the mouse. *Isr J Med Sci* 1974; 10: 532–4.
88. Knox WF. Restricted feeding and human intestinal plasma cell development. *Arch Dis Child* 1986; 61: 744–9.
89. Crabbé PA, Nash DR, Bazin H, Eyssen H, Heremans JF. Immunohistochemical observations on lymphoid tissues from conventional and germ-free mice. *Lab Invest* 1970; 22: 448–57.
90. Horsfall DJ, Cooper JM, Rowley D. Changes in the immunoglobulin levels of the mouse gut and serum during conventionalisation and following administration of *Salmonella typhimurium. Aust J Exp Biol Med Sci* 1978; 56: 727–35.
91. Lodinova R, Jouja V, Wagner V. Serum immunoglobulins and coproantibody formation in infants after artificial intestinal colonization with *Escherichia coli* 083 and oral lysozyme administration. *Pediatr Res* 1973; 7: 659–69.
92. Moreau MC, Ducluzeau R, Guy-Grand D, Muller MC. Increase in the population of duodenal immunoglobulin A plasmocytes in axenic mice associated with different living or dead bacterial strains of intestinal origin. *Infect Immun* 1978; 121: 532–9.
93. Lodinová-Žádniková R, Cukrowská B. Influence of oral colonization of the intestine with a non-enteropathogenic *E. coli* strain after birth on the frequency of infectious and allergic diseases after 10 and 20 years [Abstract]. *Immunol Lett* 1999; 69: 64.
94. Wijesinha SS, Steer HW. Studies of the immunoglobulin-producing cells of the human intestine: the defunctioned bowel. *Gut* 1982; 23: 211–14.
95. Reynolds JD, Morris B. The influence of gut function on lymphoid cell populations in the intestinal mucosa of lambs. *Immunology* 1983; 49: 501–9.
96. Nagao AT, Pilagallo MIDS, Pereira AB. Quantitation of salivary, urinary and faecal sIgA in children living in different conditions of antigenic exposure. *J Trop Pediatr* 1993; 39: 278–83.
97. Kaila M, Isolauri E, Soppi E, Virtanen E, Laine S, Arvilommi H. Enhancement of the circulating antibody secreting cell response in human diarrhea by a human *Lactobacillus* strain. *Pediatr Res* 1992; 32: 141–4.
98. Kaila M, Isolauri E, Saxelin M, Arvilommi H, Vesikari T. Viable versus inactivated *Lactobacillus* strain GG in acute rotavirus diarrhoea. *Arch Dis Child* 1995; 72: 51–3.
99. Isolauri E, Joensuu J, Suomalainen H, Luomala M, Vesikari T. Improved immunogenicity of oral D × RRV reassortant rotavirus vaccine by *Lactobacillus casei* GG. *Vaccine* 1995; 13: 310–12.
100. Yasui H, Kiyoshima J, Ushijima H. Passive protection against rotavirus-induced diarrhea of mouse pups born to and nursed by dams fed *Bifidobacterium breve* YIT4064. *J Infect Dis* 1995; 172: 403–9.
101. Malin M, Suomalainen H, Saxelin M, Isolauri E. Promotion of IgA immune response in patients with Crohn's disease by oral bacteriotherapy with *Lactobacillus* GG. *Ann Nutr Metab* 1996; 40: 137–45.
102. Prokesová L, Ladmanová P, Çechová D, *et al.* Stimulatory effects of *Bacillus firmus* on IgA production in humans and mice [Abstract]. *Immunol Lett* 1999; 69: 55–6.
103. Green F, Heyworth B. Immunoglobulin-containing cells in jejunal mucosa of children with protein energy malnutrition and gastroenteritis. *Arch Dis Child* 1980; 55: 380–3.
104. Wade S, Lemonnier D, Alexiu A, Bocquet L. Effect of early postnatal under- and overnutrition on the development of IgA plasma cells in mouse gut. *J Nutr* 1982; 112: 1047–51.
105. McDermott MR, Mark DA, Befus AD, Baliga BS, Suskind RM, Bienenstock J. Impaired intestinal localization of mesenteric lymphoblasts associated with vitamin A deficiency and protein-calorie malnutrition. *Immunology* 1982; 45: 1–5.
106. Wiedermann U, Hanson LA, Holmgren J, Kahu H, Dahlgren UI. Impaired mucosal antibody response to cholera toxin in vitamin A–deficient rats immunized with oral cholera vaccine. *Infect Immun* 1993; 61: 3952–7.
107. Stephensen CB, Moldoveanu Z, Gangopadhyay NN. Vitamin A deficiency diminishes the salivary immunoglobulin A response and enhances the serum immunoglobulin G response to influenza A virus infection in BALB/c mice. *J Nutr* 1996; 126: 94–102.
108. Beatty DW, Napier B, Sinclair-Smith CC. Secretory IgA synthesis in kwashiorkor. *J Clin Lab Immunol* 1983; 12: 31–6.
109. Watson RR, McMurray DN, Martin P, Reyes MA. Effect of age, malnutrition and renutrition on free secretory component and IgA in secretion. *Am J Clin Nutr* 1985; 42: 281–8.

110. Grdic D, Hörnquist E, Kjerrulf M, Lycke NY. Lack of local suppression in orally tolerant CD8-deficient mice reveals a critical regulatory role of CD8+ T cells in the normal gut mucosa. *J Immunol* 1998; 160: 754–62.
111. Kim P-H, Eckmann L, Lee WJ, Han W, Kagnoff MF. Cholera toxin and cholera toxin B subunit induce IgA switching through the action of TGF-β_1. *J Immunol* 1998; 160: 1198–203.
112. Strobel S, Mowat AM. Immune responses to dietary antigens: oral tolerance. *Immunol Today* 1998; 19: 173–81.
113. Söltoft J, Söeberg B. Immunoglobulin-containing cells in the small intestine during acute enteritis. *Gut* 1972; 13: 535–8.
114. Agus SG, Falchuk ZM, Sessoms CS, Wyatt RG, Dolin R. Increased jejunal IgA synthesis *in vitro* during acute infectious non-bacterial gastroenteritis. *Am J Dig Dis* 1974; 19: 127–31.
115. Silbart LK, Keren DF. Reduction of intestinal carcinogen absorption by carcinogen-specific secretory immunity. *Science* 1989; 243: 1462–4.
116. Rasmussen MV, Silbart LK. Peroral administration of specific antibody enhances carcinogen excretion. *J Immunother* 1998; 21: 418–26.

DISCUSSION

Dr. Lentze: An association is seen between IgA deficiency and autoimmune disease, for instance in celiac disease. Is this because of defective immune protection or immune exclusion in the gut, for instance for gluten molecules, or what is the mechanism?

Dr. Brandtzaeg: This could indicate that mucosal tolerance is more easily disrupted in IgA deficiency; but a genetic link might also exist as the HLA-DQ molecules are so important for the association with both celiac disease and some of the autoimmune diseases as well as with IgA deficiency. At present, it is not possible to say which of these two factors is operative, abrogation of tolerance or genetic link. These patients have a very good compensatory secretory IgM response in their gut that uses the same receptor-mediated pump as dimeric IgA. We used to believe that compensation was a paradox because we thought that IgM was an excellent complement activator, and that would mean a phlogistic secretory immune system existed rather than the quiet IgA system that does not activate complement. It turns out that this is wrong, because the only IgM that can use the polymeric Ig receptor (pIgR) is a pentameric molecule that has its J chain incorporated in the same way as dimeric IgA. It is the J-chain-deficient hexameric form of IgM that has a fantastic complement-activating capacity, whereas the pentamers have little or no such activity.

Dr. Black: I was intrigued by your argument about reduced SIgA barrier function in Western societies. What would you suggest as a technique to improve that?

Dr. Brandtzaeg: This involves a controversial probiotic discussion. Several studies are promoting the use of probiotics—lactobacilli and so on—and five or six reports have shown that they will enhance IgA production in the gut (1–5). Another report shows that this effect is T-cell–dependent (6), which fits with what goes on in the Peyer's patches, wherein we have the whole textbook of immunology with T cells and B cells and so on. A recently reported Czech study (7) showed that this protection is long term, in that several years after the subjects had been fed a nontoxogenic strain of *E. coli* early in childhood they had less food allergy than other children from the same population. So, maybe it reflects a strengthening of the barrier function.

Dr. Seidman: You said that IgA is needed to swim in the Ganges. Is the inverse of that statement true? If you do swim in the Ganges, do you have more IgA and, therefore, are you less likely to develop allergy, for example? A clinical suggestion is that perhaps less food allergy and atopy are found in the developing world, because the children are either malnourished and their immune system does not have the luxury of developing an allergic Th2 type of reaction, or perhaps because their gut immune system is so stimulated from early on in life that they develop a higher level of tolerance. Are there any animal models to prove this? If you induce enteric infection early in life in an animal model, can you stimulate a secretory IgA response and prevent the development of allergy?

Dr. Brandtzaeg: This covers the same ground as the previous question on probiotics. The only clinical study I have seen is that Czech study previously mentioned. The data seemed fairly convincing, although an abstract is always difficult to judge. Nevertheless, it gives some hope for probiotic treatment. I do not know of any reports of animal models. The problem is that we have changed our world so much in such a short time in the industrialized countries, it is horrifying to contemplate the millions of years that genes have evolved to create the mechanisms of immune exclusion and immune tolerance, and then to see that we have changed around everything in our environment in about 100 years. It is no surprise that something must go wrong in the mucosal immune system. Even the high wheat diet involved in the pathogenesis of celiac disease has only been around for 1,000 years or so, and that is nothing compared with the gathering and hunting period of our ancestors.

Dr. Marini: We have done several experiments in preterm babies formula fed giving different kinds of probiotics. We found that in the first few days, we obtain very good colonization. Later on, the infants develop very high specific IgA and IgM and they kill all the administered probiotics (8–11). On the other hand, we were able to achieve persistent colonization with bifidobacteria, when oligosaccharides were added to the formula, similar to that observed in babies fed with human milk. Can you comment about that?

Dr. Brandtzaeg: It is the nature of the secretory IgA system to eliminate the stimulatory bacteria. That is exactly the problem that has plagued people who have been trying to develop live recombinant vaccines. Because when a recombinant organism is made to colonize the Peyer's patches to induce the production of an immunogen for a vaccine, it takes some time, and then the carrier will be eliminated by the IgA response against the recombinant *Salmonella* or whatever organism was used. That is exactly what is seen with a new probiotic—the "take," so to say, will be reduced after some time, because an IgA response has occurred in the gut. Thus, either compensation is made by changes with various bacteria, or one has to be found that is less immunogenic, which is probably what you alluded to with bifidobacteria. The reason that our normal flora survive in the gut is partly that it is changing phenotype all the time. Individual bacterial flora probably changes their immunogenic surface repertoire of antigens every 2 weeks or so, and the immune system develops tolerance against stable and less stimulatory antigenic determinants of the autologous indigenous micobiota.

Dr. Marini: Do you feel that intermittent administration of probiotics is likely to be better than continuous administration?

Dr. Brandtzaeg: It could be for reasons just mentioned, but I have no personal experience in this field.

Dr. Marini: You say that changing the intestinal flora can be good for the prevention of atopy. But so far, no clear demonstration shows that this works. In fact, only one epidemiologic study (from Estonia) looked at the change in lifestyle in that country, and although an increase in allergy was predicted, the opposite was found (12). I have not yet seen any prospective study showing that by changing the flora, the risk of allergy is really reduced in babies from high risk families. We need such studies.

Dr. Brandtzaeg: I agree that epidemiologic studies are difficult to interpret, but I think what has been done by Björkstén et al. in Sweden is pretty convincing (13,14): comparing the Baltic countries with Sweden, it was shown that a change had occurred in the bacterial flora in the gut in Sweden; the Baltic countries now have a gut flora similar to that of the

Swedish population just after World War II, and they have less allergic disease. Data also relate to the East German migration to the West after the wall came down, showing that these people have less allergy than a cohort of the same age who lived in West Germany in infancy (15). Thus, several epidemiologic studies indicate that the bacterial flora is important for the maturation of the immune system in the gut, both in terms of tolerance and also of the IgA system.

Dr. Zoppi: From your presentation, I presume that oral vaccines do enhance the secretion of IgG and IgM. Is that correct?

Dr. Brandtzaeg: Yes, that is correct. In many vaccine experiments, it has been shown that giving an oral vaccine increases the titer of the correct IgA antibodies in gut fluid and, to some extent, also in tears, saliva, and the respiratory tract. But, we do not yet understand the molecules involved in homing of primed B cells outside the gut, because the adhesion molecules have not been identified. Some of intestinal type may be expressed in the lactating breast, but not in the glands of the nose, the tear glands, and salivary glands. Other homing molecules must exist that are not yet understood. Some evidence indicates that B cells originating from the tonsils will try to stay in these upper regions—they do not like going into the gut mucosa. So, some sort of regionalization exists in the mucosal homing mechanisms that may be important when designing local vaccines. Importantly, however, nasal vaccines usually increase production of systemic IgG antibodies in addition to stimulating a secretory IgA response.

Dr. Alpers: This is a very interesting scheme, but is IgA really the most important factor? I am unaware of any evidence that IgA-deficient nursing mothers have infection-prone newborn infants. So, if IgA is the major protective factor, that is inconsistent with the evidence. Is there sufficient secretory IgM in these cases?

Dr. Brandtzaeg: Yes, in the gut lots of secretory IgM is produced in IgA deficiency and transported by this same polymeric Ig receptor–dependent mechanism as dimeric IgA, even into breast milk.

Dr. Alpers: So SIgM is enough? SIgA is not needed?

Dr. Brandtzaeg: It is well known that patients with selective IgA deficiency have more problems both with autoimmune disease and with infections and allergy. That has been well established, especially in the upper respiratory tract where most of the problems occur. Secretory IgM, which to a large extent may replace IgA in the gut, does not replace IgA in the upper respiratory tract nearly so consistently, although those patients who could compensate with IgM have been shown to have fewer problems than those who could not. Those who did not compensate with IgM for a lack of IgA had more otitis media, more recurrent tonsillitis, and some even developed pneumonia (16). This shows that IgA deficiency can be a problem, and a need exists for compensation. In the gut is seen fairly consistent compensation with pentameric secretory IgM using the pIgR or polymeric Ig receptor. I do believe in the secretory IgA system: the mucosal B-cell induction and homing with access to the mammary gland is such a complex scheme that it would not have developed if it were of no use for the baby.

Dr. Lionetti: The incidence of inflammatory bowel disease is greater in the developed world than in the developing world, and this seems to parallel the decreased number of gastrointestinal infections early in infancy. Would you speculate whether the decreased number of infections play a role in the increased response of the mucosal immune system, especially the T cells?

Dr. Brandtzaeg: That would fit in with what has been discussed in relation to allergy. Early microbial stimulation of the mucosal immune system appears to be important for subsequent immune regulation, the so-called ''hygiene'' hypothesis. Also, unpublished data from Lennart

Hammarström at Huddinge Hospital in Sweden indicate a 20 times increase of Crohn's disease in selective IgA deficiency, which is something quite new.

Dr. Mäki: Is uptake of antigen always via M cells? What about cases of increased permeability or a disease such as celiac disease?

Dr. Brandtzaeg: M cells are known to be keen to take up particulate antigens and various types of pathogens. No good evidence supports that food antigens use the M cells for entrance, although, in experimental systems, horseradish peroxidase can go via the M cells into the immune system. However, most likely, food antigens will mainly enter the immune system through the large surfaces at the so-called "mucosal effector sites" and primarily induce tolerance there, as in intestinal mucosa.

Dr. Yamashiro: It takes nearly 1 month after birth until plasma cells appear in the intestine. Does the IgA level in the saliva reflect the IgA level in the intestine?

Dr. Brandtzaeg: Actually, a little more IgA is found in saliva than in the gut fluid initially. A few plasma cells are seen in salivary glands earlier than in the gut. That is strange, but it may be related to antigens in the amniotic fluid, and the fetus is swimming in this fluid. Also, the tonsils develop quite early as inductive sites, and plasma cells can be seen below the crypt epithelium only a few days after birth. However, these are minor differences and in both regions it takes months or even years before the IgA system at the mucosal secretory effector sites is fully developed to an adult level (17).

REFERENCES

1. Kaila M, Isolauri E, Soppi E, *et al.* Enhancement of the circulating antibody secreting cell response in human diarrhea by a human *Lactobacillus* strain. *Pediatr Res* 1992; 32: 141–4.
2. Kaila M, Isolauri E, Saxelin M, Arvilommi H, Vesikari T. Viable versus inactivated *Lactobacillus* strain GG in acute rotavirus diarrhoea. *Arch Dis Child* 1995; 72: 51–3.
3. Isolauri E, Joensuu J, Suomalainen H, Luomala M, Vesikari T. Improved immunogenicity of oral D × RRV reassortant rotavirus vaccine by *Lactobacillus casei* GG. *Vaccine* 1995; 13: 310–12.
4. Yasui H, Kiyoshima J, Ushijima H. Passive protection against rotavirus-induced diarrhea of mouse pups born to and nursed by dams fed *Bifidobacterium breve* YIT4064. *J Infect Dis* 1995; 172: 403–9.
5. Malin M, Suomalainen H, Saxelin M, Isaoauri E. Promotion of IgA immune response in patients with Crohn's disease by oral bacteriotherapy with *Lactobacillus* GG. *Ann Nutr Metab* 1996; 40: 137–45.
6. Prokesová L, Ladmonová P, Cechová D, *et al.* Stimulatory effects of *Bacillus firmus* on IgA production in humans and mice [Abstract]. *Immunol Lett* 1999; 69: 55–6.
7. Lodinová-Zádniková R, Cukrowská B. Influence of oral colonization of the intestine with a non-enteropathogenic *E. coli* strain after birth on the frequency of infectious and allergic diseases after 10 and 20 years [Abstract]. *Immunol Lett* 1999; 69: 64.
8. Negretti F, Casetta P, Clerici-Bagozzi D, Marini A. Researches on the intestinal and systemic immunoresponses after oral treatments with *Lactobacillus* GG in the rabbit. *Dev Phisiopath Clin* 1997; 7: 15–21.
9. Marini A, Clerici-Bagozzi D, Maglia T, Casetta P, Negretti F. Microbiological and immunological observations in the stools of preterm neonates orally treated with probotics products. Note I: Treatment with *S. boulardii. Dev Phisiopath Clin* 1997; 7: 29–37.
10. Marini A, Clerici-Bagozzi D, Maglia T, Casetta P, Negretti F. Microbiological and immunological observations in the stools of preterm neonates orally treated with probiotic product. Note II: Treatment with *B. subtilis. Dev Phisiopath Clin* 1997; 7: 79–86.
11. Marini A, Clerici-Bagozzi D, Maglia T, Casetta P, Negetti F. Microbiological and immunological observations in the stools of preterm neonates orally treated with probiotic products. Note III: Treatment with *Lactobacillus* GG. *Dev Phisiopath Clin* 1997; 7: 87–94.
12. Björkstén B, Dumitrascu D, Foucard T, *et al.* Prevalence of childhood asthma, rhinitis and eczema in Scandinavia and Eastern Europe. *Eur Respir J* 1998; 12: 432–7.

13. Sepp E, Julge K, Vasar M, *et al.* Intestinal microflora of Estonian and Swedish infants. *Acta Paediatr* 1997; 86: 956–61.
14. Björkstén B, Naaber P, Sepp E, Mikelsaar M. The intestinal microflora in allergic Estonian and Swedish 2-year-old children. *Clin Exp Allergy* 1999; 29: 342–6.
15. von Mutius E, Fritzsch C, Weiland SK, Roll G, Magnussen H. Prevalence of asthma and allergic disorders among children in united Germany: a descriptive comparison. *BMJ* 1992; 305: 1395–9.
16. Brandtzaeg P, Karlsson G, Hansson G, *et al.* The clinical condtition of IgA-deficient patients is related to the proportion of IgD- and IgM-producing cells in their nasal mucosa. *Clin Exp Immunol* 67: 626–636, 1987.
17. Brandtzaeg P, Nilssen DE, Rognum TO, Thrane PS. Ontogeny of the mucosal immune system and IgA deficiency. In: MacDermott RP, Elson CO, eds. Mucosal immunology I: Basic principles. *Gastroenterol Clin North Am* 1991; 20: 397–439.

Gastrointestinal Functions, edited by Edgard E. Delvin and Michael J. Lentze. Nestlé Nutrition Workshop Series, Pediatric Program, Vol. 46, Nestec Ltd., Vevey/Lippincott Williams & Wilkins, Philadelphia © 2001.

Development of the Structure and Function of the Neuromusculature of the Gastrointestinal Tract

Peter Milla

Gastroenterology Unit, Institute of Child Health, London, UK

DEVELOPMENT OF THE GASTROINTESTINAL TRACT

The structure and function of the gut results from a complex interplay between various cell types and components that is regulated by growth factors and hormones together with immune and neural inputs (1). The gut develops from three germ layers: the endoderm, which supplies the epithelial cells of the mucosa; the splanchnic mesoderm, providing the mesenchymal cell types (e.g., the muscle layers); and the ectoderm, the origin of the neural components. In recent years, the importance of the formation of endodermal mesenchymal cell assemblages to generate form and cytodifferentiation of the mucosa has been appreciated (2), as has the establishment of the intrinsic nervous system of the gut by neural crest cell migration and differentiation (3). In the formation of the mucosa and the enteric neuromusculature, adhesive and other interactions between cells and the extracellular microenvironment are crucial. The extracellular microenvironment consists of a labile and developmentally regulated group of interacting molecules. Some of these will be located at the interface between endoderm-derived and mesenchyma-derived cells, where they are capable of directing specific cell behavior. Another group of interacting molecules, which is found associated with the extracellular matrix (ECM) of the muscle coats of the gut, is implicated in the morphogenetic steps in the migration, homing, and differentiation of both neural cells and smooth muscle cells.

Three major phases of development occur in the human gastrointestinal tract: (a) an early period of proliferation and morphogenesis; (b) an intermediate period of differentiation when many different and distinctive cell types appear; and (c) a later period of maturation that results in a bowel capable of transporting luminal contents and digesting and absorbing nutrients (4–11).

The gastrointestinal tract first appears at 4 weeks of gestation as a tube of stratified epithelium extending from the mouth to the cloaca, which can be divided into three distinct parts:

- Foregut (esophagus, stomach, proximal duodenum, liver, and pancreas)
- Prececal gut (small intestine through to the cecum)
- Postcecal gut

Endoderm–Mesenchymal Interactions

Interactions between epithelial and mesenchymal cells may have important implications for the development of the nerves and muscle layers of the gut. Close contacts between endodermal and mesenchymal cells in the fetal intestine and between crypt epithelial cells and myofibroblastic cells of the ECM in the adult organ have been reported, and play an important role in directing morphogenesis and cytodifferentiation and in the maintenance of the steady state of the stem cell compartment in the mature gut (12). Each of the intestinal endodermal and mesenchymal tissue components exerts an effect on the development of its associated counterparts and the contacts required to allow expression of the reciprocal, permissive interaction (13).

The basal surface of the intestinal epithelium is in contact with a basement membrane or ECM that is assembled from a variety of specialized molecules. More than 50 different proteins with many domains and multiple binding sites for other matrix molecules have been described over the last 15 years. It is now clear that ECM molecules are dynamic effectors in morphogenesis and in the generation and maintenance of epithelial cell polarity (14). The matrix interacts with cell surface receptors such as integrins which transduce information from the cell environment to the intracellular component. In the intestine, the subepithelial basement membrane has been shown to contain laminin-1 type IV collagen, nidogen, and perlecan (15). Besides the basement membrane, the ground substance of the intestinal stroma comprises many fibrillar collagens (types 1 and 3), fibrinectin, and tenascin. Also found are proteoglycans composed of various types of sulfated glycosaminoglycans and unsulfated hyaluronic acid (15). It is of interest that isolated intestinal epithelial cells are unable to differentiate when cultured *in vitro* unless they are in close contact with mesenchymally derived cells. Experimentally, in culture conditions, a precise chronology of events occurs:

1. Heterologous cell contacts
2. Polarized basement membrane molecules deposited at the epithelial–mesenchymal interface
3. Epithelial cell polarization and differentiation

Thus, cell interactions between embryonic epithelial (endoderm) and stromal cells (mesenchyma) are a prerequisite for intestinal morphogenesis and differentiation (16–19). Such interactions must play an important role in the developing enteric neuromusculature.

Development of the Enteric Nervous System

It has been known since the 1950s, following a series of *in ovo* microsurgical ablations of the dorsal neural primordium of chick embryos, that the enteric nervous system is derived from the neural crest (20). The neural crest arises on the dorsal midline as part of the neural tube which later goes on to form the central nervous system. The neural crest gives rise to enteric neurons and their support cells, pigment cells, and sympathetic nervous tissue together with the adrenal medulla. More recently, much smaller scale ablations have suggested that the neural crest between somites 3 and 5 is particularly important for enteric nervous system development (21). The cell labeling techniques in chicken quail chimeric embryos used by Le Douarin and Teillet (3) confirmed that the enteric neurons arise from the vagal neural crest and that they colonize the gut in a rostrocaudal migration. However, some neural crest cells appeared to arrive in the hindgut from the lumbosacral level by a caudorostral wave of colonization.

More recent studies in mice confirm these avian findings that the gut is colonized largely by vagal neural crest cells but that some cells in the hindgut appear to arrive from a lumbosacral origin (22,23). The most recent of these studies (in the mouse) shows that the enteric neuroblasts are derived from three distinct neural crest cell lines that express the control gene *Sox 10* and *Hox B5* and the transmembrane tyrosine kinase receptor *c-ret*. At the headfold stage embryo (E8.5) *Sox 10* and *c-ret* were expressed in neural crest cells, with *c-ret* only being expressed in rhombomere 4 of the hind brain and *Sox 10* in rhombomeres 2 and 4. In contrast, *Hox B5* first appeared later at E9.5 and only occurred at the level of rhombomere 7. The cells from the vagal neural crest arrive at the gut by two pathways from the neural crest: one a dorsolateral route in a cell-free ECM between the epidermis and the somites, and a ventral route percolating through the sclerotomal mesenchyme of the somites. In mice, the neural crest cells reach the foregut after passing through branchial arches 4 and 6. *Hox B5*–expressing cells only appear to arrive in the gut at the level of the stomach, most probably following the ventral route, whereas the *Sox 10*– or *c-ret*–expressing cells appear to follow the dorsolateral route and enter by way of the primitive esophagus. Cells expressing these three genes coalesce in the environment of the gut and by day 12.5 in the embryo (E12.5) many primitive neuroblasts are expressing all three genes.

The foregut gives rise to the gut down to the duodenum and, given the compressed scale of the gut compared with the neural axis in these early developmental stages, the vagal neural crest cells require virtually no longitudinal movement to populate the gut down to the level of the second part of the duodenum. Caudal to this, the neural crest cells that have colonized the foregut migrate longitudinally within the gut mesenchyme in a caudal direction favoring the region close to the serosal surface. The vanguard of cells colonizing the gut primordium advance at a rate of about 40 μm/h (24) and the cells immediately behind the vanguard are found just outside the developing circular muscle layer; that is, they are already in position to form the myenteric plexus (25). The cells that are going to form the submucous plexus are not seen until later and it is not clear whether they are derived from a secondary migration from local myenteric cells or are a separate wave of immigrants. The sacral neural crest cells migrate ventrally through the adjacent somites before entering the hindgut at the cloaca near the stalk of the allantois; they then migrate rostrally in the gut mesenchyme.

In the human, the vagal timetable appears to start at around 3 to 4 weeks and is complete by week 12. The presumed sacral input timetable is unknown. Those vagal neural crest cells that migrate and colonize the gut are committed to becoming neuroblasts or neuronal support cells (glioblasts). Differentiation into neurons and glial cells appears not to take place until they have reached their final resting places in the gut, and their further movement through the gut mesenchyme, survival in the gut, and differentiation into mature cells are strongly influenced by contacts with the microenvironment, consisting of other cells in the mesenchyme, neural crest, and the ECM (26).

The extracellular matrix components give directional clues to migrating neural crest cells and, together with neighboring cells, provide some of the signals for crest cell differentiation. In humans, for example, the appearance of neural crest cells in the gut is preceded by expression of ECM molecules and these may play a role in migrational cues (27) or promote neuronal growth (28). Other factors (e.g., glial-derived neurotropic factor) ensure survival of committed neuroblasts (29). Several transgenic knockout mouse models and naturally occurring strains of mice with particular genetic abnormalities have provided valuable evidence of some of the factors involved. Lethal spotted and piebald spotting mice (30,31) have defects in the endothelin signaling pathway that result in an alteration of the microenvironment in which the neural crest cells find themselves. This curtails neural crest migration in the distal colon and is associated with localized overexpression of ECM molecules (32).

Intrinsic properties of the neural crest cells themselves are also important for migration survival and differentiation. Two knockout mouse models (29,33) and the human condition Hirschsprung's disease now have known genetic defects (34,35); they provide powerful evidence for these intrinsic properties. The neural crest cells express a transmembrane tyrosine kinase receptor at the cell surface, the *Ret* proto-oncogene. A transgenic knockout model in the mouse of *Ret* (33) shows a total absence of the enteric nervous system, suggesting that normal enteric nervous system migration and the survival of migrating cells are dependent on the functional integrity of this tyrosine kinase receptor and its ligand. We now know that the ligand for the *Ret* tyrosine kinase receptor is a glial-derived neurotrophic factor and a knockout model of this gene shows a similar lack of expression of enteric neurons (29). In Hirschsprung's disease, defects in chromosome 10q11.2 (34,35) (which specify the *Ret* gene) have been found, and the defects extend all along the gene. It is of interest that other abnormalities of the *Ret* gene result in multiple endocrine neoplasia type 2A and 2B, but these only occur at specific sites. In multiple endocrine neoplasia type 2B, an association is seen with hyperplasia of enteric neurons resulting in enteric ganglioneuromatosis (36). Abnormalities of *Ret* are found in some 30% of patients with Hirschsprung's disease and in families with this disorder there is incomplete penetrance of the genetic abnormality. Although abnormalities of *Ret* appear to account for a moderate number of Hirschsprung cases, other neural crest cell abnormalities (e.g., the provision of glial-derived neurotrophic factor) account for only a very small proportion. A series of experiments (37) has suggested that a glial-derived neurotrophic factor is required for survival and differentiation of the vagal neural crest cells once they arrive in the gut, and some have suggested that the lumbosacral outflow into the gut is largely of cells that will become glial cells, producing factors such as glial-derived neurotrophic factors to ensure that the migrating cells survive once they arrive in the hindgut.

The number of vagal neural crest cells colonizing the gut also seems to be important as gross reduction in numbers leads to the development of the enteric nervous system in the rostral levels of the gut but a complete absence at caudal levels (20). However, this information also suggests that perhaps some specification of different segment identity occurs to potential enteric neurons before they leave the vagal neural crest, and this may be dependent on the correct microenvironment in the gut primordium during the process of migration and ultimately differentiation. It has been suggested that spatially restricted differential expression of homeobox-containing regulatory genes along the hind brain may be responsible for this.

Developmental Control Regulatory Genes

Homeobox genes are a group of developmental control genes implicated in the positioning and patterning of organs in the embryo. These evolutionarily conserved genes encode transcription factors that self-regulate their own transcription or the transcription of other downstream effector genes in developing embryos, ranging from *Drosophila* to humans.

A group of genes that has been extensively studied are the antennapedia class of homeobox genes, the so-called "*Hox*" genes. *Hox* genes are evolutionarily highly conserved and derived from a common ancestral cluster. They are organized into four clusters A, B, C, and D on four separate chromosomes in mammals, composed of some 38 genes in total (38). The genes are numbered 1 to 13 by virtue of their 3' to 5' position along each chromosome, the lowest number being at the 3' end and the highest number at the 5' end. A given gene can have up to three related genes in equivalent positions on the other three clusters, and such a group of genes has sequence homology, forming a so-called "paralogous group" (39).

Such paralogs can display equivalent expression domains and, therefore, may have common functions during development, resulting in some functional redundancy. It is significant that *Hox* genes are expressed in precise patterns during early embryogenesis, particularly during critical periods of fate specification within a given morphogenetic field such as a limb. The expression domains of the various groups overlap to differing extents within any particular field, leading to the concept that *Hox* genes have a combinatorial mode of action (40).

Along the body axis, these genes are generally expressed with discrete rostral cut-offs, which coincide with either existing or emergent anatomic landmarks. Therefore, it has been suggested that they serve to specify component parts of the vertebrate body plan and this is particularly clear in segmented structures such as the branchial arches and the vertebral column (41). Significantly, at least in these structures, the rostrocaudal sequence of the cut-offs maps precisely with the 3′ to 5′ sequence of *Hox* genes within their respective cluster and with the order in which these genes are expressed. This phenomenon is known as spatial and temporal co-linearity (42). However, it is also clear that nonovertly segmented structures (e.g., limbs or internal organs) are also specified by *Hox* genes; thus, *Hox* genes could be upstream regulatory genes for the morphogenesis of the embryonal gut, for the migration and maturation of neural crest cells and, possibly, splanchnic mesoderm.

Hox genes from the 5′ paralogous groups 12 and 13 are known to be involved in patterning of the hindgut (43); *Hox* genes from paralogous groups 4 and 5 seem to be particularly good candidates as regulators of gut neuromusculature of at least the foregut and midgut, because they are expressed in the developing hind brain at the level of rhombomeres 6 to 8 from where a proportion of vagal neural crest cells migrate through the branchial arches into the intestine and differentiate into enteric ganglia (44). In segmented structures such as the branchial arches, the branchial *Hox* code defined by the patterns of combinatorial *Hox* gene expression has been interpreted as a developmental strategy whereby positional specification made axially within the neural tube is transmitted to the periphery through the migrating neural crest and is seen as an integral part of the mechanisms whereby the embryo develops an organ such as the head and face or the gut (45).

Preliminary data of the expression of 3′ *Hox* genes in the gut of developing mouse embryos along the length of the gut primordium show nested expression domains (46).

Further studies have delineated different spatial, temporal, and combinatorial expression patterns in different morphologic regions: foregut; prececal gut; cecum, and postcecal gut (47). Two dynamic gradients, rostral and caudal, were coordinated with nested expression domains along the gut primordium. Region-specific domains were present in the stomach and cecum. The *Hox* gene transcripts in the mesoderm of the gut primordium were spatially colocalized to the same layer of outer mesoderm clearly preferred by migrating neural crest cells and the developing intestinal muscle coats. It was of particular interest that in the postcecal gut, the appearance of enteric neuronal precursors was clearly preceded by the early presence of *Hox D4*, *C4*, and *C5* transcripts in this region of the gut primordium between E9.75 and E12.5. This important study shows that specific spatial and temporal combinations of *Hox* genes are involved in the control of morphogenesis of the gut and that they are expressed in the form of an enteric *Hox* code (47). The code provides correct positional information for migratory cells and for a permissive environment, and for the differentiation of developing tissues, particularly for the developing enteric neuromusculature. A few isolated observations of transgenic mouse models also suggest that *Hox* genes do indeed play an important role in gut morphogenesis. A transgenic knockout of *Enx, Hox 11L1* (48), causes increased innervation of the hindgut, and overexpression of *Hox A4* is associated with a megacolon (49). Destruction of *Hox C4* severely affects the morphology of esophageal smooth muscle, whereas knockout of *Hox D13* affects anal sphincters (50). It is clear that this family of genes is of importance within the genetic hierarchy of gut morphogenesis, and delineation of those genes comprising the human gut *Hox* code and of their spatiotemporal patterns of expression is an essential and integral part of understanding the molecular events underlying gut dysmorphogenesis in humans.

FUNCTIONAL DEVELOPMENT OF THE FOREGUT

Intolerance to feeds, evident as regurgitation and vomiting, occurs commonly in the very preterm infant and limits the amount of enteral nutrition that can be given. These symptoms are a consequence both of gastroesophageal reflux and of functional gastric outlet obstruction. It is assumed that these phenomena occur as a result of immature gastrointestinal motor activity. Gastrointestinal motor activity results from the integrated activity of the gastrointestinal smooth muscle, the enteric nervous system modulated by extrinsic innervation from the central nervous system, and the endocrine and paracrine environment of the gut wall. We and others have previously shown that small intestinal gastric and esophageal motor activity develop (51–53) according to an ontogenic timetable that occurs as a result of the development of these control systems. As immature development of the foregut motor apparatus prejudices the ability to feed preterm infants and may result in considerable morbidity from aspiration, pneumonia, apnea, and esophagitis, knowledge of the developmental profile of the foregut motor apparatus is of value to neonatologists. Over the last 10 years, increasingly sophisticated studies have been done of the esophagus and the small intestine.

The Esophagus

By 8 weeks of gestation, the human fetal esophagus is identifiable as a hollow, epithelium-lined tube with primitive nerve and muscle precursors. Over the next 8 weeks, maturation of the muscle layers and innervation occurs until fetal swallowing begins at about 16 weeks of gestation. An anatomic study of the developing human esophagus showed nerve synapses present from 10 weeks of gestation but nerve cell size increased from 6 μ at 8 weeks' gestation to a near maximal 20 μ at term, and that numbers of cells and nerve density peaked at around 20 weeks of gestation.

Unfortunately, functional studies of esophageal motor activity are restricted to premature infants over the age of 30 weeks' gestation. One very recent study showed that nonperistaltic motor patterns were common in premature infants between 33 and 37 weeks postconceptional age, that all infants had a high pressure zone at the lower esophageal sphincter, and that the pressure exerted increased from 3.8 mm

Hg at 29 weeks' gestation to 18.1 mm Hg at term (51). Observations of the behavior of the lower esophageal sphincter showed that both swallow-related and transient lower esophageal sphincter relaxations occurred, and that after 33 weeks' gestation the motor events associated with lower esophageal sphincter relaxation were similar to those seen in healthy adults. However, the relative preponderance of nonperistaltic pressure wave sequences in esophagi of premature infants means that they will have poorer acid clearance when reflux episodes occur and, thus, are more likely to develop esophagitis. Endoscopic studies of premature infants appear to indicate that this is indeed the case.

The Stomach

The stomach acts as an initial reservoir for feeds, and the process of digestion starts in the stomach with the secretion of acid and pepsin. In addition, the stomach secretes mucus and mucoproteins, intrinsic factor, and the polypeptide hormones gastrin and somatostatin. Gastrin is important in the regulation of acid secretion; in the neonatal period, however, it is often present at high levels. Neonatal hypergastrinemia, its duration, magnitude, and probable mechanisms have been reviewed by Lichtenberger (54). Somatostatin is important for the modulation of fasting motor activity in the stomach and appears to be present from about 34 weeks and later (55).

Gastric Motor Function

Studies of gastric function in premature infants show, in the very preterm infant, that gastric emptying is poor and, in the fasting state, that pressure generated in the gastric antrum at approximately 26 to 27 weeks of gestation is as low as 5 mm Hg (~0.7 kPa), as compared with levels of 30 mm Hg (4 kPa) by term. Paradoxically, such studies of gastric emptying that have been carried out have shown no association between longer half-emptying times and increasing prematurity; however, such studies have been limited to infants able to tolerate relatively large amounts of feed (30 ml/kg/feed or more) (56). In healthy premature infants, human milk empties faster than an adapted milk formula containing 0.7 kcal/ml and having the same casein-to-whey ratio as human milk (56). Siegal et al. observed the effects of altering the carbohydrate source of glucose—lactose versus polycose—and fat source—long chain triglyceride (LCT) versus medium chain triglyceride (MCT)—on gastric emptying profiles (57). The inhibition produced by LCT was much greater than that of MCT; alterations in carbohydrate source, by contrast, had minimal effects on gastric emptying rate. Others have shown that posture, volume, and feed temperature appear to have little effect on gastric emptying, but various pathologic conditions are clearly associated with delayed gastric emptying, including cardiovascular disease, respiratory distress syndrome, and gastroesophageal reflux. In a study of the emptying of

TABLE 1. *Stages of fasting motor activity (51)*

Pattern	Gestational age (weeks)	Complex (length) (min)	Complex interval (min)	Propagation velocity (cm/min)
Random	28–32	0	0	0
Clustered phasic	30–35	1–20	4–35	0–5
Prolonged phasic	34–36	5–40	4–30	1–5
Migrating motor complex	37–42	3–7	18–45	2–7.5

From Omari TI, Miki K, Fraser R, et al. Oesophageal body and lower oesophageal sphincter function in healthy premature infants. *Gastroenterology* 1995;109:1757–64; with permission.

different formulas in older infants with gastroesophageal reflux, it was clearly shown that the fastest half-emptying times were obtained with human milk and a whey protein hydrolysate (58). It is no surprise to neonatologists that human milk is tolerated by premature infants best; in its absence, a whey protein peptide hydrolysate containing some MCT might also be considered.

Small Intestinal Motor Activity

Over the last 10 years, various studies have been done of the development of small intestinal motor function, all of which have identified four stages in the development of fasting motor activity (52,53): (a) a disorganized stage; (b) clusters of phasic activity; (c) prolonged phasic activity; and (d) a regular cyclical migrating motor complex (MMC) pattern. These data are summarized in Table 1 and Fig. 1.

It seems clear that the development of intestinal motor activity changes toward a more mature pattern with increasing postconceptional age. The initiation of clustered phasic activity, which then becomes more prolonged, may be humorally mediated as the secretion of various polypeptide hormones involved in motor activity occurs at this gestational age (59). Propagation and the subsequent shortening of the duration of prolonged phasic contraction with the emergence of MMC activity, however, is much more likely to be caused by the development of inhibitory networks in the enteric nervous system and their interface with the central nervous system. In animal studies, similar patterns have been observed and the increase in cycle length of the MMC has been associated with the development of serotinergic neurons in the proximal small intestine (60). Similarities were also seen between these gestationally determined changes and the effects of total vagotomy on adult patterns of fasting activity. This, together with observations of the timing of maturation events determined by the central nervous system and the correlation between cyclical timing of the electrical activity in the enteric and central nervous systems of animals, suggests that not only do events in the enteric nervous system determine the nature of the pattern of fasting motor activity but also that central control systems that may modulate enteric activity develop in parallel (61).

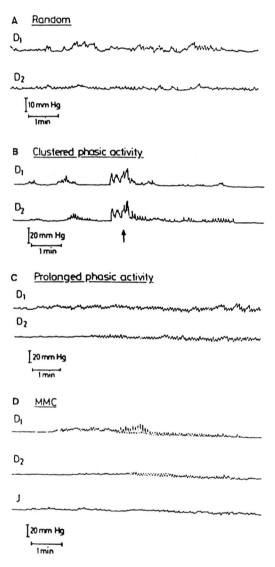

FIG. 1. Small intestinal pressure recordings at antrum (A), duodenum (D1 and D2), and jejunum (J).

In the older child and adult, cyclical fasting motor activity is disrupted after a meal and replaced by continuous activity that promotes mixing and segmentation of the luminal contents. This is required for efficient processing of feeds. A modicum of information is available regarding the development of the motor response to food in the human infant, in particular the detection of particular motor events and feed factors that determine tolerance to enteral feeds. Bisset et al. (62) showed that the length of postprandial activity and the disruption of the cyclical pattern of fasting activity were dependent on the length of time that the infant had spent taking feed. Berseth and Nordi (63) showed that tolerance to enteral feeds was closely correlated with the development of a continuous pattern of activity in response to food and with the development of cyclical clustered phasic activity in the fasting state. These initial observations have received more support recently since the demonstration of the polypeptide hormone response and its effect on motor activity in preterm infants who had been able to tolerate enteral feeds (64). Thus, postprandial events appear to be dependent on the nature of the humoral response to food, provided that the muscle coats of the gut and the enteric nerves have developed sufficiently to respond to the hormones secreted. The nature of these maturational changes, however, remains poorly explored, although knowledge in this area is allowing more logical feeding regimens to develop.

REFERENCES

1. Lucas A. Programming by early nutrition in man. In: Bock GR, Whelan J, eds. *The childhood environment in adult disease*. Chichester: John Wiley & Sons, 1991: 38–55.
2. Haffen K, Kedinger M, Semon-Assmann P. Cell contact dependent regulation of entericyte differentiation. In: Lebenthal E, ed. *Human gastrointestinal development*. New York: Raven Press, 1989: 19–39.
3. Le Douarin NM, Teillet MA. The migration of neural crest cells to the wall of the digestive tract in avian embryo. *J Embryol Exp Morphol* 1973; 30: 31–48.
4. Moxey PC, Trier S. Specialised cell types in the human fetal small intestine. *Anat Rec* 1978; 191: 269–86.
5. Colony PC, Conforte JC. Morphogenesis in the fetal rat proximal colon: effects of cytoclasin D. *Anat Rec* 1993; 235: 241–52.
6. Winton DJ, Ponder BAJ. Stem cell organisation in mouse small intestine. *Proc R Soc Lond* 1990; 23: 13–18.
7. Suh E, Traber PG. An intestine specific homeobox gene regulates proliferation and differentiation. *Mol Cell Biol* 1996; 16: 619–25.
8. Louvard D, Kedinger M, Hauri HP. The differentiating intestinal epithelial cells. Establishment and maintenance of functions through interactions between cellular structures. *Annu Rev Cell Biol* 1992; 8: 157–95.
9. Duluc I, Jost B, Feund JN. Multiple levels of control of the stage and region specific expression of rat intestinal lactase. *J Cell Biol* 1993; 123: 1577–86.
10. Henning SJ, Ruben DC, Schulman RJ. Ontogeny of the intestinal mucosa. In: Johnson LR, ed. *Physiology of the gastrointestinal tract*. New York: Raven Press, 1994: 571–610.
11. Maiuri L, Rai AV, Potter J, *et al.* Mosaic pattern of lactase expression by villous enterocytes in human adult type hypolactasia. *Gastroenterology* 1991; 100: 359–69.
12. Valentich JD, Powell DW. Intestinal sub-epithelial myofibroblast and mucosal immuno physiology current opinions. *Gastroenterology* 1994; 10: 645–51.
13. Hathen K, Lacroix B, Kedinger M. Inductive properties of fibroblastic cell cultures derived from rat intestinal mucosa on epithelial differentiation. *Differentiation* 1983; 23: 226–33.
14. Howlett AR, Bissell MJ. The influence of tissue micro environment (stroma and extracellular matrix) on the development and function of memory epithelium. *Epithelial Cell Biology* 1993; 2: 79–89.
15. Simon-Assmann P, Kedinger M, De Arcangelis A, Russo V, Symo P. Extracellular matrix components in intestinal development. In: Ekblom P, ed. *Extracellular matrix in animal development*. Amsterdam: Experentia, 1995: 65–82.
16. Kedinger M, Bouziges F, Simon-Assman P. Influence of cell interactions on intestinal brush border

enzyme expression. In: Kotic A, Skoda J, Paces V, Kosca V, eds. *Highlights in modern biochemistry.* Zeist: VSP International Science Publishers, 1989: 1103–12.

17. Probstmeier R, Martini R, Schachner M. Expression of J1 tenascin in the crypt villous unit of adult mouse small intestine. Implications for its role in epithelial cell shedding. *Development* 1990; 109: 313–21.

18. Chawengsaksophak KR, James V, Hammond F, Kontgen F, Beck F. Homeostasis and intestinal tumours in *Cdx₂* mutant mice. *Nature* 1997; 385: 84–7.

19. Lorentz O, Duluc I, De Arcangelis A, Simon-Assmann P, Kedinger M, Froynd JN. Key role of the *Cdx₂* homeobox gene in extracellular matrix mediated intestinal cell differentiation. *J Cell Biol* (in press).

20. Yntema CL, Hammond WS. The origin of intrinsic ganglia of trunk viscera from vagal neural crest in the chick embryo. *J Comp Neurol* 1954; 101: 515–41.

21. Peters Van de Sanden MGH, Kirby ML, Gittenberger de Groot AC, Tibboel D, Mulder MP, Meijers C. Oblation of various regions within the avian vagal neural crest has differential effects on ganglion formation in the fore, mid and hind gut. *Dev Dyn* 1993; 196: 183–94.

22. Serbedzija GN, Burgan S, Fraser SE, Broner Fraser M. Vital dye labelling demonstrates a sacral neural crest contribution to the enteric nervous system of chick and mouse embryos. *Development* 1991; 111: 857–66.

23. Pitera J, Smith VV, Milla PJ. Neurotrophic factors and neural crest cell receptors in the developing murine enteric nervous system. *J Pediatr Gastroenterol Nutr* 1999; 28: 565.

24. Allan IJ, Newgreen DF. The origin and differentiation of enteric neurons of the intestine of the foul embryo. *Am J Anat* 1980; 157: 137–54.

25. Tucker GC, Siment G, Thiery JP. Pathways of avian neural crest cell migration in the developing gut. *Dev Biol* 1986; 116: 430–50.

26. Pham TD, Gershon MD, Rothman TP. Time of origin of neurons in the murine enteric nervous system sequence in relation to phenotype. *J Comp Neurol* 1991; 314: 789–98.

27. Fujimoto T, Harter J, Yokoyama S, Mitomi T. A study of the extracellular matrix protein as the migration pathway of neural crest cells in the gut: analysis in human embryos with special reference to the pathogenesis of Hirschsprung's disease. *J Pediatr Surg* 1989; 24: 550–6.

28. Trupp M, Arinas E, Fainzibla M, Nilson AS, Sieber VA, Grigoriou M. Peripheral expression and biological activities of GDNF, a new neurotropic factor for avian and mammalian peripheral neurons. *Nature* 1996; 381: 789–93.

29. Schuchardt A, D'Agati V, Larsson-Blomberg L, Constantini F, Pachnis V. Defects in the kidney and enteric nervous system of mice lacking the tyrosine kinase receptor *ret. Nature* 1994; 367: 380–3.

30. Kapur RP, Yost C, Palmiter RD. A transgenic model for studying the development of the enteric nervous system in normal and aganglionic mice. *Development* 1992; 116: 167–75.

31. Hosoda K, Hammer RE, Richardson JA, Baynesh AG, Cheung JC, Giaida A. Targeted and natural pie bald lethal mutations of endothelin B receptor gene produce megacolon associated with spotted coat colour in mice. *Cell* 1994; 79: 1267–76.

32. Payette RF, Tennyson VM, Pomeranz HD, Pham TD, Rothman TP, Gershon MD. Accumulation of components of basal laminae: association with the failure of neural crest cells to colonise the presumptive aganglionic bowel of LS/LS mutant mice. *Dev Biol* 1988; 125: 341–60.

33. Sanchez MP, Selos Santiago I, Frezen J, Bin He, Lira SA, Barbacid M. Renal agenesis and the absence of enteric neurons in mice lacking GDNF. *Nature* 1996; 382: 70–3.

34. Edery P, Lyonnet S, Mulligan LM, Pelet A, Dow E, Abel L. Mutation of the *ret* proto oncogene in Hirschsprung's disease. *Nature* 1994; 367: 378–80.

35. Lyonnet S, Bellono A, Pelet A, *et al.* A gene for Hirschsprung's disease maps to the proximal long arm of chromosome 10. *Nature Genet* 1993; 4: 346–50.

36. Eng C, Smith DP, Mulligan LM, *et al.* Point mutation within the tyrosine kinase domain of the *ret* proto oncogene in multiple endocrine neoplasia type 2B and related sporadic tumours. *Hum Mol Genet* 1994; 3: 237–41.

37. Moore MW, Klein RD, Farinas I, *et al.* Renal and neuronal abnormalities in mice lacking GDNF. *Nature* 1996; 382: 76–9.

38. Manak JR, Scott MP. A class act: conservation of homeo domain protein functions. *Development* 1994; (suppl): 61–77.

39. McGuinness W, Krumlauf R. Homeobox genes and axial patterning. *Cell* 1992; 68: 283–302.

40. Hunt P, Krumlauf R. *Hox* codes and positional specification invertebrate embryonic axis. *Annu Rev Cell Biol* 1992; 8: 227–56.
41. Kessel M, Gruss P. Murine development control genes. *Science* 1990; 249: 374–9.
42. Duboule D, Dollae P. The structural and functional organisation of the murine *hox* gene family resembles that of *Drosphila* homeotic genes. *EMBO J* 1989; 8: 1497–505.
43. Dolle P, Izpisua-Belmonte JC, Bonchonelli E, Deboule D. The *hox* 4.8 gene is localised at the '5 prime' extremity of the *hox* 4 complex and is expressed in the most posterior parts of the body during development. *Mech Dev* 1991; 36: 3–13.
44. Wilkinson DG, Bhatt S, Cook M, Bonchonelli E, Krumlauf R. Segmental expression of *hox* 2 homeobox containing genes in the developing mouse hind brain. *Nature* 1989; 341: 405–9.
45. Hunt P, Gulisano M, Cook M, *et al.* A distinct *hox* code for the branchial region of the vertebrate head. *Nature* 1991; 353: 861–4.
46. Pitera J, Smith VV, Milla PJ. Normal expression of *hox* genes in the developing gastrointestinal tract: a basis for understanding abnormalities in enteric neuromusculature [Abstract]. *Gastroenterology* 1997; 112: A895.
47. Pitera J, Smith VV, Thorogood P, Milla PJ. Coordinated expression of 3' *Hox* genes during murine embryonal gut development: an enteric *Hox* code. *Gastroenterology* 1999; 117: 1339–51.
48. Shirasawa S, Yunker AM, Roth KA, Brown GA, Orning S, Korsmeyer S. ENX (*hox* L11 1) deficient mice develop myenteric neuronal hypoplasia and mega-colon. *Nature Med* 1997; 3: 646–50.
49. Wolgemuth DJ, Beringer RR, Mostola MP, Brinster RL, Palmiter RD. Transgenic mice overexpressing the mouse homeobox containing gene *hox* 1.4 exhibit abnormal gut development. *Nature* 1989; 337: 464–7.
50. Kondo T, Dolle P, Zakany J, Duboule D. Function of posterior *hox* D genes in the morphogenesis of the anal sphincter. *Development* 1996; 122: 2651–9.
51. Omari TI, Miki K, Fraser R, *et al.* Oesophageal body and lower oesophageal sphincter function in healthy premature infants. *Gastroenterology* 1995; 109: 1757–64.
52. Bisset WM, Watt JB, Rivers RPA, Milla PJ. Ontogeny of fasting small intestinal motor activity in the human infant. *Gut* 1988; 29: 453–88.
53. Berseth CL. Gestational evolution of small intestine motility in preterm and term infants. *J Pediatr* 1989; 115: 646–51.
54. Lichtenberger L. A search for the origin of neonatal hypogastroanemia. *J Pediatr Gastroenterol Nutr* 1984; 3: 161–6.
55. Marchini G, Uvnas-Moberg K. Levels and molecular forms of gastrin and somatostatin in plasma and in gastric contents of infants after section delivery. *J Pediatr Gastroenterol Nutr* 1992; 14: 406–12.
56. Cavell B. Gastric emptying in preterm infants. *Acta Paediatr Scand* 1979; 68: 725–30.
57. Siegal M, Lebenthal E, Krantz B. Effect of choloric density on gastric emptying in premature infants. *J Pediatr* 1984; 104: 118–22.
58. Billeaud C, Guillet J, Sandler B. Gastric emptying in infants with or without gastro-oesophageal reflux according to the type of milk. *Eur J Clin Nutr* 1990; 44: 577–83.
59. Lucas A, Adrian TE, Kristophades N, Bloom SR, Aynsley-Green A. Plasma motilin gastrin and enteroglucagon and enteral feeding in the human newborn. *Arch Dis Child* 1980; 55: 673–7.
60. Ruckebusch Y. Development of digestive motor patterns during perinatal life: mechanisms and significance. *J Pediatr Gastroenterol Nutr* 1986; 5: 523–36.
61. Wozniak ER, Fenton TR, Milla PJ. The development of fasting small intestinal motor activity in the human neonate. In: Roman CE, ed. *Gastrointestinal motility*. Lancaster: MTP Press, 1984: 265–70.
62. Bisset WM, Watt JB, Rivers RPA, Milla PJ. Postprandial motor response of the small intestine to enteral feeds in preterm infants. *Arch Dis Child* 1989; 64: 1356–61.
63. Berseth CL, Nordi CK. Manometry can predict feeding readiness in preterm infants. *Gastroenterology* 1992; 103: 1523–8.
64. Baker J, Berseth CL. Post natal change in inhibitory regulation of intestinal motor activity in human and canine neonates. *Pediatr Res* 1995; 38: 133–9.

DISCUSSION

Dr. Zlotkin: I take it that the morphologic development can be a postnatal as well as a prenatal phenomenon, as in your discussion of the preterm infant and the physiology of the development of their gut. Perhaps you could elaborate on that?

Dr. Milla: It is clear that both in the enteric neuromusculature and the mucosa of the bowel, many of these developmental control genes will continue to be expressed. Walters has shown in adult epithelium that *Hox* genes continue to be expressed, and are probably very important in repair and maintenance processes in the bowel. A hiatus has occurred in our understanding of what happens in the latter part of gestation, when the enteric neuromusculature starts to become functional. That is largely because it is rather difficult to do the physiologic experiments on fetal mice. We really do not understand very well how these developmental processes fit in, but are beginning to find that distinct pathways exist coding for particular nerve functions; for example, some neurons will express nitric oxide and vasoactive intestinal peptide, which involve the co-stimulatory molecules to net. When we understand the role of persephin and artemin—the other net co-stimulatory molecules—we will find that those are probably the signaling systems to tell neurons to express different neurotransmitters. The unanswered question is why is it, at about 26 weeks of gestation in the human, when topographically the enteric neuromusculature looks as though it ought to be able to function—it has nerves that contain the appropriate neurotransmitters and it has structured relationships that suggest it ought to work—it works in such a disorganized fashion. Kenton Sanders would have us believe that it has all to do with the rate at which interstitial cells of Cajal develop, and that they act as the transducers and pacemakers, which result in ordered activity. That is probably the currently favored explanation.

Dr. Brandtzaeg: I wonder about the regulation of these *Hox* genes. It must be extremely finely tuned. The regulation is at the transcriptional level, but what is known about transcription factors and how these are produced?

Dr. Milla: I wish I knew. What we do know is that induction of their expression is largely controlled by morphogens: for the caudal related genes—things such as D13—right down at the bottom end of the gut, sonic hedgehog and Indian are important; higher up the gut, it is believed that BMP4 is important. People are now looking at aberrantly expressing those particular genes by exposing them to morphogens in increased quantities, and for the mesenchymal *Hox* genes, retinoic acid seems to be an important substance. We are in the middle of some experiments in which we take fetal mouse intestine, culture it *in vitro*, and show that the intestine will grow and express its control genes in the appropriate way at the appropriate place and time; if it is then exposed to retinoic acid, the whole schedule can be advanced so that it can be brought forward in time. So, we are beginning to understand some of the controlling factors but it is all at a very early stage.

Dr. Black: To follow up the question that Dr. Zlotkin has posed with respect to the gut of the premature infant, I would like your opinion on how best to stimulate normal growth and development of the gut in the infant. Do we not feed the child, or do we feed the child? If so, how?

Dr. Milla: It seems clear that there is a tight schedule of development, but within narrow windows things can probably be moved one way or another. Certainly, one can influence the secretion of polypeptide hormones by endocrine cells, which are there ready to act. And some of the polypeptide hormones involved—particularly motilin, NPY, and gastrin—will have an effect on the primitive gut of that premature infant at certain windows in time. For example, if erythromycin is used as a motilin agonist, contractile activity can be produced after about 30 weeks of gestation. Before that, as much can be given as possible, and it does absolutely nothing—that is because no receptors are there. That is why I believe that within narrow windows of time things can be done that might have an effect. Similarly, by putting food into the gut—as we know from the studies of Aynsley, Green, and Lucas—surges of polypeptide hormones can be produced to a remarkable degree when they are first feed. If they are not fed at all, no increase in secretion of those hormones is produced. Some of them are very important for gut nerve and muscle function. So, feeding the infant is important, and feeding them with boluses seems to have a better effect than feeding them continuously. Using glucocorticoids will also influence contractile activity. Some very old data were produced by Barbero long before we understood about fasting motor activity of the bowel (1). He just measured a motility index (i.e., the numbers of contractions). He showed that dexamethasone given to mothers in the last trimester increased contractile activity. Nobody seems to do that today, or even to remember the studies. I suspect, however, that it is actually doing something quite dramatic. I do not know of any information about the use of retinoic acid or any of its analogs, or any other substances that might have an influence. What I think can be done is to influence the normal course of events by moving them slightly. No magic answers exist because we are dealing with a series of processes that are very tightly controlled developmentally.

Dr. Delvin: Do you know of any imprinted genes related to the development of the gut? Intrauterine growth retardation has been associated to some extent with parental imprinting. Does parental imprinting occur in some instances in gut dysplasia?

Dr. Milla: I do not know. Maybe someone else knows.

Dr. Lyonnet: I think chromosome 7 would be interesting to look at, because it has been shown to be involved in both disomy (which is also found in children with cystic fibrosis) and imprinting in several children with growth retardation. However, this is a very rare form of disomy. Most cases of intrauterine growth retardation that are related to isodisomy have been found in chromosomes 11 and 16, where no *Hox* genes are found. Surprisingly, so far only overexpression of *Hox A4* in the mouse has been involved in an intestinal phenotype that resembled megacolon. Do you know of knockout experiments that have resulted in the same features for the *Hox* genes?

Dr. Milla: Not megacolon, but knockout of *Hox C4* results in marked abnormality of the esophageal musculature.

Dr. Goulet: I know you are involved with the problem of chronic intestinal pseudo-obstruction syndrome in children, which is a neuronal disorder of the gastrointestinal tract. At least two types of cells are involved in this disorder: the argyrophilic neuron and the argyrophobic neuron; and one other type of cell such as the Cajal cell may be involved. Would you speculate on any relationship between the genes you described and these types of cell? According to the Hirschsprung's disease model, mutation of the *Ret* gene involves a lack of ganglion cells, so what relationship might exist between the gene you described and the pathophysiology?

Dr. Milla: Argyrophilia and argyrophobia are merely reflections of the neurofilamentous content of the cells and, to an extent, they just indicate the state of differentiation. They do not relate to specific populations of cells. They do not help us in understanding the developmental processes that cells go through, and simply dividing them into argyrophilia and argyrophobia does not help in understanding whether particular populations of cells are abnormal or not. So, silver staining is just a means of looking at the morphology of cells. The famous series of cases in which there was said to be deficiency of argyrophilic neurons is a misnomer; I think all they were describing were infants under the age of 1 in whom argyrophobic neurons might be expected. Whether the illnesses those children had were caused by neuronal disease, I do not know. I think they just did not understand at the time what silver staining of neurons meant.

As to the second part of your question, interstitial cells of Cajal exist in association with myenteric neurons and smooth muscle cells, and they form a plexus under the innermost circular muscle layer. Good evidence indicates that they act as pacemakers and as transducers between enteric neurons and muscle cells. Also, evidence shows, in piebaldism, that they are responsible for loss of connection between enteric neurons and muscle cells, and that is the mechanism of the marked constipation in piebaldism. In hypertrophic pyloric stenosis, a certain amount of evidence also suggests that the Cajal cells associated with the myenteric neurons in that area are also abnormal. So, we are beginning to learn how these cells might fit into the individual pathologies that cause pseudo-obstruction.

Dr. Memon: Is there any modulating role of folic acid in the enteric neurons?

Dr. Milla: I do not know of a role for folic acid, but I would be surprised if there was none. I told you what I know about what might induce these developmental control genes, which although is minimal, is actually the state of knowledge at the moment. We just do not understand what induces those things to occur when they occur.

Dr. N. Wright: Sonic hedgehog is expressed in mouse intestinal endoderm all the way down. A paper in *Current Biology* about 2 years ago showed that if topically expressed sonic hedgehog is found in the pancreas, the pancreas goes through a partial intestinal differentiation program, including goblet cell differentiation (2). But, the interesting thing was that intestinal mesoderm differentiation also occurred in the pancreas, complete with interstitial cells of Cajal. What are the developmental cues for these interstitial cells of Cajal? How do they differentiate, and how do you think sonic hedgehog is involved in them?

Dr. Milla: Interstitial cells of Cajal are mesodermally derived. They probably branch off from the pathway of smooth muscle cell development relatively early on. The experiments to which you refer provide good evidence for a morphogen that might induce the mesenchymal *Hox* cell genes. What is not known at the moment is which ones might be involved, because any number of mesenchymal *Hox* genes exist.

Dr. Black: For a nonspecialist in this area, some genes have very odd names. For example, what is the origin of the name ''sonic hedgehog''?

Dr. Milla: I do not know. Can anyone help?

Dr. Nanthakumar: All these weird gene names are names for *Drosophila* mutants. When they are embryonic, they look like hedgehogs, so that was the name they were given. When a mammalian homolog was found, then there were three hedgehogs, so they were called ''sonic hedgehog,'' ''Indian hedgehog,'' and some other hedgehog!

If I remember correctly, knockout of one thyroid hormone receptor gene results in a severe defect of gut motility. This was shown a few years ago (3,4). Do you have any comment on how thyroid hormone might contribute to gut motility?

Dr. Milla: We know that thyroid hormone will have an effect on interstitial cells of Cajal and on smooth muscle cells, and in looking at smooth muscle from hypothyroid or hyperthyroid individuals, the frequency of slow wave activity of the smooth muscle cells is clearly altered: in hypothyroidism, this activity is very slow and in hyperthyroidism it is very fast. If sufficiently fast and sufficiently slow, electromechanical uncoupling occurs. From a physiologic point of view, it is easy to understand why this happens.

Dr. Lentze: Is there a neuronal stem cell in the gut which then develops into different neuronal cells? That is certainly the case in the central nervous system.

Dr. Milla: I am sure this is the case and I was trying to indicate that when I pointed out that the neural crest cells originated from different rhombomeres in the hind brain, and that at least by the time they have left the hind brain, they exhibit different markers. Little work has looked specifically at the very early neural crest cells that are going to become enteric neurons, but likely one single stem cell progenitor then divides and acquires other characteristics.

REFERENCES

1. Barbero GJ, Kim IC, Davis J. Duodenal motility patterns in infants and children. *Paediatrics* 1985; 22: 1054–63.
2. Apelqueist A, Ahlgren U, Edelund H. Sonic hedgehog directs specialised mesoderm differentiation in the intestine and pancreas. *Curr Biol* 1997; 7: 801–4.
3. Fraichard A, Chassande O, Plateroti M, *et al.* The T3R alpha gene encoding a thyroid hormone receptor is essential for post-natal development and thyroid hormone production. *EMBO J* 1997; 16: 4412–20.
4. Gauthier K, Chassande O, Plateroti M, *et al.* Different functions for the thyroid hormone receptors TRalpha and TRbeta in the control of thyroid hormone production and post-natal development. *EMBO J* 1999; 18: 623–31.

Gastrointestinal Functions, edited by Edgard E. Delvin and
Michael J. Lentze. Nestlé Nutrition Workshop Series, Pediatric
Program, Vol. 46, Nestec Ltd., Vevey/Lippincott Williams &
Wilkins, Philadelphia © 2001.

Fuels For Intestinal Cells

David H. Alpers

*Department of Internal Medicine, Washington University School of Medicine, St. Louis,
Missouri, USA*

The mucosa lining the small and large intestine needs fuel to maintain energy
metabolism, to express genes, to allow growth during the process of rapid cell
turnover, and for nutrient transport and absorption. Not all potential fuels provide
equal support for all of these needs. Thus, the ''proper'' fuel depends, in part, on
the endpoint measured, for example oxygen uptake and consumption, carbon dioxide
or lactate production, gene expression or growth, or nutrient transport and absorption.
Moreover, the status of the whole organism can affect the need for various energy
substrates. Factors that can affect the use of a substrate include feeding pattern
(fasted or fed), diet composition, site of nutrient presentation (luminal vs. vascular,
small bowel vs. colon, jejunum vs. ileum), stage of development (suckling, lactation,
old age), or presence of pathology (e.g., malnutrition, sepsis, infection, bowel resection, diabetes). Most of the conditions studied have involved the small intestinal
mucosa, as it is more responsive to changes in experimental and natural variables,
and more specific markers are available as surrogate endpoints for cellular function.

NATURALISTIC DELIVERY OF SUBSTRATES TO THE SMALL INTESTINAL MUCOSA

The simultaneous delivery of substrates from lumen and blood, as well as the
vertical gradient of cell differentiation, creates a unique anatomic route for the provision of nutrients. When amino acids are provided intraluminally, the outer two thirds
of the villus are preferentially fed, whereas the lower one third receives the major
portion of intravenous amino acids (1). Most of the luminal amino acids (and glucose)
traverse the enterocyte and are absorbed intact. However, although amino acids in
the extracellular pool are not the direct precursor for enterocyte protein synthesis,
they pass through an intracellular pool that is in equilibrium with the cellular protein
(2). *In vivo*, in the rat, when glutamine is provided both intraluminally and intravenously, the amount of glutamine utilized is the sum of what is extracted from each
delivery route (3), although that from the lumen is more oxidized to lactate (3) or
carbon dioxide (4).

Glucose is not a major oxidative fuel for the small intestine, and most is absorbed
intact, when provided in the presence of the major amino acids oxidized by the

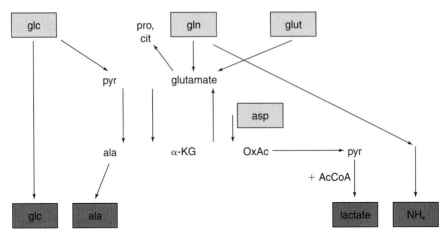

FIG. 1. Fuel oxidation in human small intestine. The three dietary amino acids that provide most of the oxidative substrate are glutamine (gln), glutamate (glut), and aspartate (asp). Most of these are provided in the lumen, although some glutamine released from muscle is provided arterially. Blood glucose serves as another source of alanine carbon. Other end products of amino acid metabolism include lactate, NH_4, and CO_2. α-KG, α-ketoglutarate; AcCoA, acetylCoA; ala, alanine; cit, citrulline; OxAc, oxaloacetate; pro, proline; pyr, pyruvate.

mucosa, namely glutamine, glutamate, and aspartate. Of the total carbon dioxide produced by rat small intestine, 80% is derived from these three amino acids (5). About two thirds of the glutamine and nearly all of the aspartate are metabolized in the rat jejunum, whereas nearly all intraluminal glucose is recovered intact (4). However, the proportion of glucose to lactate varies from approximately 33% to 100%, depending on the site of infusion, nutritional status of the animal, presence or absence of other substrates, and perfusion conditions (4). Arterial glucose is metabolized to carbon dioxide three times better than intraluminal glucose, but still much less than arterial glutamine (6). Some glycolysis does occur, however, so that the major source of the carbons in portal vein alanine is luminal glucose (5) (Fig. 1).

FACTORS AFFECTING THE UTILIZATION OF SUBSTRATES BY THE SMALL INTESTINE

Feeding has a marked effect on the utilization of mixed substrates. During fasting, in the rat, ketones are the major fuel oxidized to carbon dioxide by jejunal enterocytes (7). After feeding, however, amino acids (glutamine, glutamate, and aspartate) provide 77% of the carbon dioxide. Major differences are seen in fuel oxidation in the small and large intestine (Table 1). In the rat, a gradient of resting oxygen uptake is found that decreases from duodenum to ileum, presumably reflecting oxidation of endogenous substrates (8). However, a similar gradient is not present in the guinea

TABLE 1. *Relative importance of potential gut fuels*

Fuel	Lumen	Blood
Glutamine Glutamic acid, aspartic acid	Major: 80% of total	Major: 20% of total
Glucose	Low	Low
Fatty acids	Low (small bowel) High (colon)	Low
Ketones	Low	Major (fasting rat) Moderate (fasting human)
Polyamines	??	??
Nucleotides	??	??

pig (8). Butyrate is oxidized in the rat colon to carbon dioxide at a rate 10 times that of glutamine and 50 times that of glucose, and a very shallow gradient is seen, with the lowest oxidation in the ascending colon and the highest in the descending colon (9).

Significant species differences occur in utilization of fuels by the small intestinal mucosa (Table 2) (4,10–15). The use of ketones, glutamine, glucose, and arginine differs considerably in different species. Arginine is an essential amino acid in the cat and to a lesser degree in the dog (14), and the use of glutamine differs in rats and pigs (11,15). The rat differs from the human in its use of ketones and glucose (4,10), and the dog extracts much more glucose than the rat, and more glucose than glutamine (12), suggesting that glutamine may be much less important for dog than for rat intestine. The rat has been found to develop mucosal atrophy of the small intestine during short-term (3-day) fasting, and many studies have been performed to determine the optimal conditions for parenteral feeding that would restore small intestinal mucosal mass. However, very limited data examine instead of document a similar phenomenon in humans, and the available data support only a limited loss of mucosal tissue, even after prolonged total parenteral nutrition (16).

TABLE 2. *Species differences in small bowel utilization of fuels*

Species	Observation	Reference
Rat	Glycolysis from glucose > human	4
Rat	Ketone use > human during fasting	10
Rat	Glutamine use > pig	11
Dog	Glucose extraction > human	12
Cat, dog	Arg is essential amino acid	13
Pig, weaning	Arg production > arg metabolism	14
Pig, birth	Glutamine, glucose as fuels > glutamine for amino acid synthesis	15

Arg, arginine.

METHODOLOGIC ISSUES

The mucosal cell in the intestine exists in a special milieu between the lumen and the lamina propria, supplied from both sides by nutrients. In addition, the cells comprising the mucosa are moving along a vertical axis from undifferentiated crypt cells to mature villous cells; in some species a horizontal functional gradient is seen from duodenum to ileum, or from ascending to descending colon. The various preparations used to study fuel utilization in the intestinal mucosa inevitably disrupt this complex hierarchy, including isolated segments *in vivo*, *in vitro* segments perfused vascularly or luminally, everted sacs, cross-sectional rings, and isolated enterocytes or colonocytes.

The problems seen with studies of these systems include loss of polarization in isolated cells, loss of vascular supply in rings and sacs, use of single substrates in the absence of other major fuels, and loss of vertical and horizontal gradients. It is not surprising, therefore, that even in a single species (rat), the rate of oxygen uptake has varied by at least three- to fourfold (even up to 400-fold), depending on the preparation used (17). If oxygenation varies, so does the extent of glycolysis (lactate production) (18). Adenosine triphosphate (ATP) production was compared with carbon dioxide production in rat enterocytes, and was found to occur mainly from glucose through the anaerobic pathway (19), and glycolytic flux was six to seven times higher in jejunal cells than in ileal cells. In isolated cells, however, the glucose absorbed into and removed from the enterocyte cannot be distinguished, and both apical and basolateral surfaces of the cell are exposed to the nutrient, rather than just the one surface. The rate of oxidation of some nutrients is greater in isolated cells than in the intact organ, especially in the case of the colonocyte where cell viability is not so compromised by isolation. Thus, many studies reflect more the potential of the isolated cell for fuel metabolism than the function of the intact organ.

GLUCOSE METABOLISM

Although a large amount of free glucose is ingested or made available from starch metabolism, rather little is metabolized *in vivo* by aerobic glycolysis in the mammalian small intestinal mucosa (6). About 50% to 60% of the glucose that is metabolized results in lactate through the glycolytic pathway, and the amount of this glycolysis increases as the oxygen tension decreases. Such glycolysis products appear as lactate secreted into the portal vein. Alanine synthesis by glycolysis accounts for only 3% of the absorbed glucose (5). Although starvation reduces the metabolism of glucose in the mucosa, glucose metabolism is unchanged by the presence of ketone bodies. As noted above (19), in isolated rat small and large bowel mucosal cells, maximal utilization rates are similar for glucose and for glutamine (10). Ketone bodies are much less readily oxidized. When glucose and glutamine were present together, no increase in oxygen consumption was noted (10,20,21). However, when glucose, glutamine or both were added to acetoacetate, an increased oxygen consumption was noted (10). These data confirm the potential of the entero-cyte and colonocyte for glucose oxidation, but the degree to which this occurs *in vivo* varies greatly according to the experimental conditions.

AMINO ACID METABOLISM

The available data suggest that amino acids (mostly glutamine, glutamate, and aspartate) account for the major energy source of the small intestine. The measured oxygen consumption from those three amino acids by human intestinal jejunum accounts for approximately 80% of the predicted consumption (5) (Table 3). Gluta-mate is metabolized to a much greater extent than most other amino acids (86% vs. 10% to 35% for leucine, lysine, phenylalanine, and threonine), but all are incorpo-rated rather equally into mucosal protein (22). Dietary, not vascular, amino acids appear to be preferred for protein synthesis, at least in the pig (23). A recurring issue is whether glutamine is a preferred fuel for the enterocyte. The classic study by Windmueller and Spaeth (24) showed that oxidation of luminal glutamate (79%) was even greater than for glutamine (59%) in the intact rat small intestine. The utilization of glutamine by the intestine requires its deamidation to glutamate when delivered arterially (25,26). It seems likely, however, that most of the glutamate (or glutamine) used preferentially by the enterocyte is derived from the lumen. More than 90% of enteral glutamine is catabolized (27), but enteral glutamate is oxidized in humans even better than glutamine (28). The catabolism of enteral glutamine in pigs exceeds the rate of uptake of arterial glutamine fivefold (29). Finally, enteral glutamate is the major source of glutamate in glutathione, not the glutamate that is metabolized within the mucosa (30).

Thus, glutamine may be only a precursor for glutamate, especially when delivered luminally, where the capacity for uptake of glutamine is greatest. In humans, 54% of glutamine nitrogen and 78% of the carbon skeleton (28) is extracted on first pass, showing that glutamine is converted to glutamate in the process. The extraction rates from the lumen equal those from the blood, but glutamine accounts for only 7% of total intestinal protein synthesis (28). Glutamine, therefore, seems to be used more extensively for energy metabolism than for protein synthesis. The calculated rates of glutamine synthesis far exceed those for plasma glutamine turnover, which is

TABLE 3. *Amino acids are the quantitatively dominant fuels for small intestine*

Tissue	O₂ consumption (mmol/d)	
	Total	From amino acids
Skeletal muscle	12,000	900
Splanchnic bed	1,800	
Jejunum [Gln (lumen + blood) + Glut & Asp (lumen)]	450–550	400

Data from Jungas RL, Halperin ML, Brosnan JT. Quantitative analysis of amino acid oxidation and related gluconeogenesis in humans. *Physiol Rev* 1992;72:419.

consistent with the compartmentalization of glutamine in the splanchnic bed where it is metabolized and utilized (27,28).

Glutamine has been considered an essential amino acid for the intestine, and this view has received support from its trophic effects in experimental animals. Partial reversal of the atrophy induced by total parenteral nutrition (TPN) has been shown with 2% glutamine in rats with transplanted small intestine (31), and complete reversal with 1% glutamine in suckling pigs (32). However, glucose produced nearly as much reversal. In a study on rats, the addition of intravenous lipid to parenteral amino acids was necessary to achieve 75% to 85% reversal of small bowel atrophy induced by TPN (33). Moreover, neither glutamate nor aspartate has been used as control for glutamine, so the specificity of the response to glutamine is more apparent than real. It seems likely that any three of those major sources of amino acid oxidation in the small intestine should be capable of supporting growth in that organ. Thus, it is not clear that glutamine is uniquely important in restoring mucosal mass. It is worth remembering also that the atrophy seen in animals occurs much less strikingly in humans, if at all (16).

In humans, glutamine has been considered by some to be conditionally essential. However, approximately 60% of glutamine production represents *de novo* synthesis (34,35). The carbon skeleton for glutamine, α-ketoglutarate, is a Krebs cycle intermediate and can be made from carbohydrate, fat, or amino acids. Moreover, glutamine metabolism is higher in lymphocytes than it is in enterocytes (331 vs. 230 μmol/h/g dry weight) (36), and glutamine has effects on immune function as well as on correction of acidosis and neurotransmission. Thus, its clinical benefits, if indeed confirmed, may result from actions other than as a unique fuel for the intestine.

SHORT CHAIN FATTY ACIDS

Starches and dietary fiber not absorbed in the small intestine enter the colon of nonruminants, where colonic bacteria convert the carbohydrate to short chain fatty acids (SCFA). Absorption of these nutrients allows the colon to salvage considerable energy that would otherwise be lost in the stool. SCFA, especially butyrate, supply the substrate for 5% to 30% of the basal metabolic rate of the intact organism (37,38). The highest figures have been obtained in herbivores, such as rabbits. The wide variation in part may be related to differences in methodology used. More energy from short chain fatty acids could be available in nonruminants if dietary fiber could be digested in the small intestine. In humans, in developed countries, short chain fatty acids provide approximately 6% to 10% of energy requirements in the body (38).

Butyrate, the preferred large intestinal fuel, accounts for approximately 80% of the total oxygen consumption (39). Its oxidation exceeds that of glutamine and glucose 10 and 70 times, respectively (40). It is absorbed in the proximal and distal colon by passive diffusion and in the proximal colon by active transport mechanisms that are linked to various ion exchange transporters (41). It is possible that the regulation of fluid and electrolyte fluxes demonstrated in the presence of butyrate is related to an energy-generated effect, but this fuel effect has not been well substantiated. Butyrate also has many effects that may not be related to its role as a fuel. These include protection against neoplasia, regulation of colonic motility and blood flow, and a possible effect on colonic healing in various colitides.

Short chain fatty acids and ammonia are both bacterial metabolites that are used by the colon, but they have opposite effects on glucose metabolism by colonocytes. When both are present, more glycolysis occurs in pig colonocytes. Acetate is preferentially oxidized, and butyrate produces ketones (42). Ammonia decreases butyrate (not acetate) utilization, and increases glycolysis from glucose. In germ-free animals (i.e., in the absence of colonic microflora), the capacity to oxidize butyrate was increased (43). Thus, it may be difficult to assess the use of butyrate in the colon *in vitro* in the absence of other luminal colonic contents.

OTHER FUELS

Only a fraction of a percent of oleic acid is metabolized to carbon dioxide by rat small intestinal explants (44). Gut bacteria produce large amounts of polyamines, and polyamine-deficient diets in rats cause gut hypoplasia of the small and large bowel (45). Moreover, 30% of arterial putrescine is metabolized to succinate, and up to 70% in fasted rats (46). It is not clear, however, if these compounds are quantitatively significant sources of energy for the intestinal mucosa. Glutamine and pyrimidine metabolism are linked biochemically through the enzyme carbamoyl phosphate synthetase II in the production of endogenous pyrimidines (45). However, it is not known whether dietary nucleic acids are necessary over and above *de novo* pyrimidine synthesis, or whether parenteral nucleotides have any effect on enterocytes.

SUGGESTIONS FOR FUTURE RESEARCH

Studies should be carried out in a situation as close to that of the intact organ as possible, and in a species with intestinal physiology that reflects that of the human. These requirements are difficult to achieve in practice. Moreover, some nutrients (e.g., glutamine and butyrate) may have trophic or other functions that are not strictly related to their oxidative potential. Table 4 lists some of the recent controlled clinical studies that have been reported with glutamine supplementation, but using surrogate endpoints as diverse as intestinal permeability, nitrogen balance, mortality rates, and polymorphonuclear cell function. Only one study actually measured those variables (small bowel morphology, nutrient absorption) that might be considered direct endpoints for assessing the effect of glutamine as an intestinal fuel. The results of these experiments are not very supportive of a clinical deficiency in glutamine, or of a role for glutamine supplementation, even measuring a variety of endpoints unrelated to intestinal function. Future experiments should be designed to distinguish real nutritional endpoints from other effects, which, if reproducible, may reflect other

TABLE 4. *Controlled clinical studies of glutamine (gln) supplementation (1992–99)*

Study design	Surrogate endpoint and result	Reference
BM transplants ± gln/TPN	↓ Infection, ↑N balance	*Ann Intern Med* 1992;116:821
BM transplants ± gln/TPN	Shorter hospital stay, no other differences	*JPEN* 1993;17:407
Burn patients ± gln/TPN	↑ Bactericidal function of PMNs	*JPEN* 1994;18:128
16 trauma patients ± gln/EN	N balance, plasma gln same	*J Trauma* 1996;40:97
17 postoperative patients ± gln/EN	N balance, plasma gln same	*Am J Clin Nutr* 1997;65:977
28 abdominal surgery patients ± ala-gln/TPN	Less negative N balance	*Ann Surg* 1997;227:302
19 CABG patients ± ala-gln/TPN	Endotoxemia incidence same	*Acta Anesth Scand* 1997;41:385
14 CD patients ± oral gln	Gut permeability unchanged	*JPEN* 1999;23:7
84 ICU patients ± gln/TPN	Lower mortality	*Nutrition* 1997;13:295
78 ICU patients ± gln/EN	Mortality same	*Nutrition* 1997;15:108
34 surgical patients ± ala-gln/TPN	Lower postoperative complications	*Langenbecks Arch Chir* 1998;115:605
14 pancreatitis patients ± gln/TPN	Lower IL-8 release from WBC, same IL-6, and TNF release	*Nutrition* 1998;14:261
65 chemotherapy patients ± oral gln	Diarrhea and clinical response same	*Nutrition* 1997;13:748
8 short bowel patients ± GH, gln crossover	Small bowel morphology same, micronutrient absorption same	*Gastroenterology* 1997;113:1074

ala, Alanine; BM, bone marrow; CABG, coronary artery bypass graft; CD, Crohn's disease; EN, enteral nutrition; GH, growth hormone; ICU, intensive care unit: PMNs, polymorphonuclear leukocytes; TNF, tumor necrosis factor; TPN, total parenteral nutrition; WBC, white blood cells.

functions of the added nutrient. To do this, variables reflecting both nutritional utilization (e.g., substrate oxidation, carbon dioxide production, cell growth) and functional effects (immune response, cell differentiation) should be measured, and a clear distinction made between the two types of endpoint.

The uniqueness of a nutrient for an intestinal organ can be assessed only if it is compared with other compounds that are readily available and possibly also important *in vivo*. Thus, glutamine should be compared with glutamate or aspartate, and butyrate should be tested in the presence of other colonic luminal compounds such as acetate or ammonia. Moreover, attention should be given to whether the experimental model reflects a fasting or fed state. In interpreting published reports, be alert to the complexity of intestinal biology in the intact organism and make cautious applications of experimental results in small rodents and isolated cells, for example, to clinical situations in intact human organs.

REFERENCES

1. Alpers DH. Protein synthesis in intestinal mucosa: the effect of route of administration of precursor amino acids. *J Clin Invest* 1972; 51: 176–3.
2. Alpers DH, Their SO. Role of the free amino acid pool of the intestine in protein synthesis. *Biochim Biophys Acta* 1972; 262: 535–45.
3. Hanson PJ, Parsons DS. Factors affecting the utilization of ketone bodies and other substrates by rat jejunum: effects of fasting and of diabetes. *J Physiol (Lond)* 1978; 278: 55–67.
4. Porteous JW. Intestinal metabolism. *Environ Health Perspect* 1979; 33: 25–35.
5. Jungas RL, Halperin ML, Brosnan JT. Quantitative analysis of amino acid oxidation and related gluconeogenesis in humans. *Physiol Rev* 1992; 72: 419–48.
6. Windmueller HG, Spaeth AE. Respiratory fuels and nitrogen metabolism *in vivo* in small intestine of fed rats. *J Biol Chem* 1980; 255: 107–12.
7. Duee P-H, Darcy-Vrillon B, Blachier F, Morel M-T. Fuel selection in intestinal cells. *Proc Nutr Soc* 1995; 54: 83–94.
8. Sherratt HSA. The metabolism of the small intestine. Oxygen uptake and L-lactate production along the length of the small intestine of the rat and guinea pig. *Comp Biochem Physiol* 1968; 24: 745–61.
9. Chapman MAS, Grahn MF, Giamundo P, *et al.* New technique to measure mucosal metabolism and its use to map substrate utilization in the healthy human large bowel. *Br J Surg* 1993; 80: 445–9.
10. Ashy AA, Ardawi MSM. Glucose, glutamine, and ketone-body metabolism in human enterocytes. *Metabolism* 1988; 37: 602–9.
11. Vaugelade P, Posho L, Darcy-Vrillon P, Bernard F, Morel M-T, Duee P-H. Intestinal oxygen uptake and glucose metabolism during nutrient absorption in the pig. *Proc Soc Exp Biol Med* 1994; 207: 309–16.
12. Cersosimo E, Williams PE, Radosevich PM, Hoxworth BT, Lacy WW, Abumrad NN. Role of glutamine in adaptations in nitrogen metabolism during fasting. *Am J Physiol* 1986; 250: E622–8.
13. Morris JG. Nutritional and metabolic responses to arginine deficiency in carnivores. *J Nutr* 1985; 115: 524–31.
14. Wu G, Knabe DA, Flynn NE, Yan W, Flynn SP. Arginine degradation in developing porcine enterocytes. *Am J Physiol* 1996; 271: G913–19.
15. Wu G, Knabe DA, Yan W, Flynn NE. Glutamine and glucose metabolism in enterocytes of the neonatal pig. *Am J Physiol* 1995; 268: R334–42.
16. Alpers DH, Stenson WS. Does total parenteral nutrition–induced intestinal mucosal atrophy occur in humans and can it be affected by enteral supplements? *Curr Opin Gastroenterol* 1996; 12: 169–73.
17. Pritchard PJ, Porteous JW. Steady-state metabolism and transport of D-glucose by rat small intestine *in vitro*. *Biochem J* 1977; 164: 1–14.
18. Hutchison JD, Undrill VJ, Porteous JW. Glucose translocation and metabolism in the rat jejunum perfused in once-through mode *in vitro*. *Biochim Biophys Acta* 1994; 1200: 129–38.
19. Fleming SE, Zambell KL, Fitch MD. Glucose and glutamine provide similar proportions of energy to mucosal cells of rat small intestine. *Am J Physiol* 1997; 273: G969–78.
20. Watford M, Lund P, Krebs HA. Isolation and metabolic characteristics of rat and chicken enterocytes. *Biochem J* 1979; 178: 589–96.
21. Ardawi MSM, Newsholme EA. Fuel utilization in colonocytes of the rat. *Biochem J* 1985; 231: 713–19.
22. Fuller MF, Reeds PJ. Nitrogen cycling in the gut. *Annu Rev Nutr* 1998; 18: 385–411.
23. Stoll B, Burrin DG, Henry J, Jahoor F, Reeds PJ. Phenylalanine utilization by the gut and liver measured with intravenous and intragastric tracers in pigs. *Am J Physiol* 1997; 273: G1166–75.
24. Windmueller HG, Spaeth AE. Intestinal metabolism of glutamine and glutamate from the lumen as compared to glutamine from blood. *Arch Biochem Biophys* 1975; 171: 662–72.
25. Weber FL, Veach GL. The importance of the small intestine in gut ammonium production in the fasting dog. *Gastroenterology* 1979; 77: 235–40.
26. Weber FL, Friedman DW, Fresard KM. Ammonia production from intraluminal amino acids in canine jejunum. *Am J Physiol* 1988; 254: G264–8.
27. Battezzati A, Brillon DJ, Matthews DE. Oxidation of glutamic acid by the splanchnic bed in humans. *Am J Physiol* 1995; 269: E269–76.
28. Matthews DE, Marano MA, Campbell RG. Splanchnic bed utilization of glutamine and glutamic acid in humans. *Am J Physiol* 1993; 264: E848–54.

29. Reeds PJ, Burrin DG, Jahoor F, Wykes L, Henry J, Frazer EM. Enteral glutamate is almost completely metabolized in first pass by the gastrointestinal tract of infant pigs. *Am J Physiol* 1996; 270: E413–18.
30. Reeds PJ, Burrin DG, Stoll B, *et al.* Enteral glutamate is the preferential source for mucosal glutathione synthesis in fed piglets. *Am J Physiol* 1997; 273: E408–15.
31. Frankel WL, Zhang W, Afonso J, *et al.* Glutamine enhancement of structure and function in trans-planted small intestine in the rat. *JPEN* 1993; 17: 47–55.
32. Wu G, Meier SA, Knabe DA. Dietary glutamine supplementation prevents jejunal atrophy in weaned pigs. *J Nutr* 1996; 126: 2578–84.
33. Bark T, Svenberg T, Theodorsson E, *et al.* Glutamine supplementation does not prevent small bowel mucosal atrophy after total parenteral nutrition in the rat. *Clin Nutr* 1994; 13: 79–84.
34. Payne-James JJ, Grimble GK. The present status of glutamine. *Curr Opin Gastroenterol* 1995; 11: 161–7.
35. Buchman AL. Glutamine: is it a conditionally required nutrient for the human gastrointestinal system? *J Am Coll Nutr* 1996; 15: 199–205.
36. Newsholme EA, Carrie A-L. Quantitative aspects of glucose and glutamine metabolism by intestinal cells. *Gut* 1994; (suppl 1): S13–17.
37. Bugaut M, Bentejac M. Biological effects of short-chain fatty acids in nonruminant mammals. *Annu Rev Nutr* 1993; 13: 217–41.
38. Pouteau E, Piloquest H, Maugeais P, *et al.* Kinetic aspects of acetate metabolism in health humans using [1-^{13}C] acetate. *Am J Physiol* 1996; 270: E58–64.
39. Roediger WEW. Utilization of nutrients by isolated epithelial cells of the rat colon. *Gastroenterology* 1982; 83: 424–9.
40. Clausen MR, Mortensen PB. Kinetic studies on colonocyte metabolism of short chain fatty acids and glucose in ulcerative colitis. *Gut* 1995; 37: 684–9.
41. Velazquez OC, Lederer HM, Rombeau JL. Butyrate and the colonocyte. Production, absorption, metabolism, and therapeutic implications. *Adv Exp Med Biol* 1997; 427: 123–34.
42. Darcy-Vrillon B, Cherbuy C, Morel M-T, Durand M, Duee P-H. Short chain fatty acid and glucose metabolism in isolated pig colonocytes: modulation by NH4$^+$. *Mol Cell Biochem* 1996; 156: 145–51.
43. Cherbuy C, Darcy-Vrillon B, Morel MT, Pegorier JP, Duee PH. Effect of germfree state on the capabilities of isolated rat colonocytes to metabolize n-butyrate, glucose, and glutamine. *Gastroenter-ology* 1995; 109: 1890–9.
44. Alpers DH, Bass NM, Engle MJ, DeSchryver-Kecscremeti K. Intestinal fatty acid binding protein may favor differential apical fatty acid binding in the intestine. *Biochim Biophys Acta* 2000; 1485: 352–62.
45. Loser C, Eisel A, Harms D, Folsch UR. Dietary polyamines are essential luminal growth factors for small intestinal and colonic mucosal growth and development. *Gut* 1999; 44: 12–16.
46. Bardocz S, Grant G, Brown DS, Pusztai A. Putrescine as a source of instant energy in the small intestine of the rat. *Gut* 1998; 42: 24–8.

DISCUSSION

Dr. Ghoos: One thing about glutamine remains very intriguing: in maternal milk of all mammals, glutamine is the amino acid present in the highest concentration. Do you know of a reason why infants should need such a high intake of glutamine?

Dr. Alpers: I do not know the answer to that. However, I showed how plasma glutamine rises more than other amino acids after feeding in humans, because the release of glutamine from the large muscle mass is greater than that of any other amino acid. To some extent then, what comes out in the milk will be a reflection of what is circulating in the bloodstream at the time the mother nurses. So I could easily say that the high glutamine concentration is a reflection of what is in the blood. I do not know whether those studies are done in fasted or fed mothers. I doubt very much if they fasted them, so they probably were fed. That still does not mean that some special need might not exist for glutamine in the newborn, but I do not know of one. I do not think it could be said *a priori* that the level in the milk was high because the newborn needed it.

Dr. Ghoos: Is glutamine a stimulator of immunologic function?

Dr. Alpers: Much literature is available on the uptake of glutamine by immune cells. It is definitely taken up by a variety of cells in the immune system, and to levels that are somewhere from 50% to 80% as high as in the intestine. The intestine is still the most active as far as I know. Because of that, many people have felt that the clinical benefits of glutamine may be related to alterations in immune function, and immune function has been examined in these studies. But again, that is starting with the assumption that glutamine is important. Immune cells definitely do use glutamine and I think they metabolize it to glutamate.

Dr. Brandtzaeg: Again on the issue of glutamine and the immune system, I believe some interest is seen in this in sports medicine, in relationship to infections in elite competitors. Do you know anything about that?

Dr. Alpers: I suspect that most of those controlled studies—if they were indeed controlled—are in the vaults of the companies that promoted the idea. Do not misinterpret what I am saying: I am not saying that glutamine is necessarily bad or not a good fuel, but all the evidence so far is that for the intestine it is no better than glutamate. Is glutamate better than anything else? Again, the studies have not been done comparatively to the same degree. For example, the study I mentioned in the rat, where glutamine was compared with proline, serine, alanine, and so on, showed that those amino acids are not metabolized to the same extent as glutamate. When comparing something that is normally metabolized twice as much with something that is metabolized half as much, of course a difference is seen. A need is seen to go back to experiments comparing substrates that are equally metabolized.

Dr. Brandtzaeg: My specific question was whether those experiments showed a reduced frequency of upper respiratory tract infections in elite competitors.

Dr. Alpers: The data on the use and function of glutamine in elite athletes are mixed and inconclusive. Amino acid patterns have been examined in a few studies following intense training. One study reported a persistent change in plasma amino acids (valine and threonine increased <10%, but significantly; glutamine and histidine decreased 20%) in athletes with chronic fatigue and infection (1). However, when these athletes received glutamine supplement for 3 weeks, only 6 of 10 returned to their training, and there was no control group. Another study found no difference in plasma glutamine concentration in overtrained swimmers with or without upper respiratory infections (2). Glutamine supplementation given to marathon runners and elite male rowers after intense training with low plasma glutamine (20%) increased the T-lymphocyte helper-to-suppressor ratio and decreased subsequent infection, but infections were detected by questionnaire alone (3). In marathon runners studied by the same group, plasma concentrations of glutamine, alanine, and branched chain amino acids, and T-lymphocytes were decreased in the first hour after the race, and returned to normal after 16 hours, but glutamine supplementation had no effect on lymphocyte distribution (4). Another group found that decreased plasma glutamine concentrations postexercise in marathon runners were not responsible for the decrease in killer T-cell activity (5).

Dr. Zoppi: Among the factors that are important for fuel oxidation in the small bowel, what is the role played by ions such as zinc and copper in humans for the metabolism of fuel?

Dr. Alpers: It is a very difficult question to answer. Zinc is important for all cells and for a variety of enzymes. I believe that zinc deficiency would be deleterious for a cell that was in less than optimal condition, but I do not have any specific information on this.

Dr. Bjarnason: If glutamine is a fuel for Krebs' cycle, then of course, if Krebs' cycle is fed with glutamine and go one circle, you end up with glutamine again, so I cannot see how it can be the main fuel by that mechanism?

Dr. Alpers: Glutamate is being generated from other substrates. If exogenous glutamate is labeled, it is completely metabolized. If it is kept within the cell some of it might eventually end up as remade glutamate, but other substrates have come in to make glutamate as well. So, although it looks as though nothing has been accomplished, there should be an additive effect of metabolizing the exogenous glutamate together with other exogenous substrates.

Dr. Parsons: I have a question that has to do with other roles for glutamine and glutamate. First, I think that good evidence supports that glutaminase exists in the gastrointestinal tract and it can be upregulated, so therefore glutamine will go to glutamate, but what about the role of glutamate in the formation of citrulline and then arginine? In the rat with resected intestine, arginine becomes an essential amino acid. In newborn infants, where arginine is limited as it is used for the urea cycle, does glutamine play a role in citrulline production and reconversion back to arginine through the kidney?

Dr. Alpers: It might. In the newborn pig, the metabolism of arginine is different from later in life. If glutamate is available along with aspartate—and these data have been obtained in humans—more glutamate will be metabolized. If they are present in physiologic concentrations, wherein is much more glutamate than aspartate, both are metabolized 100%. If the same amount of aspartate as glutamate is put in, I think that it would still be 100% metabolized, because it goes through a similar mechanism inside the cell. But ordinarily, not nearly as much aspartate as glutamate is seen when proteins are broken down. So, I think they are both good fuels.

Dr. Marini: My question concerns the use of very long chain fatty acids (LCFA) soon after birth. A paper by Carlson showed that if LCFA was added, especially docosahexavoic acid (DHA), the incidence of necrotizing enterocolitis can be reduced (6). I was impressed by this work. Although the infants appear to have a very much higher incidence of necrotizing enterocolitis than we do, nevertheless they were able to reduce that incidence by almost half.

Dr. Alpers: I do not have any experience with that. I think any substrate that the intestinal cell can handle has the potential to be useful, but to show that it is actually useful requires a lot of patients. Most of these studies are very small and it is not known what else has been going on. However, I do not think long chain fatty acids should be eliminated as a possible fuel for the intestine.

Dr. Lentze: I have a clinical question. You mentioned twice that TPN-related atrophy in the human might not exist. Can you be more explicit about that? For many years we have been teaching, and were taught ourselves, that a child on TPN needs fuel to feed the gut to avoid intestinal atrophy. I still think that is very important.

Dr. Alpers: No data in humans support this belief. One or two studies in just a few patients have tried to show morphologic changes in measurements in postoperative patients, but the changes were very small (7,8). One study did show a convincing change, although only in three patients with chronic pancreatitis who were probably protein malnourished (9). When these patients were treated with TPN, the villus height fell. However, no data are available for postoperative patients. I reviewed this subject in detail a few years ago (10). All the existing data had been taken from the rat, on the assumption that the rat was a similar model to humans. But, in fact it is not. This theory has been around for a long time, so if data were available to show atrophy of the human intestine with that kind of feeding, I think it would have come to light by now.

Dr. Delvin: If we study fuel intake in a wider sense than just glutamine or glutamate and look at other fuels, and also look at variables other than oxygen consumption, what is the effect of the different fuels on energy storage, and how would the energy be stored? In essence, what is the effect of the type of energy intake or fuel intake in terms of energy storage?

Dr. Alpers: Are you referring to energy storage within the enterocyte?

Dr. Delvin: Partly yes, and also what is being secreted through the basolateral membrane.

Dr. Alpers: I do not really know of a mechanism whereby the enterocytes store energy. They take in a tremendous amount of lipid, as you know, but that lipid is almost entirely secreted, mostly in the lymphatics, but some in the portal vein as well. A small amount is metabolized. The same is true of glucose—much of it goes through, but some is metabolized—and also for many amino acids. Amino acids in the portal vein increase after a meal, except for glutamate which is 100% metabolized. So not much is stored; in the intestine, a small amount may be held in short-term reserve for these cells that only live 3 days, in case of a little starvation. But even that is not necessarily true: I could imagine that if one were not getting anything in from the lumen, one would start breaking down from the liver and muscle, and substrates are then made available in the bloodstream for utilization by the intestine. In fact, animal experiments show that the intestine uses a greater proportion of those circulating substrates in the fasting state than does the rest of the body. So, the intestine is protected from starvation. I know of no storage pool. Do you know of any?

Dr. Delvin: No. The question I really wanted to ask is whether the fact that different fuels might be given would result in the presence of different substrates, either extruded from the cell into the lymph pathway or remaining in the cell.

Dr. Alpers: It is hard to do such experiments *in situ* in the whole animal. I simply do not know of any data on that point.

Dr. Goulet: I agree with most of your comments, except maybe one. Do you not think that a place for glutamine may exist in the severely stressed patient? From my review of the literature, I believe this has been shown. In looking carefully at the provision of glutamine in severely stressed patients, it not only increases the nitrogen balance but it also decreases the rate of infection. Intensivists know that mortality in patients in the intensive care unit mainly results from multiple organ failure related to increased intestinal permeability and bacterial translocation. I do not believe glutamine has any value in normally nourished patients or in unstressed patients. I am somewhat interested in the data that seem to show that glutamine given to neonates in parenteral or to enteral nutrition solutions results in a decrease in the duration of ventilation, but not enough data are available to draw firm conclusions. However, I do believe glutamine is of value in the stressed patient.

Dr. Alpers: Let me reiterate my conclusions. I have nothing against glutamine or glutamate, but would like to propose the proper experiment that should be done. Accept that the clinical data are not terribly impressive: some studies appear to show an effect and others that do not. The properly controlled experiment would be to take glutamate, or some other amino acid that is also a good substrate for the intestine, and give it in equal amounts, in terms of oxidative substrate, to the added glutamine in the other limb of the experiment. What I think is happening now is that an easily oxidized substrate is being compared with a less easily oxidized substrate, and even then the difference shown is not terribly striking. In looking at nonoxidative outcomes, such as bacterial translocation, increased bacterial translocation has been observed in animal models that has been attributed to poor nutritional status. When this same endpoint (bacterial translocation) has been studied in humans, no relationship to poor nutritional status has been observed (11). So again, we have this difference in animals versus humans, preventing easy extrapolation to clinical conditions. In answering the question, ''I give glutamine to my patients and I think they do better; should I stop giving glutamine?'' I would say no, not if it works. But do not assume that glutamine is special or unique. It could well be that another substrate, given in an appropriate amount, would also be oxidized and would turn out to be just as good. That is the only concept that I am trying to get across.

Dr. Goulet: I agree, but we know that glutamine requirement increases in stressed patients with severe muscle catabolism. In the particular situation of the burned or otherwise traumatized patient, glutamine needs are not the same as in other patients. One could imagine that bowel physiology changes in that situation.

Dr. Alpers: Let me put this in another way. Of course, as most of the glutamine comes from muscle, in a situation such as you mentioned, if enough oxidized substrate is not given to the body, the usual amount of glutamine will not be released from muscle. So, it will look as though it is conditionally essential. But, from the kind of evidence I presented, I would just repeat that I know of no real evidence that glutamine is a conditionally essential amino acid.

Dr. Goulet: But one missing piece of the puzzle is glutamine synthesis during this situation.

Dr. Alpers: If not enough carbon backbone is given to the organism, it will not make as much; if enough is given it will. I am not trying to convince you, I am just trying to produce a little skepticism!

Dr. N. Wright: This may be a rat-specific phenomenon, but it is nonetheless interesting: if a 75% proximal resection is done and the rat is fed orally, an adaptation occurs in the ileal remnant. If that rat is isocalorically fed, that adaptation does not occur. So, food in the lumen is a stimulus to growth. This has been called "luminal nutrition," but I do not know what that means. Could you speculate on what luminal nutrition means—how absorption or mucosal work is translated into mucosal growth?

Dr. Alpers: This must mean that in the resected rat, for whatever reason, the amino acids supplied in the bloodstream do not penetrate high enough up the villus so that the bulk of the cells on a villus get sufficient substrate. On the other hand, in a normal rat, we showed a long time ago that amino acid precursors can be supplied all the way up the villus. Nobody has done this similar experiment in the resected animal, but I believe that it does not happen to the same degree. That is the best I can do.

REFERENCES

1. Kingsbury KJ, Kay L, Hjelm M. Contrasting free amino acid patterns in elite athletes: association with fatigue and infection. *Br J Sports Med* 1998; 32: 25–32.
2. Mackinnon LT, Hooper SL. Plasma glutamine and upper respiratory tract infection during intensified training in swimmers. *Med Sci Sports Exerc* 1996; 28: 285–90.
3. Castell LM, Newsholme EA. The effects of oral glutamine supplementation on athletes after prolonged, exhaustive exercise. *Nutrition* 1997; 13: 738–42.
4. Castell LM, Poortmans JR, Leclercq R, *et al.* Some aspects of the acute phase response after a marathon race, and the effects of glutamine supplementation. *Eur J Appl Physiol* 1997; 75: 47–53.
5. Rohde T, Asp S, MacLean DA, Pedersen BK. Competitive sustained activity in humans, lymphokine activated killer cell activity, and glutamine—an intervention study. *Eur J Appl Physiol* 1998; 78: 448–53.
6. Carlson SE, Montalto MB, Ponder DL, Werkmann SH, Korones SB. Lower incidence of NEC in infants fed a protein formula with egg phospholipids. *Pediatr Res* 1998; 44: 491–8.
7. Pironi L, Paganelli GM, Miglioli M, *et al.* Morphologic and cytoproliferative patterns of duodenal mucosa in two patients after long-term total parenteral nutrition: changes with oral refeeding and relation to intestinal resection. *JPEN* 1994; 18: 351–4.
8. Buchman AL, Moukearzei AA, Bhuta S, *et al.* Parenteral nutrition is associated with intestinal morphologic and functional changes in humans. *JPEN* 1995; 19: 453–60.
9. Groos S, Hunefeld G, Luciano L. Parenteral versus enteral nutrition: morphological changes in human adult intestinal mucosa. *J Submicrosc Cytol Pathol* 1996; 28: 61–74.
10. Alpers DH, Stenson WH. Does total parenteral nutrition–induced intestinal mucosal atrophy occur in humans and can it be affected by enteral supplements? *Curr Opin Gastroenterol* 1996; 12: 169–73.
11. Sedman PC, Macfie J, Sagar P, *et al.* The prevalence of gut translocation in humans. *Gastroenterology* 1194; 107: 643–9.

Gastrointestinal Functions, edited by Edgard E. Delvin and Michael J. Lentze. Nestlé Nutrition Workshop Series, Pediatric Program, Vol. 46, Nestec Ltd., Vevey/Lippincott Williams & Wilkins, Philadelphia © 2001.

Gastric Digestive Function

Daniel Ménard and Jean-René Basque

Department of Anatomy and Cell Biology, Faculty of Medicine, University of Sherbrooke, Québec, Canada

The gastric epithelium not only has a protective barrier function (against hydrochloric acid, peptidases, *Helicobacter pylori*, and so on) and a primary role in epithelial restitution (ulcer healing), but it also has specific digestive functions. The gastric mucosa is responsible for the secretion of luminal compounds such as mucus, hydrochloric acid, pepsinogen, and lipase.

One of the main purposes of gastric secretion is the digestion of dietary proteins. This involves the release of different pepsinogens (Pg1-5) by the fundic and antral gastric glands (1). These inactive proenzymes are synthesized and packaged into secretory granules of surface or glandular epithelial cells. Under acidic conditions, these secreted proenzymes are autocatalytically cleaved to generate their active form—pepsins (pepsin, prochymosin, progastricsin)—which are representative members of a group of proteolytic enzymes classified as aspartic proteases (2). In humans, pepsinogen 5 (Pg5), which is specifically synthesized and secreted by zymogenic chief cells, plays a primary role in the initiation of protein digestion and the proteolysis of collagen (the protein component of meat).

Although pepsinogen has been a subject of research since the 19th century (3), knowledge acquired over the last decade on the functions of the human stomach has expanded to include a significant role in fat digestion (4). In contrast to pepsin, the presence of a true gastric lipase has been the subject of a long controversy (4). In 1988, it was clearly established in humans that no lingual lipase exists, but instead a true lipase of gastric origin (5). This human gastric lipase (HGL) consists of a 379-amino acid polypeptide with a molecular weight of 49 kd. The characteristics of HGL (e.g., optimal acid pH) resistance to the acidic environment and to gastric protease action, and the ability to function in the absence of bile salts or cofactors, are advantageous in gastric lypolysis (6,7). Accumulating evidence supports that gastric digestion of triglycerides in normal physiologic situations is a prerequisite for efficient intestinal lipolysis, as free fatty acids and monoglycerides resulting from gastric lipolysis enhance subsequent hydrolysis of triglycerides by pancreatic lipase (8–10). Furthermore, the importance of gastric lipolysis increases in the context of perinatal physiology and pathologic conditions where secretion of gastric lipase could compensate, to some extent, for the depressed pancreatic activity. As HGL may have a special compensatory function in premature and newborn infants, it is important, therefore, to establish its ontogenesis and cellular localization and to understand the regulatory mechanisms controlling its synthesis and secretion.

MORPHOGENESIS OF HUMAN GASTRIC MUCOSA

The development of human gastric glands takes place very early during life (10–12 weeks of gestation) as opposed to rodent gastric glands, which mature strikingly during the last few days of gestation (11,12). At 8 to 10 weeks of gestation, human gastric epithelium is stratified and accumulation of glycogen occurs in the undifferentiated cells of the stratified epithelium (Fig. 1). At 11 to 12 weeks, the glandular pits are formed and the first differentiated epithelial cells, the parietal cells, appear. These cells are mainly located at the base of the developing glands and are already immunoreactive to intrinsic factor (13). From 11 weeks onward, the surface epithelial cells differentiate into mucous columnar cells, and the gastric glands develop further with the appearance of endocrine cells, mucous neck cells, and chief cells. Although the gastric glands will continue to grow during gestation, the thickness of the mucosa, as well as of the entire stomach wall in the newborn infant, is much less than in adults. Therefore, by 15 to 17 weeks of gestation, the fetal gastric glands are representative of the adult gastric glands and show all the morphologic compartments (foveolus, isthmus, neck, and base) in which cell lineages with different phenotypes exist.

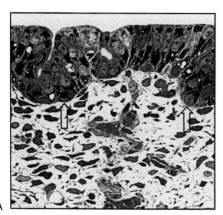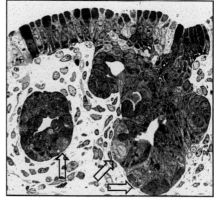

A   B

FIG. 1. Development of human gastric mucosa. (**A**) At 10 to 12 weeks of gestation, accumulation of glycogen is seen in undifferentiated cells of the stratified epithelium. Glandular buds begin to form (*arrows*) (×160). (**B**) At 17 to 20 weeks, as gastric glands develop, the surface columnar epithelium displays basal nuclei and accumulation of mucus in the apical cytoplasm. Parietal cells can be seen at the base region of gastric glands (*arrows*) (×100).

The proliferation pool responsible for the continuous renewal of all gastric epithelial cells is localized in the isthmus region. The epithelial cells leaving the proliferative zone differentiate into mucous cells during their upward migration (foveolus and surface epithelium) and into mucous, endocrine, parietal, and chief cells during downward migration (neck and glandular epithelium). During gestation, the gastric stratified epithelium, which contains scattered proliferating cells, visualized by ^{3}H-thymidine incorporation, is converted into an epithelium containing localized progenitor zones that resemble the patterns in adult gastric mucosa (11). The initial proliferation zone observed between 8 and 12 weeks is situated predominantly in the lower half of the early or pit glands. As the mucosa matures, the zone moves upward, establishing an adult location in the isthmus and neck of the glands. Thus, in the human gastric mucosa, the morphologic and proliferative compartments are already determined by 15 to 17 weeks of gestation.

ONTOGENESIS OF DIGESTIVE FUNCTIONS

Figure 2 illustrates the developmental profiles of HGL and Pg5 activities between 10 and 20 weeks of gestation, as well as the regional distribution of hydrolytic activities over the stomach. HGL activity is already present at low levels between 10 and 13 weeks of gestation and steadily increases up to 20 weeks (14). Pg5 activity is also present at 14 to 15 weeks, but does not significantly vary during the period studied. HGL activity is not evenly distributed throughout the stomach, being highest in the fundic area. Of note, HGL activity recorded in the fetal fundus at 20 weeks represents 30% of the mean lipase activity measured in the upper greater curvature in adult biopsy specimens (10). A clear, decreasing gradient is evident from the upper greater and lesser curvatures to the lower and lesser curvatures.

As opposed to HGL, Pg5 activity does not show any particular distribution over the gastric regions, although a steady increase is observed in the antrum between 16 and 20 weeks of gestation (14). These data show that the adult regional distribution of HGL activity is already in place at 15 to 16 weeks' gestation, whereas that of Pg5 is not yet established. It is obvious that the adult distribution of Pg5 over the gastric regions will occur later during development and that the adult levels of hydrolytic activities will also be in place later on. Lee et al. (9) documented the developmental profile of preduodenal lipase activity in gastric aspirates from 350 premature infants who were at various gestational ages. They reported that lipolytic activity was lower in the younger infants ($\leq$26 weeks), increased to a peak at 30 to 32 weeks, and then declined to a lower level at term ($\geq$40 weeks). Specific HGL activity determined in gastric biopsies is high in infants and children, and no significant changes occur in the age range of 3 months to 26 years (15). However, HGL activity does decrease in people aged more than 60 years. Whether this developmental profile reflects variations of the secretory capacity of the gastric mucosa or variations in the synthesis of HGL remains to be established.

A

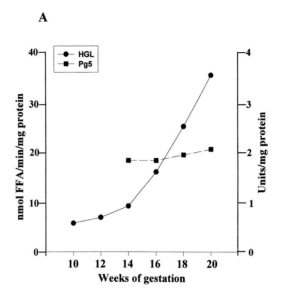

B

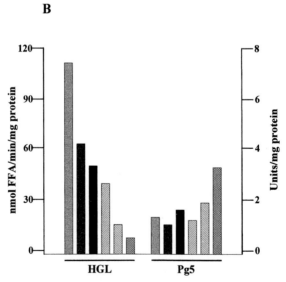

FIG. 2. Ontogeny (**A**) and tissue distribution (**B**) of human gastric digestive enzymes. (**A**) Human gastric lipase (HGL) and pepsin (Pg5) activities in gastric specimens between 10 and 20 weeks of gestation. (**B**) HGL and pepsin (Pg5) activities in the stomach of 20-week-old specimens. ■, fundus; ■, upper greater curvature; ■, upper lesser curvature; ▨, lower greater curvature; ▧, lower lesser curvature; ▨, antrum. (Adapted from Ménard D, Monfils S, Tremblay E. Ontogeny of human gastric lipase and pepsin activities. *Gastroenterology* 1995; 108: 1650–6.)

CELLULAR LOCALIZATION

Pepsinogen is synthesized and secreted by the chief cells located at the base of gastric glands of all mammals including humans. On the other hand, gastric lipase shows differential distribution among species. Indeed, gastric lipase is absent in the rat, with all lipolytic activity reported in gastric lumen being mediated by the presence of a lipase of lingual origin (4). In dog and cat models, the gastric lipase is associated with mucous-type cells of the pit compartment, whereas pepsinogen is present in chief cells located at the bottom of the fundic glands (6,16). In rabbit gastric biopsies, pepsinogen and lipase are located in a distinct zymogenic cell population in the cardiac area (17). In human gastric mucosa, HGL and Pg5 are always colocalized in chief cells of the fundic glands and never in mucous-type cells or in cells in the upper part of the gastric glands (18).

These data illustrate a unique feature for the human adult gastric mucosa regarding the cellular distribution of Pg5 and HGL. The colocalization of both digestive enzymes in human chief cells is already achieved as soon as these cells differentiate during the morphogenesis of the gastric mucosa. Indeed, the double immunofluorescence technique clearly shows that Pg5 and HGL are coexpressed in chief cells located at the glandular base of the developing fundic mucosa (Fig. 3). Furthermore, immunogold labeling demonstrates that HGL is exclusively found in the secretory granules of chief cells along the growing glands, whereas mucous and parietal cells are devoid of staining. Finally, Pg5 and HGL are colocalized in the secretory granules. These results strongly confirm the unique cellular localization of both gastric digestive enzymes in human chief cells (18). This functional specificity suggests that concepts elaborated for the regulation of digestive gastric functions in available animal models cannot be fully extrapolated to humans.

REGULATION OF PEPSINOGEN AND GASTRIC LIPASE SECRETION

Both gastric digestive enzymes are secreted very early during fetal development (14). Published studies on the control of pepsinogen secretion have used experimental models of tissue and cell preparations, including isolated gastric glands (19–21) and chief cell cultures (22–24). General agreement is found that cholecystokinin (CCK) and acetylcholine are involved in the regulation of pepsinogen secretion. However, many other candidates are also thought to participate in this regulation, namely gastrin (25), epidermal growth factor (EGF), transforming growth factor α (TGF-α) (26), and cytokines (27). Although the specific mechanisms involved in pepsinogen secretion are still little understood, it has been postulated that this process involves activation of cell surface receptors. Some evidence points to the existence of at least two separate intracellular pathways mediating the stimulus–secretion coupling of pepsinogen in chief cells; one of these involves cyclic adenosine monophosphate (cAMP) as an intracellular mediator, and the other involves the release of cytosolic calcium. Participation of cytoplasmic cAMP in the mediation of β-adrenergic stimulation is supported by the fact that forskolin, isoproterenol, and

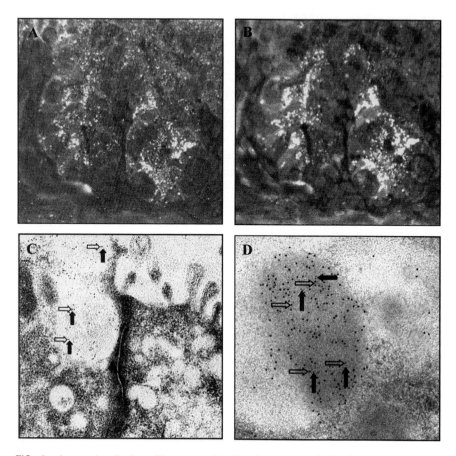

FIG. 3. Immunolocalization of human gastric digestive enzymes in fundic mucosa (20 weeks of gestation). (**A**), (**B**) Double immunolabeling was performed on 1-μm thick Lowicryl embedded tissues using guinea pig antibodies to Pg5 revealed by fluorescein-labeled immunoglobulins to guinea pig (**A**), and rabbit antibodies to human gastric lipase (HGL) revealed by rhodamin-labeled immunoglobulins to rabbit (**B**). HGL was always found coexpressed with pepsin and located exclusively in chief cells (×587). (**C**), (**D**) Immunogold-electron labeling was performed on 1-nm thick Lowicryl embedded tissues with HGL (10 nm) and Pg5 (5 nm) gold particles, respectively. Both types of gold particles are observed in apical secretory granules of chief cells (**C**). Note the secretion of both digestive enzymes in the gastric lumen (×33,000). (**D**) HGL (*blank arrows*) and Pg5 (*filled arrows*) gold particles distributed in a secretory granule (×66,000).

cholera toxin—potent stimulators of adenylyl cyclase—increase pepsinogen release in isolated gastric glands (21,23) as well as in isolated chief cells (28). However, some stimuli for pepsinogen secretion appear independent of cAMP mediation. Indeed, cholecystokinin, secretin, and vasoactive intestinal peptide do not activate adenylyl cyclase or cause cAMP elevation (29,30). It has been suggested that pepsinogen secretion stimulated by CCK and carbachol is dependent on calcium release from intracellular pools, because removal of external calcium does not affect carbachol-stimulated pepsinogen release (28,30,31). Also, in gastric chief cells, the interplay between calcium and calmodulin binding phosphorylation has a key role in modulating pepsinogen secretion (32).

It should be borne in mind that many of the actions on gastric secretion described for different factors are species specific, a concept suggesting that data taken from one species cannot be fully extrapolated to others (especially humans). Recent findings suggest that different cytokines, including growth factors, may participate in gastroduodenal repair or damage in pathologic conditions such as peptic ulceration that are partly mediated by pepsinogen secretion (33). In this regard, adequate *in vitro* models are a prerequisite for a better understanding of the effects of such peptides in the control of gastric function, including pepsinogen secretion. Serrano et al. have now shown for the first time that EGF directly stimulates basal pepsinogen secretion from dispersed human peptic cells (27). These results suggest that pepsinogen secretion induced by EGF is dependent on binding to EGF receptors, as preincubation using anti-EGF receptor antibodies inhibits the stimulation. Furthermore, the effect of EGF on pepsinogen secretion seems to involve intracellular calcium mobilization.

At present, our knowledge about the regulation of HGL secretion is scarce and limited to only a few animal species. The implications of gastrointestinal hormones in the regulatory control of preduodenal lipase secretion have been explored in the canine model. In this species, pentagastrin, together with histamine and carbachol, stimulate both lipase secretion and mucus secretion (34). Because dog gastric lipase is localized in mucous pit cells, caution is advised when extrapolating these data to humans. In dispersed rabbit gastric glands, CCK and carbachol increase rabbit gastric lipase secretion through different receptor mechanisms (35). In humans, the early observation that pentagastrin stimulates the secretion of HGL and pepsinogen in isolated glands (4) was recently confirmed by *in vivo* studies (36). In isolated human gastric glands, CCK and carbachol stimulate HGL secretion (4), but a recent *in vivo* study questioned the involvement of CCK (37). Although studies with isolated gastric glands showed a similar pattern of response to secretagogues in the secretion of lipase and pepsinogen, few studies have yet to deal with the simultaneous secretion of both these digestive enzymes (4,38). Based on species differences, cellular localization, and the diversity of the experimental models used, it is imperative to look closely at this aspect, particularly in human gastric mucosa. Increasing our knowledge of the specific regulatory mechanisms controlling the secretory process of synthesized and packaged gastric digestive enzymes will be important for understanding the pathophysiologic basis of human gastric secretion. Of equal importance, will be to understand the regulatory program governing the gene expression of these gastric enzymes.

REGULATION OF HGL GENE EXPRESSION

Because of the lack of adequate experimental models and tools, only fragmentary knowledge is available of the specific modulators involved, as well as their mechanisms of action, in the regulation of human gastric epithelial function. The unavailability of normal human gastric epithelial cell lines led researchers to focus their efforts on cell cultures generated from animals and human gastric cancers. Although organ culture techniques have substantially lengthened the period in which steady state conditions can be maintained for the study of gastric digestive function, this technique has not been found satisfactory in comparison with isolated gastric glands, because degenerative changes occur within the first 6 to 24 hours (39). However,

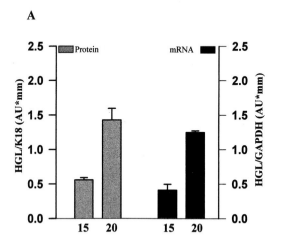

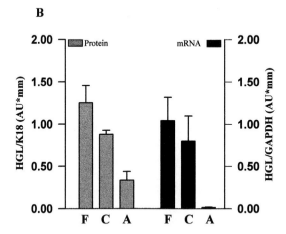

FIG. 4. Expression of human gastric lipase (HGL) during ontogeny and in different anatomic regions of the stomach. **(A)** Densitometric analysis of Western and Northern blotting experiments of HGL in gastric tissues of 15 and 20 weeks of gestation. Lipase protein (*gray columns*) and mRNA levels (*black columns*) are expressed in arbitrary units (AU) as the values of densitometric scans of autoradiographs normalized to the keratin-18 and GAPDH signals, respectively. **(B)** Representative Western and Northern blotting experiments of HGL protein (*gray columns*) and mRNA (*black columns*) in fundus (F), corpus (C), and antrum (A). Values represent the mean ± SEM of five (protein) and three (mRNA) separate and independent specimens.

we have clearly established that human fetal gastric explants can be maintained in serum-free organ culture for more than 10 days and that these explants continue to synthesize DNA, proteins, and glycoproteins (40). Thus, serum-free organ culture provides an interesting and unique tool for comparative studies on modulators and regulators of human gastric physiology.

Figure 4 shows the *in vivo* pattern of HGL expression. Between 15 and 20 weeks of gestation, a gradual increase in the relative HGL protein levels (Western blot) parallels the relative abundance of HGL mRNA levels (Northern blot). These results are consistent with the continuous increase in HGL enzymatic activity seen during the same period (Fig. 2). Furthermore, the decreasing gradient of both protein and mRNA signals from fundus to antrum is in accordance with the decreasing gradient of HGL activity (41). These data not only clearly establish that the gastric mucosa does synthesize HGL but suggest that the expression of HGL is primarily regulated at the mRNA level.

Human gastric explants in culture do synthesize and secrete HGL and Pg5, as both activities are found in gastric tissues as well as in the culture medium (Fig. 5). Indeed, a 3.8 times increase of the total activity (tissue + medium) is recorded, in accordance with the sustained or increased protein and glycoprotein synthesis reported in human fetal gastric tissues in organ culture (14). Furthermore, the analysis of HGL protein, enzymatic activity, and mRNA levels still suggests that HGL expression is regulated at the mRNA level *in vitro* (40). It is interesting to note that, although Pg5 and lipase activities show equivalently increased levels during culture, their secretion patterns differ. Indeed, although Pg5 activity rises in tissue and its secretion remains constant, tissue HGL activity diminishes drastically and is abundantly secreted into the media. These data explain the nonparallel nature of the

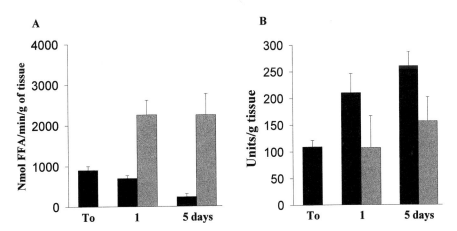

FIG. 5. Human gastric lipase (HGL) and pepsin (Pg5) synthesis and secretion profiles in cultured gastric explants. (**A**) HGL and (**B**) Pg5 activities in gastric tissues (*black columns*) and media (*gray columns*) at the beginning of culture (To) and after 1 and 5 days of culture. Data are expressed as mean ± SEM of nine independent experiments. (Adapted from Ménard D, Monfils S, Tremblay E. Ontogeny of human gastric lipase and pepsin activities. *Gastroenterology* 1995; 108: 1650–6.)

secretion of these two digestive enzymes and support the concept that Pg5 and HGL in human gastric mucosa are regulated differently.

Several hormones and growth factors are postulated to be involved in the development and maintenance of gastric functions (42). EGF, one of the best characterized growth factors, is known to play a major role in gastric physiology. EGF is involved in the maintenance of mucosal integrity because of its effects on the protection, repair, and healing processes (43,44); the inhibition of gastric acid secretion (45); and the secretion of pepsinogen (26). The fact that EGF/TGF-α receptors are ubiquitously distributed along the foveolus–gland axis (41) and, thus, in cells endowed with distinct physiologic functions, prompted us to verify its possible involvement in the regulation of Pg5 and HGL synthesis. Addition of EGF to cultured gastric explants specifically decreases tissue HGL activity without affecting its secretion, but does not modulate Pg5 activity or secretion (46). The lack of effect of EGF/TGFα on Pg5 secretion contrasts with its reported stimulation of basal pepsinogen secretion observed in isolated human peptic cells (27). This discrepancy, which could result from the different experimental conditions, stresses the need for further research. Nevertheless, these results indicate that both digestive enzymes are under different regulatory mechanisms.

The correlation between HGL activity, protein, and mRNA signals supports the concept that HGL expression is indeed downregulated at the mRNA level by EGF. Evidence provided (41) indicates that p42/p44 mitogen activated protein kinases (MAPKs) mediate the effects of EGF/TGF-α on HGL gene expression (Fig. 6). Overall, these data suggest that stimulation or inhibition of p42/p44^{MAPK} over or under a critical threshold of activity negatively regulates molecular processes that normally require MAPK activity. Interestingly, recent data also provide evidence that p42/p44^{MAPKs} mediate the effects of EGF on gastric acid secretion (47) and zymogen secretion in rat acinar (48) and guinea pig gastric chief cells (26). Therefore, the MAPK pathway would be an important effector involved in the regulatory effects of EGF/TGF-α on both synthesis and secretion of gastric digestive enzymes. Organ

---

FIG. 6. Effect of epidermal growth factor on human gastric lipase (HGL) and mitogen-activated protein kinases (MAPKs) expression. **(A)** HGL activity in gastric explants at the beginning of culture (To) and after 24 hours of culture in unsupplemented (C) and epidermal growth factor (EGF) supplemented (100 ng/ml) cultures. **(B)** Comparative effects of EGF and PD98059 on HGL mRNA. Densitometric analysis of Northern blots of HGL in gastric explants after 8 hours of culture without supplements **(C)**, with EGF nm100 ng/ml), and with PD98059 (20 nmol/L). Relative levels of HGL are expressed as arbitrary units (AU) as the values of densitometric scans of autoradiographs normalized to the GAPDH signals. **(C)** Effects of EGF and PD98049 on p42/p44^{MAPK} activity. Representative Western blot of the biphosphorylated and active forms of p42 and p44 MAPKs in gastric explants after 8 hours of culture without supplements **(C)**, with EGF (100 ng/ml), and PD98059 (20 nmol/L). Densitometric analysis shows the relative levels of active MAPKs expressed in arbitrary units (AU) as the values of densitometric scans of autoradiographs normalized to the keratin-18 signals. Values represent the mean ± SEM of four separate and independent cultures for each set of experiments. Statistically significant difference between EGF or PD compared with control (C): *$p < 0.035$. (Adapted from Tremblay E, Basque JR, Rivard N, Ménard D. Epidermal growth factor and transforming growth factor-α down-regulate human gastric lipase gene expression. *Gastroenterology* 1999; 116: 831–41.)

A

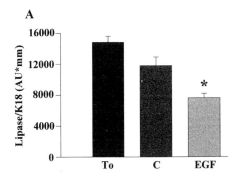

B

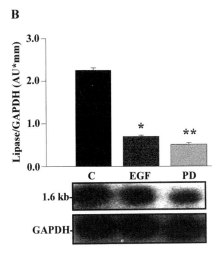

C

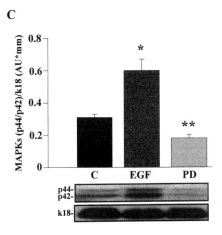

culture techniques offer a unique opportunity both to study the biological effects of a given hormone or growth factor in the synthesis and secretion of human gastric digestive enzymes and to pinpoint the molecular mechanisms involved.

CONCLUSIONS AND PERSPECTIVES

Over the last decade, it has been realized that the gastric mucosa has an important role in the digestion of both proteins and fat. The initial digestion of dietary fat or triglycerides in the stomach by a specific lipase is a prerequisite for efficient intestinal lipolysis. The importance of gastric lipolysis increases in the context of perinatal physiology and pathologic conditions (pancreatic insufficiency) because it then makes a greater contribution in the digestion of dietary triglycerides. Furthermore, the early appearance and secretion of gastric lipase supports the hypothesis that this enzyme plays a significant nutritional role during human development in hydrolyzing amniotic fluid triglycerides and providing fatty acids for intestinal metabolism.

Because the normal development of gastric lipolytic activity is essential for satisfactory digestion of fat, and because the existing information on gastric lipase is based almost exclusively on lipolytic activity in gastric juice, future studies should focus particularly on two aspects. First, based on the specificity of human chief cells that coexpress Pg5 and HGL, it is important to develop tissue and cell culture systems that allow researchers to address the synthesis and secretion of both of these digestive enzymes. The establishment of such normal human gastric epithelial cell lines, which can differentiate into chief cells, would be a great achievement. Second, with these models developed, investigations should concentrate on identifying the endocrine, paracrine, and autocrine factors involved in the upregulation and downregulation of human gastric digestive functions. Studies should also be designed to fully clarify the cellular and molecular mechanisms involved in the intricate relationship between hormones, growth factors, and cell–cell or cell–matrix interactions in normal and pathologic conditions. Overall, these data should find applications in developing new strategies to alleviate pancreatic exocrine insufficiency.

REFERENCES

1. Defize J. Development of pepsinogens. In: Lebenthal E, ed. *Human gastrointestinal development.* New York: Raven Press, 1980: 259–384.
2. Szecsi PB. The aspartic proteases. *Scand J Clin Lab Invest* 1992; 52: 5–11.
3. Davenport HW. In: *A history of gastric secretion and digestion.* Oxford: Oxford University Press, 1975: 1–401.
4. Hamosh M. In: *Lingual and gastric lipases: their role in fat digestion.* Boca Raton: CRC Press, 1990: 1–239.
5. Moreau H, Laugier R, Gargouri Y, Ferrato F, Verger R. Human preduodenal lipase is entirely of gastric fundic origin. *Gastroenterology* 1988; 95: 1221–6.
6. Carrière F, Barrowman JA, Verger R, Laugier R. Secretion and contribution of gastric and pancreatic lipases during a test meal in humans. *Gastroenterology* 1993; 105: 876–88.
7. Hernell O, Blackberg L. Molecular aspects of fat digestion in the newborn. *Acta Pediatr* 1992; 405: 65–9.
8. Hamosh M, Scanlon JW, Ganot D, Likel M, Scanlon KB, Hamosh P. Fat digestion in the newborn:

characterization of lipase in gastric aspirates of premature and term infants. *J Clin Invest* 1981; 67: 838–46.

9. Lee PC, Borysewicz R, Struze M, Raab K, Werlin ET. Development of lipolytic activity in gastric aspirates from premature infants. *J Pediatr Gastroenterol Nutr* 1993; 17: 291–7.

10. Abrams CK, Hamosh M, Dutta SK, Hubbard VS, Hamosh P. Role of nonpancreatic lipolytic activity in exocrine pancreatic insufficiency. *Gastroenterology* 1987; 92: 125–9.

11. Ménard D, Arsenault P. Cell proliferation in developing human stomach. *Anat Embryol* 1990; 182: 509–16.

12. Montgomery RK, Mulberg AE, Grand RI. Development of the human gastrointestinal tract: twenty years of progress. *Gastroenterology* 1999; 116: 702–31.

13. Aitchison M, Brown IL. Intrinsic factor in the human fetal stomach. An immunocytochemical study. *J Anat* 1988; 160: 211–17.

14. Ménard D, Monfils S, Tremblay E. Ontogeny of human gastric lipase and pepsin activities. *Gastroenterology* 1995; 108: 1650–6.

15. Dipalma J, Kirk CL, Hamosh M, Colon AR, Benjamin SB, Hamosh P. Lipase and pepsin activity in the gastric mucosa of infants, children and adults. *Gastroenterology* 1991; 101: 116–20.

16. Descroix-Vagne M, Perret JP, Daoud-el Baba M, *et al.* Variation of gastric lipase secretion in the Heidenhain pouch of the cat. *Arch Int Physiol Biochim* 1993; 101: 79–85.

17. Moreau H, Bernadac A, Tréout N, Gargouri Y, Ferrato F, Verger R. Immunocytochemical localization of rabbit gastric lipase and pepsinogen. *Eur J Cell Biol* 1990; 51: 165–72.

18. Moreau H, Bernadac A, Gargouri Y, Benkarka F, Laugier R, Verger R. Immunocytolocalization of human gastric lipase in chief cells of the fundic mucosa. *Histochemistry* 1988; 91: 419–23.

19. Kasbekar DK, Jensen RT, Gardner JD. Pepsinogen secretion from dispersed glands from rabbit stomach. *Am J Physiol* 1983; 244: G392–6.

20. Koelz HR, Hershey SJ, Sachs G, Chew CS. Cholinergic and beta-adrenergic pepsinogen release by isolated rabbit glands. *Am J Physiol* 1982; 243: G218–25.

21. Hershey SJ, Owirodu A, Miller M. Forskolin stimulation of acid and pepsinogen secretion by gastric glands. *Biochim Biophys Acta* 1983; 755: 293–9.

22. Defize J, Hunt RH. Pepsinogen synthesis and secretion in canine chief cell monolayers. *Gastroenterology* 1986; 90: 1391–9.

23. Raufman JP, Sutliff VE, Kasbekar DK, Jensen RT, Gardner JD. Pepsinogen secretion from dispersed chief cells from guinea pig stomach. *Am J Physiol* 1984; 247: G95–104.

24. Soll AH, Amirian DA, Thomas LP, Ayalon A. Secretagogue stimulation of pepsinogen release by canine chief cells in primary monolayer culture. *Gastroenterology* 1982; 82: 1184–9.

25. Wojdemann M, Norregaard P, Sternby B, Worning H, Olsen O. Low doses of pentagastrin stimulate gastric lipase secretion in man. *Scand J Gastroenterol* 1995; 30: 631–4.

26. Fiorrucci S, Lanfrancone L, Santucci L, *et al.* Epidermal growth factor modulates pepsinogen secretion in guinea pig gastric chief cells. *Gastroenterology* 1996; 111: 945–58.

27. Serrano MT, Lanas AI, Lorenke S, Sainz R. Cytokine effects on pepsinogen secretion from human peptic cells. *Gut* 1997; 40: 42–8.

28. Lanas AI, Anderson JW, Uemura N, Hirschowitz BI. Effects of cholinergic, histaminergic and peptidergic stimulation on pepsinogen secretion by isolated human peptic cells. *Scand J Gastroenterol* 1994; 29: 678–83.

29. Raufman JP, Berger S, Cosowsky L, Strauss E. Increases in cellular calcium concentration stimulate pepsinogen secretion from dispersed chief cells. *Biochem Biophys Res Commun* 1986; 137: 281–5.

30. Chew CS, Hershey SJ. Gastrin stimulation of isolated gastric glands. *Am J Physiol* 1982; 240: G504–12.

31. Fiorucci S, McArthur KE. Gastrin-releasing peptide directly releases pepsinogen from guinea pig chief cells. *Am J Physiol* 1990; 259: G760–6.

32. Tao C, Yamamoto M, Mieno H, Inoue M, Masujima T, Kajiyama G. Pepsinogen secretion: coupling of exocytosis visualized by video microscopy and $[Ca^{2+}]_i$ in single cells. *Am J Physiol* 1998; 274: G1166–77.

33. Hirschowitz BI. Mechanisms of peptic ulcer healing. In: Halter F, Garner A, Tytgat GNT, eds. *Falk symposium* Dordrecht: Kluwer Academic, 1991: 183–94.

34. Carrière F, Raphel V, Moreau H, *et al.* Dog gastric lipase: stimulation of its secretion *in vivo* and cytolocalization in mucous pit cells. *Gastroenterology* 1992; 102: 1535–45.

35. Berglindh T, Helander H, Obrink J. Effects of secretagogues on oxygen consumption, aminopyrine and morphology in isolated gastric glands. *Acta Physiol Scand* 1976; 97: 401–14.

36. Borovicka J, Schwizer W, Mettraux C, *et al.* Regulation of gastric and pancreatic lipase secretion by CCK and cholinergic mechanisms in humans. *Am J Physiol* 1997; 273: G374–80.
37. Worjdemann M, Olsen O, Norregaard P, Sternby B, Rehfeld JF. Gastric lipase secretion after sham feeding and cholinergic blockade. *Dig Dis Sci* 1997; 42: 1070–5.
38. Szafran Z, Szafran H, Popiela T, Trompeter G. Coupled secretion of gastric lipase and pepsin in man following pentagastrin stimulation. *Digestion* 1978; 18: 310–18.
39. Donaldson RM, Kapadia CR. Organ culture of gastric mucosa: advantages and limitations. *Methods Cell Biol* 1980; 21: 349–63.
40. Ménard D, Arsenault P, Monfils S. Maturation of human fetal stomach in organ culture. *Gastroenterology* 1993; 104: 492–501.
41. Tremblay E, Basque JR, Rivard N, Ménard D. Epidermal growth factor and transforming growth factor-α down-regulate human gastric lipase gene expression. *Gastroenterology* 1999; 116: 831–41.
42. Johnson LR. Functional development of the stomach. *Annu Rev Physiol* 1985; 47: 199–215.
43. Olsen PS, Poulsen SS, Kirkegaard P, Nexo E. Role of submandibular saliva and epidermal growth factor in gastric cytoprotection. *Gastroenterology* 1984; 87: 103–8.
44. Konturek SJ, Bielanoki W, Konturek JW, Oleksy J, Yamazaki J. Release and action of epidermal growth factor on gastric secretion in humans. *Scand J Gastroenterol* 1985; 24: 485–92.
45. Konturek JW, Brzozowski T, Konturek SJ. Epidermal growth factor in protection, repair and healing of gastrointestinal mucosa. *J Clin Gastroenterol* 1991; 13: S88–97.
46. Tremblay E, Monfils S, Ménard D. Epidermal growth factor influences cell proliferation, glycoprotein synthesis and lipase activity in human fetal stomach. *Gastroenterology* 1997; 112: 1188–96.
47. Nakamura K, Zhou CJ, Parante J, Chew CS. Parietal cell MAP kinases: multiple activation pathways. *Am J Physiol* 1996; 271: G640–9.
48. Dabrowski A, Groblewski GE, Schafer C, Guan KL, Williams JA. Cholecystokinin and EGF activate a MAPK cascade by different mechanisms in rat pancreatic acinar cells. *Am J Physiol* 1997; 273: C1472–9.

DISCUSSION

Dr. Brandtzaeg: Initially, you said that pepsinogen 5 was localized to the chief cells of the fundic mucosa, but later the impression was that it is evenly distributed through the whole body or corpus mucosa, all the way down to the antrum. Is that so?

Dr. Ménard: Chief cells are distributed all over the fundus and corpus mucosa, with a greater concentration at the base of the gastric glands.

Dr. Parsons: With regard to MAP kinase activity regulating human gastric lipase, it appears that p42/p44 regulates mitogenesis and the EGF regulates mitogenesis, but why does EGF not regulate both pepsinogen and the HGL?

Dr. Ménard: That is a surprise. As mentioned, it was recently shown that EGF stimulates the secretion of Pg5 by increasing the MAP kinase pathway in isolated guinea pig cells. In our system, we have intact tissue, which may be an important difference, and even though EGF stimulates the MAP kinase pathway, we were unable to see an effect on Pg5. Is this because human Pg5 has a different regulatory mechanism? Clearly, no effect whatsoever is seen on Pg5 secretion or synthesis.

Dr. Marini: What is the effect of the composition of the diet on gastric lipase production? I am thinking particularly of neonates fed human milk and different types of formula, with respect to varying protein composition.

Dr. Ménard: I have no personal experience with the use of diets in neonates. However, I doubt whether the protein portion of the diet will stimulate the release of gastric lipase. Not many studies have looked at the possible action of diets on gastric lipase.

It has been reported that differences in type of feeding (i.e., different fatty acid profiles [long chain or medium chain triglycerides], different emulsions [natural of artificial], and different fat particle size) do not affect the level of activity of gastric enzymes in preterm infants (1). However, a tendency for higher output of gastric lipase and pepsin after 2-week periods of high fat diet in healthy adult humans have been also reported (2). Therefore, a lot still needs to be learned about the regulation human gastric lipase synthesis and secretion.

Dr. Marini: How about the position of the fatty acids on the triglyceride molecule? We know that if they are in the β position on the lipase, they are better digested.

Dr. Ménard: Probably Dr. Lévy could answer this question.

Dr. Lévy: I think that human milk lipase has limited activity in the stomach—around 10% to 15%. Gastric lipase has much higher activity, approximately 30% to 40% hydrolysis, as you know. Gastric lipase is active on short, medium, and long chain fatty acids, and no problem is found with the hydrolysis of long chain fatty acids.

Dr. Marini: But the end product is mainly free fatty acids and diglycerides?

Dr. Lévy: Yes.

Dr. Endres: You mentioned TGF and EGF, but what about insulin-like growth factor (IGF)? I think IGF-1 has an important role in the growth of intestinal villi. Does it have any role in the stomach?

Dr. Ménard: We have preliminary results on the effects of IGF-1 and IGF-2, and both appear to downregulate gastric lipase activity. A short while ago, we identified for the first time a factor that increases lipase activity. This is important because it might well be clinically useful to stimulate gastric lipase activity to compensate for pancreatic insufficiency, for example. This stimulatory agent is keratinocyte growth factor (KGF), which also appears to increase Pg5. We have to confirm this, but so far it is the only growth factor known to stimulate human gastric lipase.

Dr. Ghoos: I have difficulty with the assumption that medium chain fatty acids are rapidly absorbed by the gastric mucosa, because this is the opposite of our experience using stable isotopes. Can you tell us any more about the possible uptake of nutrients by the gastric mucosa?

Dr. Ménard: Medium chain triglycerides (MCT) can be absorbed in suckling rat gastric mucosa (3–5). Moreover, it has been confirmed that MCT are absorbed directly from the human gastric mucosa and that this absorption appears to be related to age being more prolonged in the older infants (6).

Dr. Morisette: Recently, John Walsh published a paper looking at CCK gastrin receptors in the stomach (7). He was not able to visualize the CCK gastrin receptors on the parietal cells or on the chief cells in the dog and the guinea pig. According to you, at least some of the activity of chief cells is regulated by gastrin or CCK. How do you reconcile the fact that Walsh was unable to detect any CCK receptors on these cells using immunofluorescence with a specific antibody?

Dr. Ménard: I do not know how to reconcile that information. Little information has been published on the regulation of gastric lipase secretion, but researchers working with isolated human gastric glands have consistently found an effect of CCK on gastric lipase secretion. I am not aware of any study that has looked specifically at the presence of CCK receptors in the human stomach. However, one has to keep in mind that lipase and pepsinogen are associated with different gastric epithelial cell types, depending on the studied animal model, as I illustrated.

Dr. Koletzko: One of your slides showed that gastrin increases gastric lipase secretion. If gastric acid is blocked by giving proton pump inhibitors, gastrin levels increase. Has anybody looked at patients with pancreatic insufficiency—cystic fibrosis or some other pathology—to see whether gastric lipase secretion is altered by proton pump inhibitors? How does a change in pH affect lipase activity?

Dr. Ménard: In patients with pancreatic insufficiency–cystic fibrosis, dietary fat absorption ranges between 26% to 81%, although most of them did not have detectable pancreatic lipase activity. Therefore, gastric lipase activity is the responsible enzyme for fat hydrolysis. According to my knowledge, nobody has verified whether gastric lipase secretion is altered by proton pump inhibitors. Remember, although gastric lipase has an optimal acidic pH, it has a broad pH activity between 4 and 8.

Dr. N. Wright: You told us that EGF reduces gastric lipase production. Would you comment on the physiologic importance of this with respect to the local source of the EGF within the stomach? And, also, the location of EGF receptors from chief cells.

Dr. Ménard: EGF receptors are found all along the gastric glands and all gastric cell types have them. Now, is it really EGF that is acting on these cells, or is it TGF-α? That is why we have also done these studies with TGF-α, and found TGF-α mimics all the effects of EGF. What is the physiologic significance of this downregulation by EGF? We do not know. EGF appears also to have a downregulatory effect on the intestinal brush border enzymes in humans. In human fetal small intestine, it downregulates the expression of sucrase, for example, and this effect has also been shown on CaCo2 cells. So, it appears that EGF has a downregulatory action on many digestive functions in the human, but this is not the case in the neonatal mouse. For example, EGF stimulates brush border enzyme activities. So, EGF has a repressive action on gastric lipase in the human fetal stomach, although not on Pg5, and in the small intestine it also downregulates the expression of brush border enzymes.

Dr. N. Wright: In the adult, the EGF receptors are polarized to the basolateral aspect. Do you find them apically or basolaterally in the fetus?

Dr. Ménard: Always at the basolateral membrane.

Dr. N. Wright: What happens to gastrin concentrations in the stomach when you apply EGF? It has been shown very convincingly that an EGF responsive element exists in the 5′ upstream sequences of the gastrin gene (8–10) and, thus, EGF upregulates gastrin gene transcription and an increase in gastrin also occurs *in vivo*, certainly in rats. So how can you distinguish the effects of EGF on gastrin rather than the effects of EGF itself?

Dr. Ménard: We have not checked the effect of EGF on gastrin release from the gastric explants, but I think that gastrin receptors may not be present at this stage of development.

Dr. Nanthakumar: You showed that both Pg5 and gastric lipase are in the same secretory granule, but you also showed that different regulators can exist. So how do you explain, when both exist in the same secretory granule, how a differential amount is secreted into the lumen?

Dr. Ménard: We asked ourselves this same question. A similar situation occurs in the pancreas: all the pancreatic enzymes are packaged in the same granules at different levels. Is it the same in the gastric mucosa? Do we have different granules with different ratios of lipase and Pg5? We would have to do a lot of morphometric studies with double labeling with gold particles to show that. Until now, however, we have never found a granule with only one type of enzyme, so I believe that they are regulated during the packaging, and maybe some granules are more intensely packaged with lipase and others with Pg5. Although I must say that at this fetal age, Pg5 activity is very low.

REFERENCES

1. Armand M, Hamosh M, Mehta NR, *et al.* Effect of human milk or formula on gastric function and fat digestion in premature infant. *Pediatr Res* 1996; 40: 429–37.
2. Armand M, Hamosh M, DiPalma JS, *et al.* Dietary fat modulates gastric lipase activity in healthy humans. *Am J Clin Nutr* 1995; 62: 74–80.

3. Helander HF, Olivecrona T. Lipolysis and lipid absorption in the stomach of the suckling rat. *Gastro-enterology* 1970; 59: 22–35.
4. Egelrud T, Olivecrona T, Helander H. Studies on gastric absorption of lipids in the suckling rat. *Scand J Gastroenterol* 1971; 6: 329–33.
5. Lévy E, Goldstein R, Stankievicz H, Hager E, Freier S. Gastric handling of medium-chain triglycer-ides and subsequent metabolism in the suckling rat. *J Pediatr Gastroenterol Nutr* 1984; 3: 784–9.
6. Faber J, Goldstein R, Blondheim O, *et al*. Absorption of medium-chain triglycerides in the stomach of the human infant. *J Pediatr Gastroenterol Nutr* 1988; 7: 189–95.
7. Helander HF, Wong H, Poorkhalkali N, Walsh JH. Immunohistochemical localization of gastrin/CCK-B receptors in the dog and guinea-pig stomach. *Acta Physiol Scand* 1997; 159: 313–20.
8. Chupetra S, Du M, Todosco A, Merchant JL. EGF stimulates gastrin promoter through activation of Sp1 kinase activity. *Am J Physiol* 2000; 278: C697–708.
9. Merchant JL, Demeduik B, Brand SJ. A GC-rich element confers epidermal growth factor responsive-ness to transcription from the gastrin promoter. *Mol Cell Biol* 1991; 11: 2686–96.
10. Bachwich D, Merchant J, Brand SJ. Identification of a *cis*-regulatory element mediating somatostatin inhibition of epidermal growth factor–stimulated gastrin gene transcription. *Mol Endocrinol* 1992; 6: 1175–84.

Gastrointestinal Functions, edited by Edgard E. Delvin and
Michael J. Lentze. Nestlé Nutrition Workshop Series, Pediatric
Program, Vol. 46, Nestec Ltd., Vevey/Lippincott Williams &
Wilkins, Philadelphia © 2001.

Exocrine Pancreatic Function

Jean Morisset

*Department of Medicine, University of Sherbrooke, Sherbrooke,
Québec, Canada*

The control of human pancreatic enzyme secretion is still a matter of open debate,
as indicated by a recent statement by Adler:

"Human pancreatic secretion is regulated through a complicated coordination of neural,
hormonal and possibly paracrine effects. Cholinergic input is essential for full action of
any other agonist like cholecystokinin (CCK) and secretin" (1).

Indeed, confusion exists over the type of CCK receptors present on human pancreatic cells. Thus, it was suggested by *in vivo* studies in the early 1990s that exocrine
pancreatic enzyme secretion was mediated by occupation of the CCK_A receptor
subtypes (2), but more recently Tang et al. showed that the human pancreas appeared
predominantly to expresses the CCK_B subtype (3), an observation later confirmed
by Weinberg *et al.* (4). Compounding this problem, it was then reported that infusion
of postprandial concentrations of human gastrin, the natural ligand of the CCK_B
receptor, failed to stimulate human pancreatic secretion (5). As indicated recently
by Miller (6) in an editorial,

" . . . the more prominent existence of type B than type A CCK receptors within the
human pancreas raises a number of important questions such as: if the receptor resides
on the surface of the pancreatic acinar cells, why would it not be coupled to the secretory
machinery of the cell? What functional role does it play?"

These questions are still unanswered and progress has been hampered by the
difficulties in obtaining sufficient quantities of healthy human pancreatic tissue that
has not been damaged by autolysis.

In the meanwhile, pancreatic exocrine functions have been investigated in animal
models, mostly in the rat, mouse, and guinea pig, all of which are rodents. More
recently, the pig has been chosen in an effort to establish its suitability as a human
model for the study of pancreatic physiology. In this chapter, is summarized current
knowledge on pancreatic development, pancreatic enzyme synthesis, and secretion,
and the implications of CCK and its receptors for the pancreatic response to duodenal
hormone stimulation.

PANCREATIC FUNCTIONS

The exocrine pancreas supplies digestive enzymes for food digestion in the gut and ensures that the milieu of the intestine is sufficiently alkaline for maximal enzyme activity to hydrolyze the various substrates. The water needed to carry the digestive enzymes through the pancreatic duct system and the bicarbonate necessary to buffer the acidic stomach chyme are produced in and released from the pancreatic duct cells under the control of the parasympathetic nervous system and secretin. The pancreatic acinar cells, on the other hand, perform two major functions—the synthesis and secretion of the digestive enzymes. In rodents at least, the secretion of these enzymes into the intestine is controlled by the parasympathetic nervous system through acetylcholine and the gastrointestinal hormone CCK (7). The acinar cells, therefore are equipped with muscarinic (8) and CCK (9) receptors, among other receptor types.

DEVELOPMENT OF PANCREATIC COMPONENTS AND FUNCTIONS

At birth, the rat pancreatic gland is well developed and ready to assume its endocrine and exocrine functions. However, early in life, the pancreas remains in a state of active development to ensure that the strong demand for digestive enzymes to deal with the increased nutrient load necessary for proper body and organ development is

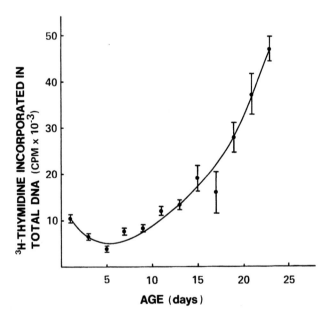

FIG. 1. ^{3}H-thymidine incorporation into pancreatic DNA with age. Pieces of pancreatic tissue excised from newborn rats up to 23 days after birth were incubated *in vitro* and ^{3}H-thymidine incorporation into DNA was measured as described in reference 47. Results are the means ± SE of six animals per point.

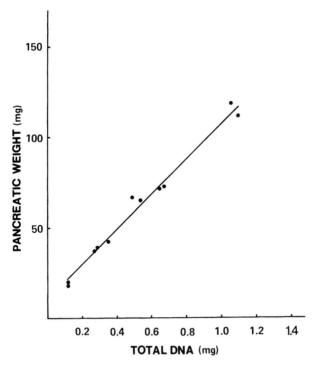

FIG. 2. Correlation between total pancreatic DNA content and pancreatic weight developments in rats. Newborn and neonatal rat pancreata obtained up to 23 days after birth were weighed and their total DNA extracted as described by Morisset *et al.* (47). These data come from the same animals used in Fig. 1.

met. As shown in Fig. 1, total thymidine incorporation, a marker of cell division, is relatively important at birth but decreases to a minimal level by day 5. From that point, an almost linear increase in DNA synthesis can be observed up to 25 days after birth. Interestingly, this active DNA synthesizing activity results in a linear increase in total DNA content when plotted against pancreatic weight, as shown in Fig. 2. From birth up to 1 year of age, development of pancreatic DNA and RNA total contents are parallel, whereas total protein content remains relatively low until weaning at 21 days, and increases tremendously thereafter, as shown in Fig. 3. The content of amylase and of chymotrypsinogen develops almost in parallel, although the pancreas is richer in amylase than in chymotrypsinogen (Fig. 4). This may result from the fact that amylase is the only enzyme responsible for starch and glycogen digestion, whereas protein digestion can be achieved by multiple proteases, including trypsinogen, procarboxypeptidases A and B, and elastases. Once the pancreatic gland has reached its full development, turnover rates of its different cell populations are comparable. Indeed, acinar cells show a labeling index of 6%, ductal cells 6%, endothelial cells 4%, interstitial cells 4% to 8%, and endocrine cells 2.5% to 4% (10).

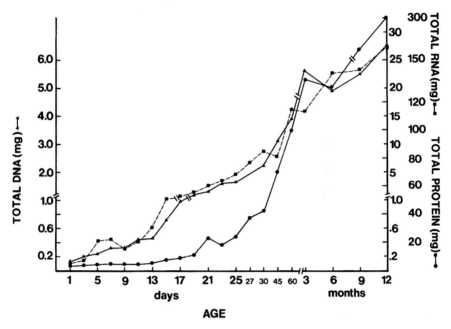

FIG. 3. Development of rat total pancreatic DNA, RNA and protein contents up to a year of age. Rats of different ages were killed and their pancreases used to evaluate DNA, RNA, and protein contents, as described by Morisset and Jolicoeur (48).

The acquisition of a secretory capacity in response to different stimuli occurs after birth. A secretory response to the muscarinic neurotransmitter acetylcholine appears after birth and reaches a maximum just before weaning in the rat (11). A good correlation has been established in the rat between acetylcholine-induced amylase output from the exocrine pancreas and the concentration of muscarinic receptors on the acinar cells (12). Premature weaning does not seem to modify the capacity of the pancreas to secrete enzymes under conditions of basal and acetylcholine stimulation or to increase its amylase and chymotrypsinogen contents (13). The secretory response to CCK is also absent in rat fetal pancreas and develops after birth (14). This lack of responsiveness to CCK in the early stage of life may result from a low binding capacity of the high-affinity component of the CCK receptor (15). In the human exists a refractoriness to secretagogs in the pancreas of young infants for which no explanation is found (16).

In adult rats, the secretory capacity of the exocrine pancreas can be either increased or severely diminished. Indeed, an increase in pancreatic weight produced by repeated injections of CCK is accompanied by proportional increases in functional capacity, as reflected by the increased maximal protein output in response to CCK (17). On the other hand, the rat secretory response to the acetylcholine analog carbamylcholine was severely impaired during the induction of acute pancreatitis by high doses of cerulein, a CCK analog (18). This pathology resulted in major decreases

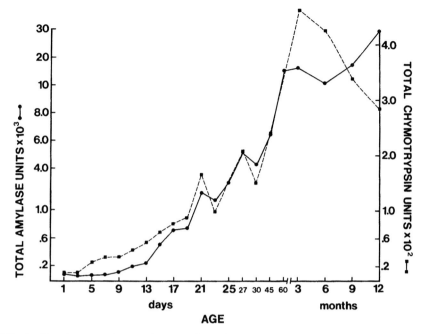

FIG. 4. Development of rat total pancreatic amylase and chymotrypsin contents up to 1 year of age. Enzyme assays were performed as described by Morisset and Jolicoeur (48).

in pancreatic amylase concentrations after 2 days of treatment, loss of acetylcholine potency and efficacy in stimulating amylase release, and an important reduction in acetylcholine muscarinic receptor concentration, although with no effect on their affinity for the agonist.

PANCREATIC ENZYME SYNTHESIS

Pancreatic enzyme synthesis—the major and most important function of the pancreatic acinar cells—concerns the replenishment of the different pancreatic digestive enzymes after their release into the duodenum. It is logical to assume that changes in the relative amounts of enzymes packaged in the zymogen granules of the acinar cells result from altered rates of specific synthesis. The capacity of the pancreatic gland to synthesize enzymes can be affected by various factors, including feeding, starvation, diet composition, and the administration of gastrointestinal hormones and cholinergic agents.

The synthesizing response of the pancreas to feeding has been studied in different animal models but little experimental evidence is seen for major variation in enzyme synthesis rate after meals. When fed rats are compared with 24-hour fasted rats, little (19) or no (20) change is seen in incorporation of labeled phenylalanine into protein as measured *in vitro*. In rats trained to eat for 1 hour every 12 hours for 3 days, and then fasted for 24 hours, refeeding for 15 minutes resulted in a small decrease in amino acid incorporation into protein *in vivo* 45 minutes after the meal, followed by a small increase 90 to 105 minutes after the meal (21). Other studies indicated that refeeding after prolonged fasting (48 hours) increased amino acid incorporation into pancreatic protein in rats (20) and depleted pancreatic stores of amylase (22).

Prolonged periods of fasting have dramatic effects on the exocrine pancreas, including major loss of protein and amylase (19,23). Under starvation conditions, amino acid incorporation into total pancreatic protein shows a marked decrease after 48 hours or more of fasting in rats (19,20), guinea pigs (24), and pigeons (25). Prolonged starvation also alters the overall protein machinery, including decreases in RNA polymerase activity (26) and RNA synthesis (27), and alterations in polysome morphology and function (28).

A fascinating aspect of the regulation of pancreatic enzyme synthesis remains the great potential of the acinar cell to adjust its specific digestive enzyme synthesis to the composition of the diet. The phenomenon was first described in the early 1940s by Grossman et al., when they observed that feeding rats a regimen rich in protein for 21 days caused a sevenfold increase in pancreatic protease activity when compared with animals fed a starch-rich diet (29). Similar increases in the pancreatic content of amylase (30) and lipase (31) were observed after feeding rats on diets rich in carbohydrates and fat, respectively.

This adaptive process is rapid, occurring within a couple of days of initiating the new diet (32,33), and involves changes in enzyme synthesis rates, as demonstrated by increases in amino acid incorporation into amylase in rats fed a starch-rich diet and into chymotrypsinogen in rats on a casein-rich diet (34).

The specific increases in pancreatic amylase synthesis in response to carbohydrate feeding seem to involve circulating glucose acting directly on the acinar cells and indirectly through the release of insulin (30).

Adaptation of the pancreatic lipase to a high fat diet occurs more efficiently on feeding long chain, unsaturated fatty acids than saturated fatty acids (33). Among the potential factors responsible for the effects of fat on lipase adaptation are gastric inhibitory peptide (GIP) (35), secretin (36), and CCK (37).

Intact dietary protein is mandatory to induce changes in proteolytic enzyme synthesis in the rat, as feeding protein hydrolysates or amino acids fails to modify pancreatic protease levels (38). This adaptation of proteases to a high protein diet may involve an intestinal factor because parenteral administration of amino acids has no effect on pancreatic protease contents (30,39); the factor is believed to be CCK, which is known to increase pancreatic proteolytic enzyme content when administered chronically (36).

The effects of acute and prolonged administration of CCK on pancreatic enzyme synthesis have been studied almost exclusively in the rat. Increases in protein synthesis *in vivo* were observed after acute CCK administration (40,41). In anesthetized rats, relatively large doses of CCK in combination with secretin resulted in an early fall in protein synthesis (within minutes) followed by an increase, with a preferential increase in chymotrypsinogen synthesis over amylase and lipase (42). Increases in pancreatic protein synthesis were also observed in response to cholinergic agonists (43). Chronic administration of CCK preferentially increases trypsinogen and chymotrypsinogen content over that of lipase and amylase, with trypsinogen increased almost threefold and chymotrypsinogen sevenfold (36). The response to secretin is different from that to CCK, as it increases lipase and chymotrypsinogen content almost equally, with little effect on amylase (36). Secretin is much less potent than CCK but it potentiates the effects of CCK when they are given together (36). Chronic administration of cholinergic agonists had only a small effect on total pancreatic protein content in one study (44), whereas others found little or no effect on individual enzyme contents (45,46).

It is clear from all these data that pancreatic protein and enzyme synthesis can be modulated by hormonal and cholinergic stimulation, and that components of the diet can control rates of synthesis of specific enzymes.

PANCREATIC ENZYME SECRETION

Pancreatic enzyme secretion can be measured either *in vitro* or *in vivo*. Several different types of *in vitro* pancreatic preparations have been used to study the secretory actions of hormones and neurotransmitters. Among these are whole pancreas, fragments of the organ, lobules, dispersed acini, and isolated cells. Each preparation from rat, mouse, or guinea pig has its advantages and disadvantages; currently, freshly dispersed preparations of acini seem to be the most reliable, consistent, and widely used model. *In vivo*, investigators have used the canulated pancreas at its duodenal junction in the anesthetized rat (49) or in conscious rats kept in Bollman type cages (50). The latter model is more physiologic because of the absence of anesthesia, and more versatile because it permits studies to evaluate the effects of meal consumption, and of various nutrient infusions either in the stomach or in the duodenum, on pancreatic volume, total protein, or specific enzyme outputs.

In Vitro Studies

Among the secretagogues recognized to increase pancreatic enzyme secretion are the cholinergic agent acetylcholine and its analogs bethanechol and carbamylcholine (49,51), the duodenal hormone CCK and its analog cerulein (52,53), the gastric hormone gastrin (54), peptides of the bombesin family (55), and members of the secretin family peptides, including secretin and vasoactive intestinal peptide (VIP) (56). By measuring amylase secretion, the response of dispersed acini was found to be substantially greater than that from isolated single cells, although comparable to that obtained with pancreatic lobules (57–59).

With preparations arranged so that multiple identical samples can be taken during a single incubation, it became possible to measure multiple cellular indices associated with the secretory process simultaneously. Indeed, in a single protocol, it is possible to monitor dose-response curves and the time course of secretion, and to measure accurately amylase release, cyclic nucleotide production, and calcium movements. Such studies showed that amylase release stimulated by CCK and bombesin was associated with phospholipase-C activation, phosphatidylinositol hydrolysis, inositol triphosphate production, and intracellular calcium release, events connected with the initiation of exocytosis (60). In these same acinar cells, stimulation by peptides of the secretin family also led to enzyme release, but through activation of adenylate cyclase and cyclic AMP production (59). The increase in enzyme secretion caused by giving a secretagogue associated with cyclic AMP production, together with one associated with calcium release, produced a potentiation of the effect that was greater than the sum of the increases caused by each secretagogue acting alone (59). These models were helpful in dissecting the intracellular events associated with the secretory processes, and are now used to investigate the early intracellular reactions implicated in cell cycle activation (61) related to the control of growth, regeneration, and differentiation of the pancreatic gland.

In Vivo Studies

Permanent fistulae fitted into the pancreatic and bile ducts in the rat (62) and the pig (63) enabled the discovery of the negative feedback control of pancreatic enzyme secretion. This mechanism functions with trypsin, chymotrypsin, or a mixture of bile and pancreatic juice in the small intestine to control enzyme secretion from the pancreas by hydrolyzing a trypsin-sensitive, CCK-releasing peptide constantly secreted from the intestine (64). Indeed, when pancreatic juice was diverted from the rat duodenum, hypersecretion of pancreatic juice and proteins was observed, associated with increased plasma CCK concentrations and concomitant pancreatic growth (65).

These permanent fistulae in rat pancreatic and bile ducts were largely responsible for the finding of a major circadian cycle of pancreatic secretion with a regular pattern, superimposed on which was a surprising regular minor cycle (66), independent of both cholinergic- and CCK-related mechanisms (67). Furthermore, it was also shown that secretion of each digestive enzyme is independently regulated and that they are differentially released, although the release of the enzymes may be strongly intercorrelated (68). This rat pancreatic model, developed by Green and Lyman (62), is the closest we can get to normal human physiology. Indeed, the pancreatic gland operates in its natural environment with its normal blood supply and natural stimuli initiated from nerves or from the gut.

CHOLECYSTOKININ AND ITS RECEPTORS IN PANCREATIC GROWTH CONTROL

Besides its known effects on pancreatic enzyme secretion, CCK has trophic effects on the pancreas of many rodents. CCK performs its numerous physiologic functions through two different receptor types: the *peripheral receptor* of the A type, CCK_A (A for alimentary), which is found in the pancreas, gallbladder, and intestine; and the *central nervous system receptor* of the B type, CCK_B (B for brain), which was described in neurons of the central nervous system (69).

Chronic occupation of the rat pancreatic CCK receptors by the CCK analog cerulein resulted in pancreatic growth characterized by acinar cell hypertrophy (70) and hyperplasia (71). This stimulated growth process involved increased rates of DNA synthesis in all cell types in the pancreas except for the endocrine cells (10,47). Pancreatic growth depends on adequate nutritional support as it does not occur in animals on a low protein diet (72). Growth of the pancreas also occurs in response to endogenous CCK release obtained either by pancreatic juice diversion (65) or by feeding rats a protein-rich diet (73). CCK-induced pancreatic growth in the rat involves occupation of the high affinity receptors of the CCK_A type because it can be reproduced by treatment with the high affinity CCK agonist JMV-180 (74), and inhibited by the CCK_A receptor antagonist L-364-718 (65). The presence of the CCK_A receptor subtype on acinar cells from rat and mouse pancreas has recently been confirmed by immunofluorescence (75). Using repeated ultrasound examinations of the pancreas, a significant increase in human pancreas size was observed 4 weeks after camostate (trypsin inhibitor) feeding, concomitant with increased plasma CCK levels (76). Although these data suggest stimulation of human pancreatic growth by endogenous CCK release, they will have to be confirmed by biochemical indices such as the protein, RNA, and DNA content. Furthermore, it will have to be established that CCK is the active growth factor operating through occupation of the CCK_B receptor subtype present in the human pancreas (3). Because access to human pancreas is almost impossible *in vivo*, future studies will probably be performed in the pig, as its pancreas possesses the CCK_B receptor subtype like the human pancreas (77).

Regeneration of the pancreatic gland has been observed following partial gland destruction after acute pancreatitis in the rat. It was stimulated by endogenous and exogenous CCK (78) and involved occupation of the CCK_A receptor subtype (79). In the human, one study seems to indicate that the pancreas does not have the capacity to regenerate after partial resection (80). On the other hand, two recent studies indicated that the pig pancreas can regenerate after partial pancreatectomy (81,82) and that bombesin could be one of the factors involved (81).

REFERENCES

1. Adler G. Regulation of human pancreatic secretion. *Digestion* 1997; 58(suppl 1): 39–41.
2. Cantor P, Olsen O, Gertz BJ, Gjorup I, Worning H. Inhibition of cholecystokinin-stimulated pancreaticobiliary output in man by the cholecystokinin receptor antagonist MK-329. *Scand J Gastroenterol* 1991; 26: 627–37.
3. Tang C, Biemond I, Lamers CBHW. Cholecystokinin receptors in human pancreas and gallbladder muscle: a comparative study. *Gastroenterology* 1996; 111: 1621–6.
4. Weinberg DS, Ruggeri B, Barber MT, Biswas S, Miknyocki S, Waldman SA. Cholecystokinin A and B receptors are differentially expressed in normal pancreas and pancreatic adrenocarcinoma. *J Clin Invest* 1997; 100: 597–603.
5. Cantor P, Petronijevic L, Pedersen JF, Worning H. Cholecystokinetic and pancreozymic effect of o-sulfated gastrin compared with nonsulfated gastrin and cholecystokinin. *Gastroenterology* 1986; 91: 1154–63.

6. Miller LJ. Does the human pancreas have a type A or B personality? *Gastroenterology* 1996; 111: 1767–70.
7. Gardner JD, Jensen RT. Regulation of pancreatic enzyme secretion *in vitro*. In: Johnson LR, ed. *Physiology of the gastrointestinal tract*. New York: Raven Press, 1981: 831–71.
8. Larose L, Poirier GG, Dumont Y, Frégeau C, Blanchard L, Morisset J. Modulation of rat pancreatic amylase secretion and muscarinic receptor populations by chronic bethanechol treatment. *Eur J Pharmacol* 1983; 95: 215–23.
9. Sankaran H, Goldfine ID, Deveney CW, Wong KY, Williams JA. Binding of cholecystokinin to high affinity receptors on isolated rat pancreatic acini. *J Biol Chem* 1980; 255: 1849–53.
10. Morisset J, Grondin G. Dynamics of pancreatic tissue cells in the rat exposed to long-term caerulein treatment. 2. Comparative analysis of the various cell types and their growth. *Biol Cell* 1989; 66: 279–90.
11. Larose L, Morisset J. Acinar cell responsiveness to Urecholine in the rat pancreas during fetal and early postnatal growth. *Gastroenterology* 1977; 73: 530–3.
12. Dumont Y, Larose L, Morisset J, Poirier GG. Parallel maturation of the pancreatic secretory response to cholinergic stimulation and the muscarinic receptor population. *Br J Pharmacol* 1981; 73: 347–54.
13. Dumont Y, Larose L, Poirier GG, Morisset J. Effect of early weaning of the neonatal rat on pancreatic acinar cell responsiveness to Urecholine. *Digestion* 1978; 17: 323–31.
14. Doyle CM, Jamieson JD. Development of secretagogue response in rat pancreatic acinar cells. *Dev Biol* 1978; 65: 11–27.
15. Leung YK, Lee PC, Lebenthal E. Maturation of cholecystokinin receptors in pancreatic acini of rats. *Am J Physiol* 1986; 250: G594–7.
16. Lebenthal E, Lee PC. Development of functional response in human exocrine pancreas. *Pediatrics* 1980; 66: 556–60.
17. Petersen H, Solomon T, Grossman MI. Effect of chronic pentagastrin, cholecystokinin and secretin on pancreas of rats. *Am J Physiol* 1978; 234: E286–93.
18. Morisset J, Wood J, Solomon TE, Larose L. Muscarinic receptors and amylase secretion of rat pancreatic acini during caerulein-induced acute pancreatitis. *Dig Dis Sci* 1987; 32: 872–7.
19. Morisset JA, Webster PD. Effects of fasting and feeding on protein synthesis by the rat pancreas. *J Clin Invest* 1972; 51: 1–8.
20. Webster PD, Singh M, Tucker PC, Black O. Effect of fasting and feeding on the pancreas. *Gastroenterology* 1972; 62: 600–5.
21. Malo C, Morisset JA. Time course of pancreatic protein synthesis following feeding. *Am J Dig Dis* 1978; 23: 6–8.
22. Morisset J, Dunnigan J. Exocrine pancreas adaptation to diet in vagotomized rats. *Rev Can Biol* 1967; 26: 11–16.
23. Viera-Matos AN, Tenenhouse A. The effect of fasting on the synthesis of amylase in rat exocrine pancreas. *Can J Physiol Pharmacol* 1977; 55: 90–7.
24. Meldolesi J. Effect of caerulein on protein synthesis and secretion in the guinea pig pancreas. *Br J Pharmacol* 1970; 40: 721–31.
25. Webster PD, Tyor MP. Effect of intravenous pancreozymin on amino acid incorporation by pancreatic tissue. *Am J Physiol* 1966; 211: 157–60.
26. Black O, Webster PD. Nutritional and hormonal effects on RNA polymerase enzyme activities in pancreas. *Am J Physiol* 1974; 227: 1276–80.
27. Webster PD, Tyor MP. Effects of fasting and feeding on uridine-^{3}H incorporation into RNA by pancreas slices. *Am J Physiol* 1967; 212: 203–6.
28. Black O, Webster PD. Protein synthesis in pancreas of fasted pigeons. *J Cell Biol* 1973; 57: 1–8.
29. Grossman MI, Greengard H, Ivy AC. The effect of dietary composition on pancreatic enzymes. *Am J Physiol* 1943; 138: 676–82.
30. Morisset J, Dunnigan J. Effects of glucose, amino acids, and insulin on adaptation of exocrine pancreas to diet. *Proc Soc Exp Biol Med* 1971; 136: 231–4.
31. Robberecht P, Deschodt-Lanckman M, Camus J, Bruylands J, Christophe J. Rat pancreatic hydrolases from birth to weaning and dietary adaptation after weaning. *Am J Physiol* 1971; 221: 376–81.
32. Ben Abdeljlil A, Desnuelle P. Sur l'adaptation des enzymes exocrines du pancréas à la composition du régime. *Biochim Biophys Acta* 1964; 81: 136–49.
33. Deschodt-Lanckman M, Robberecht P, Camus J, Christophe J. Short-term adaptation of pancreatic hydrolases to nutritional and physiological stimuli in adult rats. *Biochimie* 1971; 53: 789–96.
34. Reboud JP, Marchis-Mouren G, Cozzone A, Desnuelle P. Variations in the biosynthesis rate of

pancreatic amylase and chymotrypsinogen in response to a starch-rich and a protein-rich diet. *Biochem Biophys Res Commun* 1966; 22: 94–9.

35. Walsh JH. Gastrointestinal peptide hormones and other biologically active peptides. In: Sleisenger MH, Fordtran JS, eds. *Gastrointestinal disease*. Philadelphia: WB Saunders, 1978: 107–55.

36. Solomon TE, Petersen H, Elashoff J, Grossman MI. Interaction of caerulein and secretin on pancreatic size and composition in rat. *Am J Physiol* 1978; 235: E714–19.

37. Folsch UR, Winckler K, Wormsley KG. Influence of repeated administration of cholecystokinin and secretin on the pancreas of the rat. *Scand J Gastroenterol* 1978; 13: 663–71.

38. Grossman MI, Greengard H, Ivy AC. On the mechanism of the adaptation of pancreatic enzymes to dietary composition. *Am J Physiol* 1944; 141: 38–41.

39. Lavau M, Bazin R, Herzog J. Comparative effects of oral and parenteral feeding on pancreatic enzymes in the rat. *J Nutr* 1974; 104: 1432–7.

40. Mongeau R, Dagorn JC, Morisset J. Further evidence that protein synthesis can be decreased *in vivo* following hormonal stimulation in rat pancreas. *Can J Physiol Pharmacol* 1976; 54: 305–13.

41. Reggio H, Cailla HL. Effect of actinomycin D, pancreozymin and secretin on RNA synthesis and protein synthesis measured *in vivo* in rat pancreas. *Biochim Biophys Acta* 1974; 338: 37–42.

42. Dagorn JC, Mongeau R. Different action of hormonal stimulation on the biosynthesis of three pancreatic enzymes. *Biochim Biophys Acta* 1977; 498: 76–82.

43. Farber E, Sidransky H. Changes in protein metabolism in the rat pancreas on stimulation. *J Biol Chem* 1956; 222: 237–48.

44. Mainz DL, Black O, Webster PD. Hormonal control of pancreatic growth. *J Clin Invest* 1973; 52: 2300–4.

45. de Caro G, Ronconi I, Sopranzi N. Action of caerulein on pancreatic amylase and chymotrypsinogen in the rat. In: Mantegazza P, Horton EW, eds. *Prostaglandins, peptides, and amines*. London: Academic Press, 1969: 167–79.

46. Rothman SS, Wells H. Enhancement of pancreatic enzyme synthesis by pancreozymin. *Am J Physiol* 1969; 213: 215–18.

47. Morisset J, Chamberland S, Gilbert L, Lord A, Larose L. A study of DNA synthesis performed *in vivo* and following caerulein treatment in segments of the rat pancreas. *Biomed Res* 1982; 3: 151–8.

48. Morisset J, Jolicoeur L. Effect of hydrocortisone on pancreatic growth in rats. *Am J Physiol* 1980; 239: G95–8.

49. Morisset JA, Webster PD. *In vitro* and *in vivo* effects of pancreozymin, Urecholine, and cyclic AMP on rat pancreas. *Am J Physiol* 1971; 220: 202–8.

50. Green GM, Nasset ES. Effect of bile duct obstruction on pancreatic enzyme secretion and intestinal proteolytic enzyme activity in the rat. *Am J Dig Dis* 1977; 22: 437–43.

51. Larose L, Dumont Y, Asselin J, Morisset J, Poirier GG. Muscarinic receptor of rat pancreatic acini: [^{3}H]QNB binding and amylase secretion. *Eur J Pharmacol* 1981; 76: 247–54.

52. Jensen RT, Lemp GP, Gardner JD. Interaction of cholecystokinin with specific membrane receptors on pancreatic acinar cells. *Proc Natl Acad Sci USA* 1980; 77: 2079–83.

53. Sarfati P, Green GM, Morisset J. Secretion of protein, fluid and immunoreactive somatostatin in rat pure pancreatic juice: adaptation to chronic cerulein and secretin treatment. *Pancreas* 1988; 3: 375–82.

54. Solomon TE, Morisset J, Wood JG, Bussjaeger LJ. Additive interaction of pentagastrin and secretin on pancreatic growth in rats. *Gastroenterology* 1987; 92: 429–35.

55. Jensen RT, Moody T, Pert C, Rivier JE, Gardner JD. Interaction of bombesin and litorin with specific membrane receptors on pancreatic acinar cells. *Proc Natl Acad Sci USA* 1978; 75: 6139–43.

56. Gardner JD, Rottman AJ, Natarajan S, Bodanszky M. Interaction of secretin$_{5-27}$ and its analogues with hormone receptors on pancreatic acini. *Biochim Biophys Acta* 1979; 583: 491–503.

57. Gardner JD, Jackson MJ. Regulation of amylase release from dispersed pancreatic acinar cells. *J Physiol (Lond)* 1977; 270: 439–54.

58. Haymovits A, Scheele GA. Cellular cyclic nucleotides and enzyme secretion in the pancreatic acinar cell. *Proc Natl Acad Sci USA* 1976; 73: 156–60.

59. Peikin SR, Rottman AJ, Batzri S, Gardner JD. Kinetics of amylase release by dispersed acini prepared from guinea pig pancreas. *Am J Physiol* 1978; 235: E743–9.

60. Matozaki T, Sakamoto C, Nagao M, Nishizaki H, Baba S. G protein in stimulation of Pi hydrolysis by CCK in isolated rat pancreatic acinar cells. *Am J Physiol* 1988; 255: E652–9.

61. Rivard N, Rydzewska G, Lods JS, Morisset J. Novel model of integration of signaling pathways in rat pancreatic acinar cells. *Am J Physiol* 1995; 269: G352–62.

62. Green GM, Lyman RL. Feedback regulation of pancreatic enzyme secretion as a mechanism for trypsin inhibitor induced hypersecretion in rats. *Proc Soc Exp Biol Med* 1972; 140: 6–12.
63. Corring T, Chayvialle JA, Simoes-Nunes C, Abello J. Régulation de la sécrétion pancréatique par rétroaction négative et hormones gastro-intestinales plasmatiques chez le porc. *Reprod Nutr Dev* 1985; 25: 439–50.
64. Spannagel AW, Green GM, Guan D, Liddle RA, Faull K, Reeve UR. Purification and characterization of a luminal cholecystokinin-releasing factor from rat intestinal secretion. *Proc Natl Acad Sci USA* 1996; 93: 4415–20.
65. Rivard N, Guan D, Maouyo D, Grondin G, Bérubé FL, Morisset J. Endogenous cholecystokinin release responsible for pancreatic growth observed after pancreatic juice diversion. *Endocrinology* 1991; 129: 2867–74.
66. Maouyo D, Sarfati P, Guan D, Morisset J, Adelson JW. Circadian rhythm of exocrine pancreatic secretion in rats: major and minor cycles. *Am J Physiol* 1993; 264: G792–800.
67. Maouyo D, Guan D, Rivard N, Adelson JW, Morisset J. Stability of circadian and minor cycles of exocrine pancreatic secretion in atropine- and MK-329-infused rats. *Am J Physiol* 1995; 268: G251–9.
68. Maouyo D, Morisset J. Amazing pancreas: specific regulation of pancreatic secretion of individual digestive enzymes in rats. *Am J Physiol* 1995; 268: E349–59.
69. Innis RB, Snyder SH. Distinct cholecystokinin receptors in brain and pancreas. *Proc Natl Acad Sci USA* 1980; 77: 6917–21.
70. Solomon TE, Petersen H, Elashoff J, Grossman MI. Interaction of caerulein and secretin on pancreatic size and composition in rat. *Am J Physiol* 1978; 235: E714–19.
71. Solomon TE, Vanier M, Morisset J. Cell site and time course of DNA synthesis in pancreas after caerulein and secretin. *Am J Physiol* 1983; 245: G99–105.
72. Green GM, Sarfati PD, Morisset J. Lack of effect of caerulein on pancreatic growth of rats fed a low-protein diet. *Pancreas* 1991; 6: 182–9.
73. Morisset J, Guan D, Jurkowska G, Rivard N, Green GM. Endogenous cholecystokinin, the major factor responsible for dietary protein–induced pancreatic growth. *Pancreas* 1992; 7: 522–9.
74. Rivard N, Rydzewska G, Lods JS, Martinez J, Morisset J. Pancreas growth, tyrosine kinase, PTd Ins 3-kinase, and PLD involve high-affinity CCK-receptor occupation. *Am J Physiol* 1994; 266: G62–70.
75. Bourassa J, Lainé J, Kruse ML, Gagnon MC, Calvo E, Morisset J. Ontogeny and species differences in the pancreatic expression and localization of the CCKA receptors. *Biochem Biophys Res Commun* 1999; 260: 820–8.
76. Friess H, Kleef J, Isenmann R, Malfertheiner P, Buchler MW. Adaptation of the human pancreas to inhibition of luminal proteolytic activity. *Gastroenterology* 1998; 115: 388–96.
77. Morisset J, Levenez F, Corring T, Benrezzak O, Pelletier G, Calvo E. Pig pancreatic acinar cells possess predominantly the CCK-B receptor subtype. *Am J Physiol* 1996; 271: E397–402.
78. Jurkowska G, Grondin G, Massé S, Morisset J. Soybean trypsin inhibitor and cerulein accelerate recovery of cerulein-induced pancreatitis in rats. *Gastroenterology* 1992; 102: 550–62.
79. Jurkowska G, Grondin G, Morisset J. Involvement of endogenous cholecystokinin in pancreatic regeneration after cerulein-induced acute pancreatitis. *Pancreas* 1992; 7: 295–304.
80. Triotos GG, Barry MK, Johnson CD, Sarr MG. Pancreas regeneration after resection: does it occur in man? *Pancreas* 1999; 19: 310–13.
81. Fiorucci S, Bufalari A, Distrutti E, *et al.* Bombesin-induced pancreatic regeneration in pigs is mediated by p46^{shc}/p52^{shc} and p42/p44 mitogen-activated protein kinase upregulation. *Scand J Gastroenterol* 1998; 33: 1310–20.
82. Morisset J, Morisset S, Lauzon K, *et al.* Evidence of pancreas regeneration in the pig after subtotal pancreatectomy. *Pancreas* 1999; 19: 432.

DISCUSSION

Dr. Zoppi: I have a comment. We published a paper on pancreatic exocrine function in premature and full-term neonates (1,2). We showed that when we fed the infants with partially skimmed milk, pancreatic lipase did not increase, whereas when we gave the infants adapted formula rich in lipids, the lipase did increase. By adding starch to the feeding, we obtained an enhancement of α-amylase secretion. This was the first time anyone had shown that pancreatic function could be induced in humans by substrate.

Dr. Roy: Dr. Morisset, I have a question about your experiments where trypsin inhibition led to increased CCK and, therefore, to an increased pancreatic trypsin output: in view of the fact that CCK receptors are on the islet cells, what happened to the islet cells themselves? Did they grow? And, secondly, did the proximity of islet cells have anything to do with the proliferation of acini? In other words, does the presence of insulin in the immediate environment have anything to do with the proliferation of acini?

Dr. Morisset: This is the first demonstration by immunofluorescence that the β cells have the CCK_A type receptors. We knew that insulin release occurred if CCK was injected, but we did not know which type of receptor was involved. In humans, it seems that the receptor is of a different type; from the two studies I presented (3), the receptors over the acinar cells appear to be of the B type. The image of the pancreas we obtained was a gross image, not at the ultrastructural level, and we are not able to visualize the A type receptors on this type of picture. In the study by Friess et al. (4), whether insulin was involved was not mentioned. Possibly, it is because insulin increases the growth of CCK-stimulated cultured acinar cells (5). Probably insulin is a growth factor for the pancreas. Whether it is also involved in secretion is debatable. However, studies in the dog done some years ago (6) showed that a meal fed after immunoneutralizing the dog's insulin produced no secretory response, nor does a response occur under these conditions if CCK and secretin are injected. The conclusion was that insulin was also important in inducing the secretion of pancreatic enzymes. We do not yet know if that is a direct or an indirect effect.

Dr. Yamashiro: Recently, a Japanese group claimed that insulin plays an important role in developing amylase secretory capacity (7,8).

Dr. Parsons: I have two questions relevant to clinical care. The first has to do with the common practice of using nasojejunal feeds in the treatment of pancreatitis. A nasojejunal tube is inserted beyond the ligament of Treitz and protein, lipid, and carbohydrate are perfused on the assumption that the pancreas is being rested. My question then is, are there CCK receptors beyond the ligament of Treitz? Secondly, you show a decreased amylase output in severe pancreatitis in the rat, and I believe that it would be very similar in the human. Does that mean reduced amylase production or does it mean duct blockage and escape of enzymes into the circulatory system? I assume amylase and lipase are both very high in the plasma.

Dr. Morisset: CCK is produced in the first part of the gut; very little is found after the ligament of Treitz. So, if a patient is fed beyond the ligament of Treitz, a release of CCK should not occur. However, according to clinicians with whom I have discussed this, it seems very difficult to keep the tube down at that level. To answer your second question: it is true that when pancreatitis occurs in the human, the plasma enzyme content goes up, but this lasts only for 2 days. My studies in animals show a more long-term decrease occurs in amylase production. I do not know how long it takes to recover, and I have never evaluated the human pancreas.

Dr. Alpers: I have some comments on those questions. Not much work has been done in the human. Almost all the data come from animals, and they run the gamut to whether pancreatic enzyme secretion is up, down, or normal in pancreatitis. The data on putting the tube beyond the ligament of Treitz are simply empiric; isolated cases show that a tube can be put beyond the ligament of Treitz and patients with pancreatitis successfully fed and their condition does not worsen clinically, but others report of putting the tube in the stomach and showing the same thing (9). It has become a cult thing now to say that the tube has to go beyond the ligament of Treitz in order to rest the pancreas. Not a shred of evidence supports this; it may be true, but nothing shows it. It simply is not worth the bother of trying to keep the tube in the right place. People with pancreatitis can be fed and as soon as it can be done without pain, it is probably a good idea. I do not think it matters where the tube is put.

Dr. Lévy: What is the exact role of CCK in digestion? Do you have any patients with mutations of CCK or defective CCK showing the exact importance of CCK in digestion?

Dr. Morisset: This is an interesting question. I do not know of CCK mutation, but a mutation of the CCK receptors has been seen. A strain of rats is totally deficient in CCK_A receptors, and the curious thing is that the pancreas seems normal in these animals. They can apparently do without CCK. Probably what is happening is that other growth factors (e.g., bombesin, secretin, or acetylcholine) take care of the normal physiology of the gland. If the CCK_B receptors are knocked out in the rat, the stomach is affected: gastrin level is increased in the blood, the somatostatin population decreases, and the secretory function of the gland decreases (10). However, rodents do not necessarily need CCK, because the animals grow normally if the CCK receptor is knocked out.

Dr. Black: Could you comment on the role of CCK in appetite suppression and the mechanism behind that?

Dr. Morisset: This is a bit out of my field, but we have done some experiments in which we gave rats a CCK_A receptor antagonist and observed increased food consumption. This means that the antagonist goes to the brain and has some effect there. I cannot say whether satiety is controlled by the A or the B type of CCK.

Dr. Yamashiro: Different CCK receptors exist for each pancreatic enzyme, because the development of enzyme secretion is different. For example, amylase takes more than 10 months to reach full production, whereas trypsin develops much earlier. What is the mechanism of these differences? Are there different CCK receptors for each enzyme?

Dr. Morisset: No, I do not think so. This is the whole question of pancreatic adaptation. It was shown in the early 1950s that in an animal fed a sugar-rich or a starch-rich diet, amylase will be synthesized preferentially (11). If the gland is stimulated, more amylase comes out, because there is more in the gland in proportion to the other enzymes. On the other hand, if the animals are fed high-protein diets, the amylase goes down and the protease goes up. If the gland is stimulated, more protease than amylase will be released, because more protease is in the gland. Insulin seems to be important in the control of amylase synthesis, because in diabetic animals amylase disappears, at least in rodents. As soon as insulin is injected, amylase mRNA appears and amylase begins to be synthesized again. But insulin has nothing to do with the synthesis or the control of the other enzymes at all. It seems that CCK controls protease synthesis in the gland, because rats treated with CCK resulted in preferential synthesis of the protease over lipase and amylase, and this is a direct effect on the gland. Also, the message has to be from the gut, because animals given high concentrations of amino acids intravenously do not have this adaptation in the pancreas.

Dr. Mansbach: One of the hormones currently coming to the fore is PYY (peptide tyrosine tyrosine). Do you have any experience with PYY and its effects on either pancreatic enzyme secretion or growth?

Dr. Morisset: We have done some studies with PYY. It is released from the gut and acts as a secretory inhibitor in a negative feedback loop, so that the secretory response does not overshoot. It is mainly produced in the ileum. It may be involved in the late control of secretion—to inhibit secretion when the chyme reaches this level in the gut. Also, when somatostatin is infused into the ileum, basal pancreatic secretion increases. This means that basal release of PYY occurs, and when that release is inhibited, basal pancreatic secretion goes up. So, PYY may be involved in the basal control of pancreatic secretion, at least in the rat. With regard to growth, we found that if PYY is injected for at least 5 days, a small increase in pancreatic growth occurs, but we did not pursue these studies to determine the mechanism.

REFERENCES

1. Zoppi G, Andreotti G, Pajno-Ferrara F, Njai DM, Gaburro D. Exocrine pancreas functions in premature and full term neonates. *Pediatr Res* 1972; 6: 880.
2. Zoppi G, Andreotti G, Pajno-Ferrara F, Gaburro D. The development of specific responses of the exocrine pancreas to pancreozymin and secretin stimulation in newborn infants. *Pediatr Res* 1973; 7: 198.
3. Bourassa J, Lainé J, Kruse ML, *et al.* Ontogeny and species differences in the pancreatic expression and localization of the CCK$_A$ receptors. *Biochem Biophys Res Commun* 1999; 260: 820–8.
4. Friess H, Kleef J, Isenmann R, Malfertheiner P, Buchler MW. Adaptation of the human pancreas to inhibition of luminal proteolytic activity. *Gastroenterology* 1998; 115: 388–96.
5. Logsdon CD, Williams JA. Pancreatic acini in short term culture: regulation by EGF, carbachol, insulin, and corticosterone. *Am J Physiol* 1983; 244: G675–82.
6. Lee KY, Krusch D, Zhou L, *et al.* Effects of endogenous insulin on pancreatic exocrine secretion in perfused dog pancreas. *Pancreas* 1995; 11: 1901–5.
7. Kinouchi T, Koizumi K, Kuwata T, Yajima T. Crucial role of milk-borne insulin in the development of pancreatic amylase at the onset of weaning in rats. *Am J Physiol* 1998; 275: R1958–69.
8. Kinouchi T, Koizumi K, Kuwata T, Yajima T. Milk borne insulin with trypsin inhibitor in milk induces pancreatic amylase development at the onset of weaning in rats. *J Pediatr Gastroenterol Nutr* 2000; 30: 515–21.
9. Voitk A, Brown RA, Echave V, *et al.* Use of an elemental diet in the treatment of complicated pancreatitis. *Am J Surg* 1973; 125: 223–7.
10. Langhans N, Rindi G, Chiu M, *et al.* Abnormal gastric histology and decreased acid production in cholecystokinin-B–gastrin receptor–deficient mice. *Gastroenterology* 1997; 112: 280–6.
11. Rebout JP, Marchis-Mouren G, Cozzone A, Desnuelle P. Variations in the biosynthesis rate of pancreatic amylase and chymotrypsinogen in response to a starch-rich and a protein-rich diet. *Biochem Biophys Res Commun* 1996; 22: 94–9.

Gastrointestinal Functions, edited by Edgard E. Delvin and Michael J. Lentze. Nestlé Nutrition Workshop Series, Pediatric Program, Vol. 46, Nestec Ltd., Vevey/Lippincott Williams & Wilkins, Philadelphia © 2001.

Malabsorption

Charles M. Mansbach, II

Department of Gastroenterology, University of Tennessee William F. Bowld Hospital, and University of Tennessee Health Science Center, Memphis, Tennessee, USA

GENERAL ISSUES REGARDING STEATORRHEA

Malabsorption is a large topic that covers a variety of states in which the small intestine absorbs any nutrient incompletely. This can range from congenital malabsorptive states (e.g., Hartnup disease) in which basic amino acids are poorly absorbed, to immunologically induced problems (e.g., gluten sensitive enteropathy), to iatrogenic problems (e.g., gastric resection or radiation-induced injury), or to the ''programmed'' malabsorptive state of lactose in older children. A variety of specific nutrients can be poorly absorbed such as vitamin B_{12} in pernicious anemia, lactose in lactase insufficiency, certain amino acids in congenital states, or the more general malabsorption seen in small bowel diseases.

When considering malabsorptive states, it is most often lipid malabsorption (steatorrhea) that is meant, although concomitant protein malabsorption (creatorrhea) and carbohydrate malabsorption can also occur. The focus is on lipids because little lipid (2 g/d) is secreted into the stool on a lipid-free diet (1) so that excessive stool fat (> 6 g/d on a 100-g fat diet) can be easily demonstrated from a poorly absorbed dietary intake. The percentage of dietary fat that is absorbed each day holds true over a wide range of fat intakes. Up to 500 g/d of fat can be eaten with a 95% absorption rate (2). Protein malabsorption also occurs but the dietary component in the feces is difficult to identify because of the large amount of protein secreted into the bowel each day (3). Carbohydrate malabsorption is also difficult to quantitate because of colonic bacterial transformation of carbohydrates to short chain fatty acids. The short chain fatty acids are absorbed by the colonic mucosa, where they are used as the prime metabolic fuel of colonocytes.

Steatorrhea is inevitably accompanied by diarrhea, which is defined as a stool weight of more than 200 g/d. The cause of this is threefold (Table 1). Steatorrhea is accompanied by osmotically active particles from other malabsorbed parts of the diet, resulting in osmotically induced diarrhea as water enters the colon in response to the induced hyperosmolar load. Second, bacteria in the colon are capable of hydroxylating oleic acid, a common fatty acid in the diet, as well as other fatty acids. This produces 10-hydroxyoleate (4) from oleate, which has the same effect

TABLE 1. *Mechanisms by which steatorrhea causes diarrhea*

1. Excessive amounts of osmotically active particles from malabsorbed dietary constituents
2. Hydroxylation of oleate to 10-hydroxyoleate, which acts as a cathartic
3. Fatty acids themselves impair water and electrolyte absorption

on the bowel as the cathartic 12-hydroxyoleate, the active acyl group in tri-ricinoleic acid (castor oil). Third, fatty acids themselves inhibit fluid absorption by the colon (5).

This chapter does not cover all the malabsorptive states—only the common ones as they specifically apply to lipid malabsorption. In general, lipid malabsorption can be subdivided into that associated with impaired hydrolysis, reduced solubilization, mucosal diseases or resection, and lymphatic transport defects. One disease from each category will be examined in more detail.

IMPAIRED LIPOLYSIS

Pancreatic Insufficiency

Pancreatic insufficiency, seen in chronic pancreatitis, can cause the most severe steatorrhea found in the absence of intestinal resection. The reason for this is that triacylglycerol is not absorbed without being partially hydrolyzed. Before clinically evident malabsorption can occur, however, more than 90% of pancreatic function must be destroyed (6). Thus, steatorrhea is an insensitive indicator of pancreatic function. In the Western world, most of the cases of chronic pancreatitis are caused by chronic alcoholism. Other less common causes are pancreatic tumors or trauma, which impairs ductal drainage, or hypertriglyceridemia. In 20% of cases, no cause is known. Patients with cystic fibrosis are living longer and are now presenting to adult physicians for care. Gallstones can cause acute pancreatitis but they do not cause chronic pancreatitis.

Diagnosis

The diagnosis of chronic pancreatitis as the cause of steatorrhea is made easier if the patient is a known alcoholic and has had previous bouts of abdominal pain compatible with acute exacerbations of pancreatitis. The presence of diabetes also points to the pancreas. Often, other signs of chronic pancreatitis are seen such as a pseudocyst or calcification in the pancreas found on an x-ray film, ultrasound, or computed tomography (CT) scan of the abdomen. Instead of having high levels of lipase or amylase in the blood, as would be seen in acute pancreatitis, patients with chronic pancreatitis may have low levels of these enzymes or, better studied, reduced levels of serum trypsin(ogen) (7).

Testing for Chronic Pancreatitis

No sensitive tests exist to establish the diagnosis of chronic pancreatitis. The tests that are available can be divided into functional tests and observed anatomic abnormalities. The most sensitive *functional tests* are the secretin test and the Lundh test meal; these are only abnormal after 70% of the pancreas is destroyed. In the United States, secretin is no longer available from the manufacturer and, thus, the test meal remains the only viable option. The test requires intubation of the duodenum and special handling and testing of collected samples. It also requires a normally functioning intestinal mucosa. Tests of this complex nature are not practical in the general endoscopic laboratory and should be reserved for specialized centers. Other tests such as the bentiromide test, in which peptide-bound *p*-aminobenzoic acid is released in the intestine and secreted into the urine, and the pancreolauryl test, in which fluorescent dilaurate is ingested with a meal and fluorescein released in the intestinal lumen and secreted in the urine, are not available in the United States. The *anatomic observations* that can be made (Table 2) include an abnormal pancreatic duct on endoscopic retrograde cholangiopancreatography (ERCP), and ultrasound or CT showing a widened pancreatic duct, pancreatic calcification, or the presence of a pseudocyst. The sensitivity of ultrasound is 50% to 70% and of CT, 75% to 90%; both have a specificity of 80% or better. A scoring system (the Cambridge system) has been set up to standardize ultrasound and CT findings, which describe criteria for no, mild or moderate, and severe radiographic alterations associated with chronic pancreatitis. ERCP has a sensitivity of 75% to 95% and a specificity of more than 95%.

Two newer endoscopic/radiologic tools have been introduced in recent years, and these are still to be fully evaluated. Magnetic resonance cholangiopancreatography (MRCP) has proved useful in not only the primary diagnosis of pancreatic disease but also under postsurgical conditions where ERCP is not possible (8,9). Endoscopic ultrasonography (EUS) is being increasingly employed and, in the hands of skilled operators, it appears to be an accurate way of diagnosing pancreatic disease (10). When combined with fine needle aspiration, EUS should prove valuable in the diagnosis of pancreatic disorders, especially masses.

TABLE 2. *The diagnosis of chronic pancreatitis*

Diagnostic methods in chronic pancreatitis	Expected findings
1. Endoscopic retrograde pancreatography	Calcifications, dilated ducts, cyst*
2. Endoscopic ultrasound	Calcifications, dilated ducts, cyst*
3. Magnetic resonance cholangiopancreatography	Calcifications, dilated ducts, cyst*
4. Abdominal ultrasound	Calcifications, dilated ducts, cyst*
5. Computed tomography	Calcifications, dilated ducts, cyst*

* The cysts seen are really pseudocysts.

Steatorrhea in Chronic Pancreatitis

The steatorrhea affecting patients with pancreatic insufficiency is the most severe of all steatorrheas, with the exception of that in patients with large intestinal resections. As pancreatic exocrine dysfunction is not clinically obvious until at least 90% of the pancreas has been destroyed, small additional degrees of destruction can have major effects on function. At maximum, 70% of ingested fat can be excreted. That excretion is not greater than 70% is because of the activity of gastric lipase, which is secreted by the chief cells in the gastric pits in humans (11). This lipase, which is active in an acidic environment and which does not require colipase for its activity to be maintained in the presence of bile acids, preferentially hydrolyzes triacylglycerols at the sn-3 position (12). Further, because of the lack of pancreatic bicarbonate secretion, a more acidic environment is maintained in the duodenum (13), enabling the lipase to remain active further down the intestinal tract. In pancreatic steatorrhea, as might be expected, the fecal fat concentration in the stool is greater than in steatorrheas from other causes in patients with an intact intestinal tract (14).

Treatment

The treatment of patients with pancreatogenous steatorrhea is simple in concept but causes problems in practice. The concept is to replace the pancreatic enzymes with exogenous pancreatic extracts. The practical issues are that gastric acid irreversibly denatures a variable portion of the replaced enzymes, and proteolysis of the lipase occurs when the exogenous proteases are in a suitable milieu. This results in poor delivery of the administered enzymes to the duodenum. Only 8% of lipase given by mouth is still in active at the ligament of Treitz (15). As the percentage of active enzyme delivered to the ligament of Treitz is increased as the duodenal pH increases (16), patients resistant to replacement therapy may benefit from a reduction of gastric acid output by pharmacologic means.

REDUCED SOLUBILIZATION

Impaired Delivery of Bile Salts to the Intestine

The products of lipid hydrolysis are solubilized in the intestinal lumen by bile salts. An adequate supply of bile salts results in the most efficient rate of lipid absorption. In the absence of bile salts, most of the lipids are absorbed, but over a longer expanse of small bowel. This is especially true for the polyunsaturated fats which have more intrinsic water solubility. To maintain an adequate supply of bile salts, three events must occur. First, the liver must synthesize bile salts adequately; at steady state, the synthetic rate in the liver is the same as the rate at which bile salts are lost to the colon (~0.5 g/d). Second, the liver must be able to extract bile salts from the plasma, conjugate them with glycine or taurine if they have become unconjugated in the intestinal lumen, and secrete them into the intestine; bile salt secretion may become disordered in any liver disease in which bile excretory failure occurs. Third, the ileum must reabsorb the luminal bile salts presented to it in an efficient manner. This is accomplished primarily by the recently cloned Na^+-coupled bile salt transporter. In the case of surgical resection, ileal disease, or, rarely, congenital absence of the transporter (17), bile salts are lost to the colon where they can cause diarrhea with or without steatorrhea.

Physiology and Pathophysiology of Bile Salts and Their Absorption

Bile salts have the property of self-association to form micelles above a critical concentration called the "critical micellar concentration" (CMC). It is only bile salts in micellar form, not the intermicellar bile salts, that solubilize lipids. Thus, any reduction in bile salt concentration has a greater impact on the micellar concentration of bile salts, and on the amount of lipid that can be solubilized as a result, than might otherwise be anticipated. For example, the CMC for the mixed bile salts in bile is 1.4 mM (18) and an average postprandial concentration of bile salts in the intestinal lumen is 9 mM (19), leaving 7.6 mM in micellar form. If the bile salt concentration is reduced to 3 mM, this would leave only 1.6 mM available to solubilize the split lipids.

Bile salts are said to be in the enterohepatic space during their circulation from liver to bile duct to intestine and back to the liver in the portal vein. The system is conservative in that only 500 mg of bile salts are lost each day from a total pool of 3 g, which recirculates six times on average each day. If the system becomes dysfunctional because of impaired resorption of the bile salts by the ileum (Table 3), the liver is able to compensate by increased synthesis for a loss of up to 20% of the bile salt pool. Beyond this loss, the bile salt pool declines and stool fat increases (in the monkey) (20). In the human, the progressive loss of bile salts to the enterohepatic circulation results first in diarrhea without steatorrhea, as a result of the increased bile salts perfusing the colon, and second in steatorrhea along with diarrhea (21).

Another result of bile salt malabsorption is the compositional change that occurs in the bile salt pool. Before secretion, bile salts are conjugated with either glycine or taurine. Normally, the steroid nucleus is better conserved than the conjugates (22). In bile salt malabsorption, this is exaggerated because of the loss of bile salts to the colon, which puts a drain on the taurine pool. The result is a functional deficiency of taurine at the site of bile acid conjugation, which can be corrected by giving taurine orally. Thus, the ratio of glycine to taurine conjugates increases from its normal 3:1 to 15:1 ratio (23). Second, the perfusion of the colon with cholic

TABLE 3. *Effects of an impaired enterohepatic circulation of bile salts*

---

1. Diarrhea; or if severe, steatorrhea
2. An increased proportion of the bile salt pool conjugated with glycine *vs.* taurine
3. An increased proportion of the bile salt pool composed of deoxycholate
4. A reduced bile salt pool size

---

acid results in a dehydroxylation at the $12-$ position, producing deoxycholate which, after absorption, now forms a greater than normal part of the total bile salt pool (24).

Testing for Bile Salt Malabsorption

Testing for bile salt malabsorption can be done by the ^{75}Se-homotaurocholic acid test (SeHCAT). In this test, the SeHCAT, which is resistant to bacterial deconjugation, is given orally and whole body gamma scans are used to follow the disappearance of the tracer over time. Normally, 80% of the radiolabel is retained at 24 hours, 50% at 72 hours, and 19% at 7 days. In many patients with bile salt malabsorptive defects, even those without steatorrhea, most (95%) of the bile salt pool is lost to the colon after just one meal (25). Cholestyramine, an anion exchange resin that binds primarily dihydroxylated bile salts, may also be given as a test of bile salt malabsorption. However, if moderate to severe steatorrhea is present, the diarrhea usually continues despite treatment with the resin (26).

Treatment

Treatment of choloretic enteropathy is by cholestyramine. It is effective in the setting of no or mild steatorrhea (26). If diarrhea persists, it may be because of excessive fatty acids in the stool, not bile salts. In this case, the diarrhea is treated by lowering the amount of fat in the diet (26).

MUCOSAL DEFECTS

Celiac Disease

Clinical Features

Celiac disease, which is genetically based, affects both children and adults. If the problem appears in childhood, the disease abates during adolescence, only to recur later in life. The major issue faced by these patients is that created by malabsorption. Common symptoms include weight loss, fatigue, flatulence, and diarrhea associated with steatorrhea. Although these are the classic presenting complaints, an increasing number of patients now present with more subtle symptoms (e.g., osteopenia, folate deficiency, or iron deficient anemia not corrected by oral iron) in the absence of diarrhea. Even oral thyroid preparations can be inadequately absorbed so that large amounts are required to suppress thyroid gland function. These less overt symptoms reflect the fact that the disease is more severe proximally than distally in the intestine; thus, specific proximal intestinal functions can be affected, whereas lipid absorption may be adequate because the whole small bowel can be used for this purpose. Vitamin B_{12} deficiency occasionally occurs. Overt manifestations of the disease can be uncovered in previously asymptomatic individuals who have gastric surgery that results in enhanced gastric emptying.

TABLE 4. *Causes of steatorrhea in gluten-sensitive enteropathy*

1. The secretory state of the intestine causing a dilutive effect
2. The immaturity of the cells facing the lumen
3. A reduction of duodenal cholecystokinin able to be released in response to a meal
4. A reduced intestinal surface area

Pathophysiology

Much has been learned about why patients with celiac disease develop specific symptoms. Steatorrhea develops for four reasons (Table 4). The first involves the secretory state of the intestine. In celiac disease, the cells facing the intestinal lumen are immature because of their rapid turnover. This leads to a reduction in several of the functions expected of mature enterocytes. The first of these is that the intestine is in a secretory state, which probably reflects both an increase in the cryptal secretion of fluid and a decrease in the amount of fluid expected to be reabsorbed by the cells at the surface of the intestine (27). The increase in cryptal secretion occurs because the crypts are expanded both laterally and vertically in this disorder, so that mitotic figures appear near the intestinal lumen rather than being limited to the proximal third of the villus, as they are supposed to be. The excessive secretion of fluid dilutes the bile salts present in the intestinal lumen, reducing the concentration of bile salts that are in the aggregated or micellar form (28). This prevents the hydrolyzed products of lipid digestion from being adequately solubilized and, thus, reduces the rate at which these split lipids can be absorbed.

Second, the absorptive functions of the enterocytes are also impaired in celiac disease because of the immaturity of the cells that are at the top of the ''villi'' and, therefore, are presumably the most mature (29). Immature cells have a reduced ability to resynthesize both triacylglycerols and phospholipids (30). Both of these are important steps in the transport of lipids into the body.

A third problem is the reduction in either the number or function of the cells in the duodenum that secrete cholecystokinin (CCK). This can be shown directly by measuring CCK in biopsies of the duodenum (31) and functionally by showing much less bilirubin (a marker for gall bladder contraction) in the lumen of the intestine when essential amino acids are infused intraduodenally than in healthy individuals. If CCK is given intravenously, the gall bladder of patients with celiac disease contracts promptly (28). This shows that the problem is in signaling from the intestine for the gall bladder to contract, and not a problem in the gall bladder itself when it is appropriately stimulated.

Finally, the all too obvious reduction in villus height and the blunted nature of the microvilli in this disease severely reduce the surface area of the intestine over which nutrients can be absorbed. In addition to these abnormalities of intestinal function, the intestine of patients with celiac disease is clearly more permeable than is normal (32).

Diagnosis

The diagnosis of celiac disease has undergone a change in recent years, with the development of the endomysial antibody test (33) and, subsequently, an enzyme-linked immunosorbent assay for the presumed antigen recognized in the endomysial antibody test, tissue transglutaminase (34). In patients proved to have celiac disease, 98% have high titers of IgA against tissue transglutaminase, whereas 95% of control sera have normal titers. This improvement in diagnostic ability seems well founded in Europe, less so in the United States, for reasons that are unclear.

Pathogenesis

Even after many years of investigation, the root cause of celiac disease has not yet been defined. A major hurdle has been the lack of an animal model or cell line in which multiple samples can be tested. However, progress is being made. It was the work of Dicke that led to the original discovery of the harmful effects of wheat and certain other cereals (35). Later studies showed that an alcohol extract of wheat was harmful (36) and, to demonstrate this, the classic assay for measuring stool fat was developed (37).

Most investigators now believe that celiac disease is caused by an environmental event that triggers an immunologic response in a genetically predisposed host. The most common genetic background in celiac disease is that patients are DR3 or DR5/DR7 heterozygotes by serological testing and at the molecular biological level express $DQ(\alpha_1*0501,\beta_1*0201)$ (38). That an environmental event triggers clinical expression of the disease is suggested by twin studies in which only 70% of monozygotic twins have the disease (39). The immunologic response is suggested by many observations, but key among these is the prominence of intraepithelial lymphocytes, which are a hallmark of the morphologic picture of celiac disease. These cells are predominantly CD8 + T cells, which have a greatly increased expression of the γ/δ T-cell receptor compared with normal individuals (40).

Treatment

Treatment of celiac disease is by withdrawing all gluten from the diet. This requires careful reading of labels from prepared foods and knowledge of "hidden" sources of gluten. Support groups such as the Celiac Society are helpful sources of information. On a strict diet, the patient with celiac disease will improve clinically over several weeks, although the intestinal biopsy may lag well behind the improving clinical symptoms. If no improvement occurs with the institution of the diet, then the patient may have an additional cause of steatorrhea such as chronic pancreatitis or bacterial overgrowth. In this case, treatment of the other conditions as well as celiac disease will result in improvement. If still no improvement occurs, then the patient does not have celiac disease but a "refractory" form of sprue.

LYMPHATIC TRANSPORT DEFECTS

Abetalipoproteinemia

In abetalipoproteinemia, a syndrome caused by an autosomal recessive defect, chylomicrons cannot be formed and, thus, lipid transport into the lymph is blocked. Similarly, the liver cannot produce very low density lipoprotein (VLDL) and little is found in the blood. This results in very small amounts of plasma apolipoprotein B (apoB), which is associated with the triacylglycerol-rich lipoproteins and, thus, a reduced concentration of plasma triacylglycerol and cholesterol. Although the disease's name implies that apoB is not expressed in the liver or intestine, it is actually normally transcribed and the apoB gene is normal (41). The defect resides in the synthesis of the newly described protein, the microsomal triglyceride transport protein (MTP) (42), because of different mutations in the MTP gene (43). The lack of MTP results in the inability of the intestine and liver to form triacylglycerol-rich lipoproteins because MTP is required at an early stage of VLDL—and by extension chylomicron—formation, that is before the addition of lipids (44). Nevertheless, it is evident from transgenic mouse work that the intestine must express apoB in order for chylomicrons to be mature enough to be transported from the endoplasmic reticulum to the Golgi apparatus (45). These mice, which express no apoB in their intestines, have an increased number of chylomicrons in the endoplasmic reticulum but few in the Golgi apparatus.

Abetalipoproteinemia is a rare homozygous defect in which the principal clinical manifestations are related to the impaired absorption of fat soluble vitamins. This is especially true for vitamin E. In addition to modest steatorrhea, the patients may have acanthocytosis, a neurologic disorder similar to Friedreich's ataxia, and an atypical type of retinitis pigmentosa (46). Characteristically, the patients will have lipid-laden enterocytes on a fasting intestinal biopsy specimen (47), indicating the inability to transport triacylglycerol out of the absorptive cells. It is of particular interest that these patients do not develop severe steatorrhea, despite their inability to achieve postprandial chylomicronemia (46). Although the cause of this is speculative, evidence in the rat indicates that considerably more absorbed lipid than was previously thought is transported from the intestine in the portal vein rather than in the lymphatics (48) in cases of a large lipid load. The proportion of lipid transported in portal venous blood is reduced when the lipid load is decreased (49).

REFERENCES

1. Lewis GT, Partin HC. Fecal fat on an essentially fat free diet. *J Lab Clin Med* 1954; 44: 91–3.
2. Kasper H. Fecal fat excretion, diarrhea and subjective complaints with highly dosed oral fat intake. *Digestion* 1970; 3: 321–2.
3. Nasset ES, Ju JS. Mixture of endogenous and exogenous protein in the alimentary tract. *Nutrition* 1961; 74: 461–5.
4. Kim YS, Spritz N. Hydroxy acid excretion in steatorrhea of pancreatic and non-pancreatic origin. *N Engl J Med* 1968; 279: 1424–6.
5. Ammon HV, Phillips SF. Inhibition of colonic water and electrolyte absorption by fatty acids in man. *Gastroenterology* 1973; 65: 744–9.

6. DiMagno EP, Go VLW, Summerskill WHJ. Relations between pancreatic enzyme outputs and malabsorption in severe pancreatic insufficiency. *N Engl J Med* 1973; 288: 813–15.

7. Felder M, Vantini I, Petrillo M, *et al.* Circulating trypsin-like immunoreactivity in chronic pancreatitis. *Dig Dis Sci* 1981; 26: 532–7.

8. Adler A, Velzke W, Abou-Rebyeh H, Hammerstingl R, Vogl T, Felix R. Clinical significance of magnetic resonance cholangiopancreatography (MRCP) compared to endoscopic retrograde cholangiopancreatography (ERCP). *Endoscopy* 1997; 29: 182–7.

9. Yamaguchi K, Chijiwa K, Shimizu S, Yokohata K, Morisaki T, Tanaka M. Comparison of endoscopic retrograde and magnetic resonance cholangiopancreatography in the surgical diagnosis of pancreatic diseases. *Am J Surg* 1998; 175: 203–8.

10. Zimmerman M, Aabakken L, Tamasky PR, *et al.* Prospective assessment of the ability of endoscopic ultrasound to diagnose, exclude, or establish the severity of chronic pancreatitis found by endoscopic retrograde cholangiopancreatography. *Gastrointest Endosc* 1998; 48: 18–25.

11. Moreau H, Bernadac A, Gargouri Y, Benkouka F, Laugier R, Verger R. Immunocytolocalization of human gastric lipase in chief cells of the fundic mucosa. *Histochemistry* 1989; 91: 419–23.

12. Carriére F, Rogalska E, Cudrey C, Ferrato F, Laugier R, Verger R. *In vivo* and *in vitro* studies on the stereoselective hydrolysis of tri- and diglycerides by gastric and pancreatic lipases. *Bioorg Med Chem* 1997; 429: 429–35.

13. Nakamura T, Arai Y, Tando Y, *et al.* Effect of omeprazole on changes in gastric and upper small intestine pH levels in patients with chronic pancreatitis. *Clin Ther* 1995; 17: 448–59.

14. Bo-Linn GW, Fordtran JS. Fecal fat concentration in patients with steatorrhea. *Gastroenterology* 1984; 87: 319–22.

15. DiMagno ER, Malagelada JR, Go VLW, Moertel CG. Fate of orally ingested enzymes in pancreatic insufficiency. *N Engl J Med* 1977; 1977: 1318–22.

16. Graham DY. Enzyme replacement therapy of exocrine pancreatic insufficiency in man. *N Engl J Med* 1977; 296: 1314–17.

17. Oelkers P, Kirby LC, Heubi JE, Dawson PA. Primary bile acid malabsorption caused by mutations in the ileal sodium-dependent bile acid transporter gene (SLC10A2). *J Clin Invest* 1997; 99: 1880–7.

18. Hofmann AF. The function of bile salts in fat absorption. *Biochem J* 1963; 89: 57–68.

19. Mansbach CM, Cohen RS, Leff PB. Isolation and properties of the mixed micelles present in intestinal content during fat digestion in man. *J Clin Invest* 1975; 56: 781–91.

20. Dowling RH, Mack E, Small DM. Effects of controlled interruption of the enteroheptic circulation of bile salts by biliary diversion and by ileal reaction on bile salt secretion, synthesis, and pool size in the Rhesus monkey. *J Clin Invest* 1970; 49: 232–42.

21. Mansbach CM, Garbutt JT, Tyor MP. Bile salt and lipid metabolism in patients with ileal disease with and without steatorrhea. *Am J Dig Dis* 1972; 17: 1089–99.

22. Hepner GW, Hofmann AF, Thomas PJ. Metabolism of steroid and amino acid moieties of conjugated bile acids in man. *J Clin Invest* 1972; 51: 1889–97.

23. Garbutt JT, Lack L, Tyor MP. Physiological basis of alterations in the relative conjugation of bile acids with glycine and taurine. *Am J Clin Nutr* 1971; 24: 218–28.

24. Garbutt JT, Wilkins RM, Lack L, Tyor MP. Bacterial modification of taurocholate during enterohepatic recirculation in normal man and patients with small intestinal disease. *Gastroenterology* 1970; 59: 553–66.

25. Low-Beer TS, Wilkins RM, Lack L, Tyor MP. Effect of one meal on enterohepatic circulation of bile salts. *Gastroenterology* 1974; 67: 490–7.

26. Hofmann AF, Poley JR. Role of bile acid malabsorption in pathogenesis of diarrhea and steatorrhea in patients with ileal resection I. *Gastroenterology* 1972; 62: 918–34.

27. Fordtran JS, Rector FC, Locklear TW, Ewton MF. Water and solute movement in the small intestine of patients with sprue. *J Clin Invest* 1967; 46: 287–98.

28. DiMagno EJ, Go VLW, Summerskill WHJ. Impaired cholecystokinin-pancreozymin secretion, intraluminal digestion and maldigestion of fat in sprue. *Gastroenterology* 1972; 63: 25–32.

29. Beck IT, Dinda PK, DaCosta LR, Beck M. Sugar absorption by small bowel biopsy samples from patients with primary lactase deficiency and with adult celiac disease. *Am J Dig Dis* 1976; 21: 946–52.

30. Mansbach CM. Complex lipid synthesis in hamster intestine. *Biochim Biophys Acta* 1973; 296: 386–400.

31. Calam J, Ellis A, Dockray GJ. Identification and measurement of molecular variants of cholecystokinin in duodenal mucosa and plasma. Diminished concentrations in patients with celiac disease. *J Clin Invest* 1982; 69: 218–25.

32. Hamilton I, Cobden I, Rothwell J, Axon ATR. Intestinal permeability in coeliac disease: the response to gluten withdrawal and single-dose gluten challenge. *Gut* 1982; 23: 202–10.

33. Walker-Smith JA, Guandalini S, Schmitz J, Shmerling DH, Visakorpi JK. Revised criteria for diagnosis of coeliac disease. *Arch Dis Child* 1990; 65: 909–11.

34. Dietrich W, Laag E, Schopper H, *et al.* Autoantibodies to tissue transglutaminase as predictors of celiac disease. *Gastroenterology* 1998; 115: 1317–21.

35. Dicke WK. *Coeliac disease: investigation of the harmful effects of certain types of cereal on patients with coeliac disease* [Thesis, in Dutch]. Utrecht: University of Utrecht, 1950.

36. Van de Kamer JH, Weyers HA, Dicke KW. Coeliac Disease IV. An investigation into the injurious constituents of wheat in connection with their action on patients with coeliac disease. *Acta Paediatr* 1953; 42: 223–31.

37. Van de Kamer JH, ten Bokkel Huinink H, Weyers HA. Rapid method for the determination of fat in feces. *J Biol Chem* 1949; 177: 347–51.

38. Sollid LM, Thorsby E. HLA susceptibility genes in celiac disease: genetic mapping and role in pathogenesis. *Gastroenterology* 1993; 105: 910–22.

39. Gluten sensitive enteropathy in Spain: genetic and environmental factors. In: McConnell RB, ed. *The genetics of celiac disease*. Lancaster: MTB Press, 1981: 211–31.

40. Halstensen TS, Scott S, Brandtzaeg P. Intraepithelial T cells of the TcRdγ/δ + CD8–phenotypes are increased in coeliac disease. *Scand J Immunol* 1989; 30: 665–72.

41. Talmud PJ. Genetic evidence from two families that the apolipoprotein B gene is not involved in abetalipoproteinemia. *J Clin Invest* 1988; 82: 1803–6.

42. Wetterau J, Aggerbeck LP, Bouma M-E, *et al.* Absence of microsomal triglyceride transfer protein in individuals with abetalipoproteinemia. *Science* 1992; 258: 999–1001.

43. Sharp D, Blinderman L, Combs KA, *et al.* Microsomal triglyceride transfer protein: part II. *Nature* 1993; 365: 65–9.

44. Rustaeus S, Stillenmanrk P, Lindberg K, Gordon D, Olofsson S-O. The microsomal triglyceride transport protein catalyzes the post-translational assembly of apolipoprotein B-100 very low density lipoprotein in McA-RH7777 cells. *J Biol Chem* 1998; 273: 5196–203.

45. Hamilton RL, Wong JS, Cham CM, Nielsen LB, Young SG. Chylomicron-sized lipid particles are formed in the setting of apolipoprotein B deficiency. *J Lipid Res* 1998; 39: 1543–57.

46. Isselbacher KJ, Scheig R, Plotkin GR, Caufield JB. Congenital β-lipoprotein deficiency: an hereditary disorder involving a defect in the absorption and transport of lipids. *Medicine* 1964; 43: 347–61.

47. Dobbins WO. An ultrastructural study of the intestinal mucosa in congenital β-lipoprotein deficiency with particular emphasis upon the intestinal absorptive cell. *Gastroenterology* 1966; 50: 195–210.

48. Mansbach CM, Dowell RF, Pritchett D. Portal transport of absorbed lipids in the rat. *Am J Physiol* 1991; 261: G530–8.

49. Mansbach CM, Dowell RF. Portal transport of long acyl chain lipids: effect of phosphatidylcholine and low infusion rates. *Am J Physiol* 1993; 264: G1082–9.

DISCUSSION

Dr. Ghoos: It is very useful to give enzyme replacement therapy in cases of severe exocrine pancreatic insufficiency. The preparations used to contain bile salts but recently they have been withdrawn. What is the reason for that?

Dr. Mansbach: I did not know that bile salts were given. There was a compound called ''Carter's Little Liver Pills,'' which contained bile salts. These were ox bile salts, and they were used as a cathartic. They were withdrawn because it was found that human bile salts were altered by these ox bile salts. Perhaps that induced the notion that they were bad. I do not believe bile salts were ever included, because it would have required a very large pill and because patients with chronic pancreatitis secrete bile salts normally.

Dr. Ghoos: We found that a supplement of bile salts did increase the uptake of lipids in pancreatitis.

Dr. Mansbach: In theory, they should not. The reason is, that for bile salts to be effective, lipolysis needs to be occurring, and the amounts of diacylglycerols or triacylglycerols that are solubilized by bile acid micelles is very low, so I do not think that would be a particularly good mechanism. If supplementary bile salts are given, the trihydroxylated form is much less destructive to the tissues (e.g., gastric or small intestinal mucosa) than the dihydroxylated form.

Dr. Lentze: Just a comment. You mentioned magnetic resonance cholangiopancreatography as a new tool for imaging bile ducts and pancreatic ducts. In the pediatric age range, the technique is limited by the smallness of the structures. In small children, below 10 years of age, this method does not work as well as in adults, because the ducts are so small and so little fluid is flowing. We use the technique for children above 10 years of age with success.

Dr. Yamashiro: In Japan, this technique is well established and works well even in children below 3 years of age. Two papers on this were published recently (1,2).

Dr. Milla: As with Dr. Yamashiro, we find MRCP helpful in children. My question is about chronic pancreatitis in children. Contrary to what you said, chronic pancreatitis does occur in childhood and usually it is not genetic or inherited, and not alcoholic as far as one knows! Do you have any insight into what the etiologic factors might be? Some have invoked autoimmune disease, others loss of antioxidative defenses.

Dr. Mansbach: My notion of chronic pancreatitis in children stops with cystic fibrosis. Is this a real problem in children?

Dr. Milla: If you are unfortunate enough to have to look after them, yes.

Dr. Mansbach: One of the main problems with chronic pancreatitis is giving lipase in a form that is clinically effective. It is very difficult to do this with the materials currently available, at least in adults. I would call your attention to the work of DiMagno (3) in trying to get a bacterial lipase on to the market. This really is very efficacious, but the company that is working with him to bring it onto the market so far has not done so.

Dr. Alpers: A comment on chronic pancreatitis. It has now been shown that some patients who have mutations of the cystic fibrosis gene have chronic pancreatitis as adults (4). The hypothesis is that many cases of idiopathic pancreatitis in adults might be incomplete forms of cystic fibrosis. This possibly could be an explanation for children as well.

Dr. Milla: I think it is becoming increasingly understood that in cystic fibrosis some of the less typical mutations of CFTR will result in isolated conditions such as chronic pancreatitis or male infertility because of an abnormality of the vas deferens, rather than the more classic presentation that one associates with mutations such as Δf508.

Dr. Goulet: You mentioned that bacterial overgrowth impairs fat digestion and absorption. How does it do this?

Dr. Mansbach: More than one reason is found for the effect of bacteria on fat absorption. One is that the bile acids deconjugate. If the bile salt is conjugated, for instance, to taurine, the pKa is 1.8, and to glycine, about 4.5. Now, if they are deconjugated, the pKa then goes up to about 6.5. In the normal milieu of the upper intestine most of the bile salts will be proteinated and inactive at this pKa, unable to micellize, and unable to support the solubilization of split lipids. Another thing that happens is that the bile salts become dehydroxylated. In that case, they become toxic to the mucosa, because they are now dihydroxylated rather than trihydroxylated. The third thing is that bacterial glycosylases strip off the surface of the absorptive cells. This allows passive entry of the now protonated bile salts and causes cell damage. This can be seen electron microscopically by the dilated endoplasmic reticulum in these cells.

Dr. Spolidoro: We have seen a couple cases of intestinal lymphangiectasia in the complete form with protein-losing enteropathy. Sometimes, however, when endoscopy is done in children for other reasons, we find a similar appearance in the second part of the duodenum, with white points resembling ectasia of lymphatics. Some of these patients have no symptoms at all and are undergoing endoscopy for other reasons entirely. In reviewing these patients afterward, we find some have steatorrhea, although this is not clinically evident, whereas others have abdominal pain, which may improve when we put them on a low fat diet. What do you think causes this ectasia of the lymphatics in the second part of the duodenum? The appearances certainly are not those of classic intestinal lymphangiectasia.

Dr. Mansbach: I have not seen this appearance myself so I do not feel able to comment further. However, we did some studies years ago in which we showed that more than 80% of the lipid is absorbed by 30 or 40 cm down into the jejunum, so it is a very rapid process that takes place mostly in the upper bowel. Thus, any defect in lymphatic drainage will perhaps be most obvious in the proximal bowel.

Dr. Castro: You mentioned that, in the absence of bile salts, 60% of the fats could still be absorbed. By what pathway or mechanism are they absorbed?

Dr. Mansbach: There is a finite solubility of fatty acids in water, and the more unsaturated the lipids, the more they are solubilized in water—that is one mechanism. Another mechanism is the formation of liquid crystals as a product of lipid hydrolysis, and these become very finely dispersed in water. These may be absorbed or provide the intestine with fatty acids and monoacylglycerides. Although these mechanisms are not as efficient as those present under normal conditions, the intestine is very long if no intestinal resection has been done and, therefore, a reasonable amount of absorption can occur.

Dr. Lévy: Many years ago, Roy and I tried hard to find apoB in patients with abetalipoproteinemia but we could not detect it in intestinal biopsies. Do you think that in this situation, apoB is degraded and we are then unable to diagnose patients with abetalipoproteinemia?

Dr. Mansbach: A constitutive expression of apoB is seen, and this apoB, if not properly lipidated, is destroyed intracellularly. That may have been happening in your cases. However, as described, these patients have a normal apoB gene and it translates normally, so I do not really have an explanation for your inability to identify apoB in the biopsies of those patients.

Dr. Parsons: Have you seen polymorphisms related to fatty acid binding protein or lipase? I ask this because some cases are seen wherein fat absorption is normal, but takes place more rapidly than normal. Where are we in the process of understanding fat absorption that is more rapid rather than less than normal?

Dr. Mansbach: Some fatty acid binding protein isoforms exist, but these are not relevant to fat absorption, only to insulin sensitivity.

Dr. Parsons: I was particularly interested in apoB isoforms. This is of interest to cardiologists as some individuals seem able to assimilate chylomicrons at a much faster rate than others.

Dr. Mansbach: ApoE isoforms are really related to cholesterol absorption rather than to lipid absorption or neutral lipid absorption. Wide variation is seen in how people react to a load of fat, which is reflected in considerable variation in postprandial triglyceride levels. It is interesting that the triglyceride levels in the plasma are never really all that high. The reason for this is that the chylomicron turnover rate is so great that it keeps the plasma triglyceride levels low.

Dr. Spolidoro: The van de Kamer technique is very difficult to do in clinical practice. What method do you recommend for diagnosing steatorrhea in a patient?

Dr. Mansbach: Well, one effective way is to look at the lipid content in oil droplets in the stool under the microscope, with oil red O stain. That is a technique originally described in the early 1960s (5). It is a very good technique once sufficient experience has been acquired. The stool is heated with acetic acid so that the fatty acid becomes protonated and, therefore, able to accept the oil red O stain. Then, the size and number of oil red O positive droplets are examined.

REFERENCES

1. Shimizu T, Suzuki R, Yamashiro Y, *et al.* Progressive dilatation of the main pancreatic duct using magnetic resonance cholangiopancreatography in a boy with chronic pancreatitis. *J Pediatr Gastroenterol Nutr* 2000;30:102–4.
2. Shimizu T, Suzuki R, Yamashiro Y, *et al.* Magnetic resonance cholangiopancreaticography in assessing the cause of acute pancreatitis in children. *Pancreas* (in press).
3. Suzuki A, Mizumoto A, Sarr MG, *et al.* Bacterial lipase and high-fat diets in canine exocrine pancreatic insufficiency: a new therapy of steatorrhea? 1997; 112: 2048–55.
4. Bornstein JD, Cohes JA. Cystic fibrosis in the pancreas: recent advances provide new insights. *Curr Gastroenterol Rep* 1999; 1: 161–65.
5. Drummey GD, Benson JA, Jones CM. Microscopical examination of the stool for steatorrhea. *N Engl J Med* 1961; 264: 85–7.

Gastrointestinal Functions, edited by Edgard E. Delvin and
Michael J. Lentze. Nestlé Nutrition Workshop Series, Pediatric
Program, Vol. 46, Nestec Ltd., Vevey/Lippincott Williams &
Wilkins, Philadelphia © 2001.

Structure, Function, and Regulation of Intestinal Lactase–Phlorizin Hydrolase and Sucrase-Isomaltase in Health and Disease

Hassan Y. Naim

*Department of Physiological Chemistry, School of Veterinary Medicine Hannover,
Hannover, Germany*

Carbohydrates are essential constituents of the mammalian diet. They occur as oligosaccharides, such as starch and cellulose (plant origin), as glycogen (animal origin), and as free disaccharides such as sucrose (plant) and lactose (animal). These carbohydrates are hydrolyzed in the intestinal lumen by specific enzymes to monosaccharides before transport across the brush border membrane of epithelial cells into the cell interior. The specificity of the enzymes is determined by the chemical structure of the carbohydrates. The monosaccharide components of most of the known carbohydrates are linked to each other in an α orientation. Examples of this type are starch, glycogen, sucrose, and maltose. β-Glycosidic linkages are minor. Nevertheless, this type of covalent bond is present in one of the major and most essential carbohydrates in mammalian milk, lactose, which constitutes the primary diet source for the newborn.

The enzymes implicated in the digestion of carbohydrates in the intestinal lumen are membrane-bound glycoproteins that are expressed at the apical or microvillus membrane of the enterocytes (1–3). In this chapter, the structural and biosynthetic features of the most important disaccharidases, sucrase-isomaltase and lactase–phlorizin hydrolase, and the molecular basis of sugar malabsorption (i.e., enzyme deficiencies) are discussed.

STRUCTURE, BIOSYNTHESIS, AND POLARIZED SORTING OF INTESTINAL DISACCHARIDASES

Lactase–Phlorizin Hydrolase

Lactase–phlorizin hydrolase (LPH) (EC 3.2.1.23/62) is an integral membrane glycoprotein of the intestinal brush border membrane. The same polypeptide chain contains two major hydrolytic activities (4): (a) lactase activity, which is responsible for the hydrolysis of the milk sugar lactose, the main carbohydrate in mammalian milk; and (b) phlorizin hydrolase, which digests β-glycosylceramides, which are part of the diet of most vertebrates. Drastic reduction in lactase activity is associated with diarrhea and accompanying symptoms on drinking milk in both newborns and adults; a physiologic role of phlorizin hydrolase activity is still unknown (4).

Structural Features

The LPH protein is encoded by a completmentary DNA (cDNA) that consists of 6,274 base pairs (bp) and corresponds to 17 exons of the LPH gene, which is located on chromosome 2 (5,6). The amino acid sequence deduced from the LPH cDNA consists of 1,927 amino acids. LPH is a type I integral membrane glycoprotein with an NH_2-terminal extracellular domain followed by a transmembrane domain composed of 19 hydrophobic amino acids and a COOH-terminal cytoplasmic domain of 26 amino acids (5). Fig. 1 is a schematic representation of the structure and biosynthesis of LPH.

The extracellular domain itself consists of an NH_2-terminal cleavable signal peptide (19 amino acids) necessary for translocation into the endoplasmic reticulum (11). The LPH molecule is highly glycosylated. The primary sequence of the human enzyme contains 15 potential N-glycosylation sites (the rabbit and rat enzymes possess 14 and 15, respectively). All cloned LPH species have shown that the molecule consists of four highly conserved structural and functional regions. These domains, denoted I-IV, have co-identity of 38% to 55%. The catalytic activity of lactase is localized to glutamine 1273 in the homologous region III, and of phlorizin hydrolase to glutamine 1749 in the homologous region IV (12). Because of the four homologous regions, LPH may have arisen from two subsequent duplications of one ancestral gene (5). An evolutionary and developmental example that lends support to this notion is given by the sequence similarities of LPH and each of its homologous regions with β-glycosidases from archaebacteria, eubacteria, and fungi. These similarities suggest that LPH is a member of a superfamily of β-glucosidases and β-galactosidases. The procaryotic β-glycosidases, on the average, are approximately 50 kd in size, which corresponds to approximately one quarter of the size of full-length LPH or roughly to the size of one homologous region (I-IV).

Biosynthesis

The mode of biosynthesis and processing of LPH is very similar in the species so far investigated (1,13,14). In what follows, an account of the biosynthesis and processing of the human enzyme is provided (Fig. 1). In small intestinal epithelial cells, LPH is synthesized as a single chain, 215-kd pro-LPH precursor that undergoes core mannose-rich N-glycosylation while translocating into the endoplasmic reticulum. In the endoplasmic reticulum, pro-LPH monomers form homodimers before processing in the Golgi apparatus (15). The homodimerization event constitutes an absolute requirement for a transport-competent configuration of pro-LPH that enables it to leave the endoplasmic reticulum. The transmembrane domain is directly

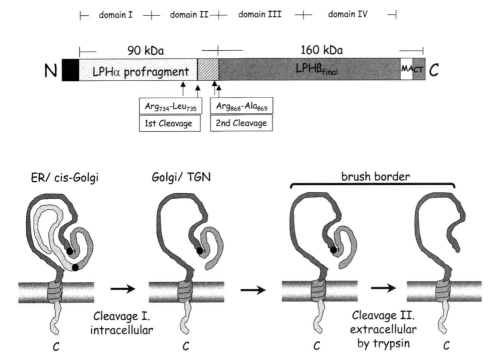

FIG. 1. Schematic representation of the structure and biosynthesis of pro-lactase-phlorizin hydrolase (pro-LPH) in human small intestinal cells. Some important structural features of pro-LPH in human small intestinal cells compiled from data which employed biosynthetic studies in human small intestinal explants (1,3,6), cDNA cloning (5), and recombinant expression in COS-1 (7–9) or Madin-Darby canine kidney (MDCK) cells (10). The *N*-terminus starts with a cleavable signal sequence (SS) (Met_1-Gly_{19}) for cotranslational translocation into the endoplasmic reticulum (ER). The ectodomain (Ser_{20} to Thr_{1882}) can be divided into four homologous domains as indicated. The membrane-anchoring domain (MA) extends from Ala_{1883} to Leu_{1902} and the cytosolic tail (CT) from Ser_{1903} to Phe_{1927}. Two proteolytic cleavage steps of pro-LPH take place: one intracellularly between Arg_{734} and Leu_{735} that generates $LPH\beta_{initial}$, which is sorted to the brush border membrane. The second cleavage step between Arg_{868} and Ala_{869} takes place in the intestinal lumen by pancreatic trypsin and generates the brush border mature enzyme, $LPH\beta_{final}$ (8,9). LPH-α is the profragment that plays a role as an intramolecular chaperone in the folding of pro-LPH.

implicated in the dimerization process. Elimination of this region results in a correctly folded pro-LPH monomer which, however, does not dimerize and is blocked in the endoplasmic reticulum and ultimately degraded.

Dimerization is not only important for efficient transport from the endoplasmic reticulum, it is crucial for the acquisition of enzymatic activity (15). Here again, correct folding of monomeric pro-LPH is not sufficient for a functional protein. During the pathway through the Golgi apparatus en route to the cell surface, the mannose-rich *N*-linked sugar chains are processed by mannosidases of the *cis*-Golgi and several types of sugars are added, resulting in a complex glycosylated protein of an approximate apparent molecular weight of 230 kd (3,7). Of particular importance, is O-glycosylation at the Ser or Thr residues in the LPH molecule. This event, which begins in the *cis*-Golgi apparatus and ends in the *trans*-Golgi network, leads to an increase in the enzymatic activity of LPH by a factor of 4 (6).

Complex glycosylated mature pro-LPH undergoes two proteolytic cleavage steps (8,9). In the first, the large profragment LPH-α is intracellularly eliminated at Arg_{734}/Leu_{735}, leaving the membrane-bound LPH-$\beta_{initial}$, which extends from Leu_{735} to Tyr_{1927}. This form is transported to the apical membrane where it is cleaved by pancreatic trypsin at Arg_{868}/Ala_{869} to LPH-β_{final} (Ala_{869}–Tyr_{1927}), which is known as mature brush border LPH of 160 kd (1,13,14). This form comprises the functional domains of the enzyme. The possible role played by the intracellular proteolytic cleavage and the large profragment LPH-α in the acquisition of transport competence and enzymatic activity has been investigated by recombinant expression of pro-LPH in heterologous cell systems. Expression of pro-LPH in the Madin-Darby canine kidney cell line (MDCK) has localized the initial cleavage step (pro-LPH to LPH-$\beta_{initial}$) to an intracellular compartment at or immediately after the *trans*-Golgi network (10). In another mammalian cell line—the simian virus–transformed COS cells—cleavage does not take place, thus providing a convenient model to address the important question of the role of cleavage in trafficking and in the function of pro-LPH. Recombinant pro-LPH in COS-1 cells is efficiently transported to the cell surface and shows enzymatic activity similar to that of the intestinal mature brush border LPH (7). Consequently, the intracellular proteolytic processing of pro-LPH in intestinal epithelial cells is not essential for the acquisition of transport competence and biological function.

Although the mature brush border form of LPH, the LPH-β_{final} species, has been extensively studied, the fate of the large profragment, which was later named "LPH-α," was obscure. In pulse chase experiments of intestinal biopsy samples and immunoprecipitation with an antibody directed against a 12 amino acid peptide immediately downstream, the signal sequence of pro-LPH, a 100-kd polypeptide, was isolated, which appears concomitantly with the appearance of LPH-β (16). Interestingly, this polypeptide is neither N-glycosylated, despite the presence of five potential N-glycosylation sites, nor O-glycosylated. The high content of hydrophobic amino acids in LPH-α and the tendency of this domain to form a compact, rigid, and trypsin-resistant structure immediately after translation, in which the N- and O-glycosylation sites may be embedded, explain the inaccessibility of the N sites to glycosyltransferases. Such structural features endow LPH-α with the characteristics of an intramolecular chaperone directly involved in the folding of the LPH-β domain. Individual expression of a cDNA encoding the LPH-β generated a protein that was not as transport competent as pro-LPH. Despite the presence of the active site in the LPH-β domain, the enzymatic activity was below detection limits in the absence of the LPH-α domain. Furthermore, trypsin sensitivity assays showed that individual LPH-β alone is readily degraded by the protease, pointing to its malfolded structure. It is clear, therefore, that LPH-α is required in the context of the correct folding of pro-LPH. Finally, despite the structural homologies between regions I, II contained in LPH-α, III, and IV, encompassing LPH-β and containing the enzymatic centers lactase and phlorizin hydrolase, no activity could be detected in LPH-α (16).

Polarized Sorting of Pro-LPH

To achieve its physiologic function, pro-LPH or its membrane-bound form must be transported to the luminal surface of epithelial cells (i.e., to the brush border membrane). The process of polarized sorting of proteins in epithelial cells is mediated by specific sorting signals in the protein and signal interacting cellular components. The sorting of proteins to the basolateral membrane has been intensively investigated. In most of the cases a tyrosine-based cryptic signal in the cytoplasmic tail of a protein mediates its targeting to the basolateral membrane (17). Usually, these signals have a dual function both as sorting and as endocytic signals, and it is thought that basolateral sorting uses a mechanism similar to that of endocytosis through clathrin-coated pits.

The sorting to the apical membrane of proteins such as LPH is not unique, and at present three types of signals for sorting proteins to the apical surface of epithelial cells or to the axon of neurons are known. Glycolipid (glycophosphatidyl inositol, GPI) anchors direct proteins to the apical surface of several types of epithelial cell (18), apparently by associating in the *trans*-Golgi network with detergent-insoluble membrane domains enriched in glycosphingolipids and cholesterol (19). Oligosaccharides on some secreted proteins appear to specify apical transport (20), although this mechanism does not apply to all secreted proteins (21). Neither of these sorting signals applies to LPH. LPH is not associated with microdomains, and processing of *N*- or *O*-linked glycans remains without effect on the sorting pattern of LPH (22–24). Neither the cleavage process nor the large profragment LPH-α that is generated on proteolytic cleavage of pro-LPH is implicated in the sorting event of LPH to the apical membrane (10). Recent observations have strongly suggested that putative sorting signals of pro-LPH are exclusively located in the domain corresponding to the brush border–associated LPH-β. The importance of the ectodomain in the intracellular transport and polarized sorting of LPH has been analyzed in deletion mutants of homologous region IV contiguous to the transmembrane domain (25). We could show that a region with features of a "stalk region" similar to that found in intestinal sucrase-isomaltase and aminopeptidase *N* is neither obligatory for intracellular transport of membrane-bound LPH nor for its polarized sorting to the apical membrane. In these studies, we were able to narrow down the region containing the sorting signals of pro-LPH. In fact, deletion of 236 amino acids containing more than one third of phlorizin-hydrolase domain (homologous region IV), including the catalytic domain, has almost no influence on LPH dimerization and transport to the plasma membrane. Although further deletion of 87 amino acids upstream in the phlorizin-hydrolase domain affected the dimerization and intracellular transport of the protein, it caused no gross structural alterations to the tertiary protein structure.

Sucrase-Isomaltase

The sucrase-isomaltase (SI) enzyme complex (SI; EC 3.2.1.48-10) is the most abundant glycoprotein in the intestinal brush border membrane. SI is an integral membrane protein that is composed of two subunits, sucrase and isomaltase (26). The isomaltase subunit is larger than sucrase ($\sim$145 kd vs. $\sim$ 130 kd), primarily because of increased O-glycosylation (2,27). Both subunits digest the most abundant class of carbohydrates in the mammalian diet, which has an α configuration. By virtue of its hydrolytic specificity, SI belongs to a super family of α-glucosidases that are found in higher organisms. Members of this family are, for example, mammalian lysosomal α-glucosidase, yeast invertase, and glucoamylase (28). Sucrase digests primarily 1,2-α- and 1,4-α-glucopyranosidic bonds. It is responsible for the terminal digestion of dietary sucrose and starch. Isomaltase, which also has maltase activity, hydrolyzes mainly α-1,6 linkages. Another brush border enzyme with similar digestive properties to isomaltase, maltase glucoamylase, contributes to the overall digestion of α-glycosidic linkages of carbohydrates. Maltase glucoamylase compensates the lack of SI in some cases of congenital sucrase-isomaltase deficiency (CSID) (see later).

Structural Features

Sucrase-isomaltase is a type II membrane glycoprotein—that is, the membrane-anchoring domain has a dual function as a provider of the signal sequence necessary for translocation of the newly synthesized protein to the endoplasmic reticulum and to retain the protein in the membrane (27). Fig. 2 shows a schematic presentation of the structure and biosynthesis of SI.

In addition to the membrane-anchoring domain, SI contains three autonomous major domains. The cytoplasmic tail contains 12 amino acid residues and may be phosphorylated *in vivo* through a conserved Ser residue (Ser_6). This raises the possibility that phosphorylation of the cytoplasmic domain may be implicated in post-translational regulatory processes. The 20 amino acid membrane anchor region is immediately followed by a Ser/Thr-rich domain, also called the "stalk region," which is considered to be part of the isomaltase subunit and is heavily O-glycosylated (27). Isomaltase ends with amino acid residue Arg_{1007}, and sucrase starts immediately thereafter with Ile_{1008}. The Arg/Ile peptide sequence between isomaltase and sucrase is a trypsin site where the mature large precursor pro-SI is cleaved in the intestinal lumen on exposure to pancreatic secretions (3). These two subunits remain associated with each other by noncovalent strong ionic interactions (2). Both subunits are heavily N- and O-glycosylated and it seems that carbohydrates can modulate the specific activities of these proteins. Recent observations have shown that the isomaltase activity is almost twofold lower when isomaltase is not properly O-glycosylated. On the other hand, reduced O-glycosylation has an opposite effect on the activity of sucrase (Naim et al, unpublished data).

Sucrase is almost as long as isomaltase without the membrane anchor and stalk

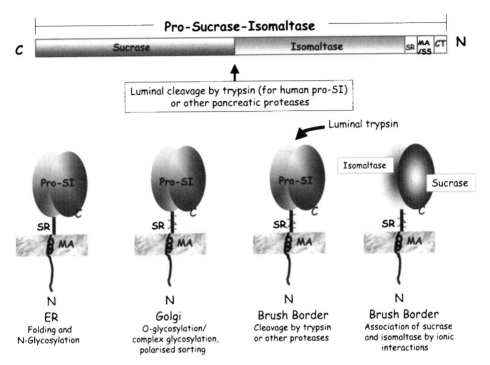

FIG. 2. Schematic representation of the structure and biosynthesis of pro-sucrase-isomaltase (pro-SI) in human small intestinal cells. Pro-SI is a type II integral membrane glycoprotein that is synthesized with an uncleavable signal sequence for translocation into the endoplasmic reticulum (ER) and consists of 1,827 amino acids. Pro-SI, therefore, has an N_{in}/C_{out} orientation. The N-terminus starts with a cytoplasmic tail (CT) (Met_1-Ser_{12}) followed by a membrane anchor (MA) that also contains the signal sequence (SS) (Leu_{13}-Ala_{32}). A Ser/Thr-rich stalk region (SR) encompasses the sequences Thr_{33}-Ser_{61} and is the site of extensive O-glycosylation of pro-SI. Isomaltase ends with amino acid residue Arg_{1007} and sucrase starts immediately thereafter with Ile_{1008}. The Arg/Ile peptide sequence between isomaltase and sucrase is a trypsin site where the mature large precursor pro-SI is cleaved in the intestinal lumen by pancreatic secretions. The human enzyme is cleaved by trypsin. Pro-SI is synthesized in intestinal epithelial cells as an uncleaved precursor that is cotranslationally N-glycosylated with mannose-rich chains. After acquisition of correct folding and transport competence in the ER, pro-SI is transported to the Golgi apparatus where O-glycosylation of the stalk region (SR) and also of other potential O-glycosylation sites in the sucrase subunit begins. Termination of the N- and O-linked glycosylation events are followed by sorting of pro-SI in the *trans*-Golgi network. Pro-SI is transported to the apical membrane with high fidelity and is cleaved by pancreatic secretions (trypsin in the case of the human enzyme and elastase for the rat enzyme). Sucrase and isomaltase remain strongly associated with each other through ionic interactions.

regions. Molecular cloning of full-length cDNAs encoding the rabbit and human species of SI has shown that 38% of the amino acid sequence of sucrase and isomaltase are identical and an additional 34% show conservative changes (27). These data have led to the belief that the SI gene has arisen by one cycle of duplication of a single gene (27). Furthermore, sequence comparison of SI with the human lysosomal α-glucosidase and also the glucoamylase from the yeast *Schwanniomyces occindetalis* suggests that these proteins have evolved from the same ancestral gene (28).

Biosynthesis

Sucrase-isomaltase is expressed and synthesized exclusively in intestinal cells. The earliest detectable form in the endoplasmic reticulum is a large, mannose-rich polypeptide precursor (pro-SI$_h$, h standing for high mannose or mannose-rich) of an apparent molecular mass of 210 kd. This form is transported at a fairly slow rate from the endoplasmic reticulum to the Golgi cisternae (t$\frac{1}{2}$ ~75 minutes) (for comparison, dipeptidyl peptidase IV and aminopeptidase N are transported at a t$\frac{1}{2}$ ~ 15 minutes and 20 minutes, respectively) (2,3). Many membrane glycoproteins form dimers, trimers, or higher order polymers as a prerequisite for acquisition of transport competence before their exit from the endoplasmic reticulum. In this respect, pro-SI is one of the exceptional cases and probably its persistence as a monomeric molecule is what determines its rate of transport to the Golgi apparatus (3). On the other hand, by virtue of the striking sequence similarities between sucrase and isomaltase, an implication of some kind of dimeric structure (e.g., pseudodimers) along the secretory pathway of pro-SI could be postulated. It is not known at present whether each of the individual subunits acquires correct folding and enzymatic activity and is already transport competent after being processed in the endoplasmic reticulum. It is worth mentioning that analysis of a phenotype of CSID provided evidence that the isomaltase subunit is transport competent and does not require the sucrase subunit for correct sorting to the apical membrane (30). However, this event occurs in the *trans*-Golgi network and, therefore, this phenotype does not answer the question of whether the isomaltase subunit alone exits the endoplasmic reticulum efficiently.

Major processing of the mannose-rich pro-SI molecule occurs in the Golgi apparatus (2). Here, the mannose-rich *N*-linked glycans are trimmed by Golgi mannosidases and different types of sugar residue are added in the medial and *trans*-Golgi, resulting in a complex type of *N*-glycosylation. Concomitant with processing of the *N*-glycans in the Golgi apparatus, pro-SI acquires *O*-glycosidically linked carbohydrates. Both the isomaltase and the sucrase subunits are *O*-glycosylated. In the human small intestine, *O*-glycosylation of the sucrase subunit is heterogeneous by virtue of the existence of at least four glycoforms of differently *O*-glycosylated sucrase species (2). By contrast, the *O*-glycosylation pattern of the isomaltase subunit is unique, suggesting a more efficient and more consistent glycosylation event for isomaltase than for sucrase. It has been proposed that the variations in the *O*-glycosylation pattern of the subunits correlate with the position of each domain within the enzyme complex (2). The isomaltase is readily *O*-glycosylated as it contains a Ser/Thr-rich stalk region that is located in immediate proximity to the membrane, whereas the sucrase is more distal (27).

The trimming of the mannose-rich chains and the start of the *O*-glycosylation event in the Golgi apparatus are temporally associated: *O*-glycosylation of pro-SI does not start before the first outermost mannose residues of the mannose-rich chains are trimmed by mannosidase I in the *cis*-Golgi (28a). Complete processing of the *N*-linked chains is crucial for the function of pro-SI, as proper *O*-glycosylation of pro-SI is required for correct targeting of pro-SI to the apical membrane to exert its function (see later), and the activity of isomaltase increases concomitantly with *O*-glycosylation. The fully glycosylated precursor (pro-SI$_c$, c standing for complex glycosylated, 245 kd) is then transported to the microvillus membrane where it is cleaved by trypsin (26) or other pancreatic proteases into its two mature, enzymatically active subunits, sucrase (S$_c$, 130 kd) and isomaltase (I$_c$, 145 kd).

Sorting of Pro-SI

Pro-SI is sorted with high fidelity to the apical membrane. At least 85% of newly synthesized pro-SI is expressed at the apical membrane and, in pulse chase experiments, pro-SI is found entirely at the apical membrane after prolonged chase periods. The partial presence of pro-SI in the basolateral membrane has led to the hypothesis that it is transported in small amounts along the transcytotic pathway to the apical membrane. Until very recently, the identity and location of the sorting signals for pro-SI were still obscure. Important information about sorting came from a few cases of naturally occurring SI mutants. These showed that the sorting mechanism is a signal-mediated event and that the isomaltase subunit is the exclusive carrier of the sorting elements (30,31). In addition, these studies have excluded a role of *N*-glycans as mediators of apical sorting. In view of this, we designed a study to localize putative sorting elements within the isomaltase subunit. One attractive region that may be involved in apical sorting is the Ser/Thr heavily *O*-glycosylated stalk region (27). It has been proposed that *O*-linked glycans are involved in sorting the neurotrophin receptor, a neuronal protein, when it is heterologously expressed in an MDCK epithelial cell line (21). However, no data were available on a potential role of *O*-linked glycans in the sorting of an endogenously expressed membrane glycoprotein in a highly polarized cell line. We evaluated the role of *O*-linked glycans on the transport and sorting of pro-SI in CaCo2 cells by employing benzyl-*N*-acetyl-α-D-galactosaminide (benzyl-GalNAc), a potent inhibitor of *O*-linked glycosylation that competes with *N*-acetyl-D-galactosamine in binding potential *O*-glycosylation sites, Ser or Thr.

A drastic reduction in its *O*-glycosylation pattern in the presence of benzyl-Gal-NAc dramatically shifts the sorting behavior of pro-SI from highly efficient targeting to the apical membrane to random delivery of the modified pro-SI glycoform to

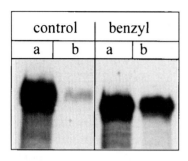

control		benzyl	
a	b	a	b

FIG. 3. Role of *O*-linked glycans in the polarized sorting of pro-SI. Colon carcinoma cells, CaCo2, differentiate spontaneously to polarized epithelial cells and typical small intestinal proteins, such as pro-sucrase-isomaltase (pro-SI), lactase-phlorizin hydrolase (LPH), dipeptidyl peptidase IV, and aminopeptidase N, become expressed. These cells were used to study the role of *O*-linked glycans in the apical sorting of pro-SI. For this, the cells were grown on membrane filters to mimic the *in vivo* situation and obtain an epithelial cell monolayer. Six days after confluence, the cells were biosynthetically labeled with ^{35}S-methionine in the presence or absence of benzyl-GalNAc ("benzyl"), a potent inhibitor of *O*-glycosylation. Pro-SI was immunoprecipitated from the apical or basolateral compartments by adding monoclonal antibody separately to either domain. The immunoprecipitates were analyzed by sodium dodecyl sulfate–polyacrylamide gel electrophoresis (SDS-PAGE) and fluorography. As shown, a substantial shift was revealed in the size of pro-SI in the presence of benzyl-GalNAc (*right two lanes*) as compared with the control sample (*left lane*), indicating that *O*-linked glycosylation was strongly impaired or inhibited by benzyl-GalNAc. Concomitant with this effect, the sorting of pro-SI was also dramatically affected. The control samples (*left two lines*) show that pro-SI is predominantly (~95%) sorted to the apical membrane ("a"), approximately 40% of pro-SI was now detected at the basolateral membrane ("b") in the presence of benzyl-GalNAc. Clearly, the inhibition or impairment of *O*-linked glycosylation is associated with a substantial loss of sorting fidelity of pro-SI, underlining the essential role of *O*-linked glycans as a signal in the context of apical sorting of pro-SI.

both apical and basolateral membranes (24) (Fig. 3). *O*-linked glycans, therefore, are directly implicated as a signal in mediating the sorting of pro-SI to the apical membrane.

The question arises as to the possible location of the *O*-glycan sorting signal within the pro-SI molecule. Deletion of the heavily *O*-glycosylated stalk region of pro-SI was associated with the loss of high fidelity of sorting, clearly demonstrating that *O*-glycans in the stalk region provide the main sorting information. The mechanism by which the sorting of pro-SI occurs is through the association of SI with detergent-insoluble membrane microdomains enriched in glycosphingolipids and cholesterol, known as lipid rafts because inhibition of sphingolipid synthesis by fumonisin results in the random delivery of pro-SI to either membrane. A direct involvement of *O*-linked glycans in the association of pro-SI with lipid rafts is likely to be the driving mechanism for apical sorting of pro-SI. How could this association be explained? One possibility is through binding of the *O*-linked glycans of pro-SI to a sorting protein in the *trans*-Golgi network, a lectin-like protein such as VIP36, which is a member of a recently characterized group of leguminous lectin-like proteins that are implicated in various steps of the secretory pathway (32).

GENE EXPRESSION OF LPH AND SI

Cell differentiation in many tissues is characterized by marked alterations in the expression of genes, which could be caused by either activation or repression of gene transcription. The gene regulation in these phases is controlled by tissue-specific transcription factors or proteins. Transcription factors are often capable of activating multiple genes in the same cell, and the expression of these genes generates novel cellular phenotypic markers that, in many cases, are associated with dramatic morphologic and functional alterations of the differentiated cell. This pattern of gene expression is best exemplified by the differentiation of intestinal crypt cells to columnar epithelial cell that reveals two structurally and functionally different domains, the apical and basolateral domains (33).

During the differentiation of intestinal cells, the genes encoding the disaccharidases LPH and SI become expressed (34). As a result of multiple studies, a generally accepted pattern of expression of SI and LPH has emerged. Functional, immunohistochemical, and *in situ* hybridization studies have shown that SI and LPH are barely detectable in the crypts, their pattern of expression reaching maximal levels between the lower and mid-villus and decreasing at the villus tip (3,35). In one study, SI was also detected in crypt cells, but it seems that this form has an altered conformation. The gene for LPH is approximately 55 kilobase (kb) and is made of 17 exons that all encode the LPH (11). Binding sites for common transcription factors such as CTF/NF-1 and AP2 were identified within 1 kb of the 5′ flanking region of the rat and human genes (36). Glucocorticoids enhance lactase activity in rats during the first weeks in life and have also been shown to regulate human lactase (37). However, glucocorticoid responsive elements in the 5′ flanking region of LPH have not been identified. Analysis of 5′ flanking sequences fused to human growth hormone (hGH) as a reporter gene in transfected CaCo2 cells (adenocarcinoma cell line) or the nonintestinal cell line HepG2 have shown the exclusive and specific function of these sequences in cells of intestinal lineage (38). Footprint analysis of the promoter region has led to the identification of a nuclear protein (NF-LPH1) that binds a 15 base pair (bp) region just upstream of the transcription site (between -54 and -40), is functional in the CaCo2 cell line, and is probably involved in regulation of lactase activity (36,39).

Much of the information accumulated so far about the structure of the SI gene has described 5′ flanking regions and their role in transcription and regulation (33). In addition to this, the structure of three exons and the corresponding intervening DNA sequences is known, along with the sequence of the full-length cDNAs of the rabbit and human species. It is perhaps unique for SI that its first exon is untranslated and the second exon starts with the initiation ATG codon.

Initial expression studies of promoter regions of the SI gene have mapped the intestine-specific promoter elements to a region between -183 and $+54$. On the other hand, several stretches within the sequence -3424 to $+54$ have an inhibitory effect on the level of transcription of SI. Assessment of the interaction of nuclear proteins with the promoter by footprint analyses has identified three specific footprints for SI (denoted SIF1, SIF2, and SIF3, for *S*ucrase-*I*somaltase *F*ootprints 1, 2, and 3, respectively). Only SIF1 was found to be intestine specific, as it was not identified in the nonintestinal cell line HepG2, in contrast to SIF2 and SIF3. Nevertheless, all three elements are implicated in the positive regulation of SI gene transcription. The nuclear protein that binds SIF2 and SIF3 has been identified as

HNF-1, a hepatocyte nuclear factor previously thought to play a role in transcription of genes in the liver (40). The expression of LPH and SI during development follows a similar pattern at the protein and mRNA levels (41).

Enzyme Deficiencies and Phenotypes

The absence of enzymatic activity for digesting carbohydrates leads in most cases to abdominal pain, cramps or distention, flatulence, nausea, and osmotic diarrhea. The reason is that the intestinal epithelium does not have mechanisms allowing the uptake of disaccharides or higher order carbohydrates through cellular membranes to the cell interior. Different types of LPH and SI deficiencies will be discussed next.

LPH Deficiency

Lactose intolerance is the most common intestinal disorder that is associated with an absence or drastically reduced levels of an intestinal enzyme. Lactase deficiency has been described in children and adults and can have a primary or a secondary cause (42). During development in almost all mammals, lactase activity is high at birth and during nursing, when milk is the exclusive nutrient. Around weaning and before adulthood, lactase activity declines drastically—from about 80% to 90% to low adult levels—in most mammals, including humans. In the human population, this decrease happens at around the age of 5 years. The exceptions to this expression profile are northern Europeans and their descendants and some isolated minorities, mainly in Africa. Of northern Europeans, 95% show autosomal dominant inheritance of a lifelong high lactose digesting capacity. The pattern of reduction of activity has been termed ''late onset of lactase deficiency'' or ''adult type hypolactasia.'' Genetic analysis of homozygotes and heterozygotes of lactase persistent and lactase nonpersistent families supported the initial idea that lactase activity is inherited as a single autosomal dominant gene. Currently, several theories attempt to explain the late onset of lactase activity. Initially, it was thought that lactase regulation may be a post-translational event, and that alterations in structural features of LPH itself, at a certain point, lead to an inactive protein or perhaps to intracellular degradation of the protein. This hypothesis was further discussed when mRNA levels of lactase in the intestine of adult rats were found to be very similar to mRNA levels in fetal rats (43). Another study used biopsy material to demonstrate that appreciable levels of lactase mRNA were detected in the intestines of hypolactasic individuals in southern Italy. These observations have led to the view that lactase protein is synthesized in adult-type hypolactasia but undergoes post-translational modifications that result in a malfolded or enzymatically inactive protein that is degraded at a relatively high rate.

A study of a race and sex balanced cohort, in which lactose tolerance, levels of jejunal lactase protein, lactase activity, and messenger RNA (mRNA) were measured, clearly showed that black heritage predicts low lactose digesting capacity, and white heritage predicts high lactose digesting capacity (44). One variable used in this study was the assessment of the lactase-to-sucrase (L:S) ratio in jejunal biopsy specimens. All subjects with a high lactose digesting capacity had an L:S ratio above 0.5, immunodetectable LPH protein, and measurably higher LPH mRNA levels than subjects with low lactose digesting capacity. Further, LPH mRNA levels were highly correlated with lactase specific activity ($r = 0.80$) and the L:S ratio ($r = 0.88$). The direct correlation between LPH mRNA levels and lactase expression argues that the gene responsible for human lactase polymorphism regulates the level of LPH mRNA. Similarly, studies in the rat small intestine found an essentially similar coordinate pattern of interrelation between mRNA and protein levels of LPH (43).

Although lactase activity was clearly dependent on the presence of LPH mRNA pattern, the regional distribution of activity did not correlate absolutely with the mRNA and protein levels along the proximal to distal axis. This suggests that additional secondary mechanisms, perhaps post-translational, influence lactase activity. *O*-glycosylation, for example, a post-translational event that starts in the *cis*-Golgi, increases the activity of LPH fourfold (6). The interesting aspect of this observation is that variations in the quantities of *O*-glycans reflect the differentiation state of intestinal cells to polarized enterocytes. These events are associated with dramatic alterations in the gene expression of intestinal proteins and the coordinated synthesis of typical intestinal markers such as SI, LPH, and a number of glucosyl transferases that affect the glycosylation pattern of glycoproteins. Despite this, the major regulatory mechanism of LPH is transcriptional as most of the accumulated data have clearly shown that adequate levels of LPH mRNA must be present to detect LPH activities (44–46).

Work from the Noren and Sjöström laboratory has identified a specific region in the LPH promoter, CE-LPH1, which interacts with an intestinal- and LPH-specific *trans*-acting nuclear factor, NF-LPH1, that is strongly associated with the regulation of gene transcription of LPH (39,47). However, clear differences in the promoter region of LPH between individuals with low and high lactose digesting capacity have not yet been found. Likewise, no data describe variations in the absence or presence of transcription factors associated with changes in lactose-digesting capacity.

Minor forms of lactose intolerance are also seen, for example congenital lactase deficiency, a rare autosomal recessive trait that is characterized by the absence of active LPH (48). Here, as in the case of congenital SI deficiency (see later), post-translational mechanisms may be crucial in the regulation of the activity. Lactase deficiency occurs also as a primary event in premature infants because of immature intestinal development. Other forms of lactase deficiency are secondary and are caused by mucosal injury from infectious gastroenteritis, celiac disease, parasitic infection, drug-induced enteritis, and Crohn's disease.

SI Deficiency

The pattern of expression of SI is different from that of LPH; essentially, it is the opposite to LPH. The activity of sucrase increases during weaning and persists at high levels in adulthood. Although the mechanisms for the regulation of LPH are still not elucidated, much more progress has been made in this respect with SI. As shown above, the regulation of SI activity is a transcriptional event that implicates several SI-specific and intestine-specific nuclear factors. However, rare conditions of SI deficiency are a result of impaired, defective, or abnormal post-translational processing of an otherwise normally expressed SI protein. Congenital sucrase-isomaltase deficiency belongs to this category.

Inherited as an autosomal recessive trait, CSID is clinically manifested as a watery osmotic-fermentative diarrhea on ingestion of di- and oligosaccharides (49). In addition to its clinical relevance, CSID has been used as a promising approach to characterizing various steps in the biosynthesis, transport, and sorting of SI as a general model for cell surface membrane proteins and highly polarized proteins in epithelial cells. Enterocytes of patients with this disease lack the sucrase activity of the enzyme SI, whereas the isomaltase activity can vary from absent to practically normal.

Substantial progress has been made in elucidating the molecular basis of CSID. We and others have initially proposed that different molecular defects or mutations in the SI gene are responsible for CSID. In fact, investigations of intestinal biopsy samples from patients with this disorder at the subcellular and molecular level have led to the identification of five different phenotypes of SI in CSID (30,31) (Table 1).

In *phenotype I*, a normal protein is synthesized that rests in the endoplasmic reticulum as a mannose-rich glycosylated protein. Partial misfolding of SI in this phenotype prevents conformational maturation of SI. Transport out of the endoplasmic reticulum is prevented and the SI protein is eventually degraded in the organelle.

Phenotype II is characterized by an intracellular accumulation of a mannose-rich SI in the endoplasmic reticulum, the endoplasmic reticulum/*cis*-Golgi intermediate

TABLE 1. *Structural and biosynthetic features of sucrase-isomalase (SI) in phenotypes of congenital sucrase-isomaltase deficiency*

Phenotype	Biosynthetic features
I	Accumulation of pro-SI in the ER and subsequent degradation
II	Retention in the ERGIC, *cis*-Golgi, and *trans*-Golgi
	Recycling between the ER and Golgi? Quality control beyond the ER?
III	Inactive enzyme, but normal intracellular trafficking and sorting
IV	Missorting of pro-SI to the basolateral membrane
V	Abnormal intracellular cleavage of pro-SI: degradation of sucrase and normal apical sorting of isomaltase

ER, endoplasmic reticulum.

compartment, and the *cis*-Golgi. Transport of the SI protein to the medial and *trans*-Golgi occurs in a related phenotype. Phenotypes I and II both express an enzymatically inactive protein.

Phenotype III is the opposite of the previous two, as an enzymatically inactive but transport competent SI is expressed that reaches the apical membrane correctly. In this phenotype, the catalytic site of sucrase is not functional whereas that of isomaltase is normal.

One of the most interesting phenotypes—with implications for the sorting mechanisms and targeting of SI in particular and proteins in general in polarized epithelial cells—is *phenotype IV*. In this phenotype, SI is expressed as a partially folded, mannose-rich SI molecule that is missorted to the basolateral membrane. It is thought that a point mutation in SI could be responsible for this defect, and the identification of the region containing this putative point mutation may provide important clues about the role of specific protein domains of SI in the sorting process and the particular mechanisms implicated.

Finally, *phenotype V* is an SI species that undergoes intracellular degradation, leaving behind the isomaltase subunit that is correctly targeted to the brush border membrane (30). This phenotype is important as it shows that the isomaltase contains everything necessary for apical transport of SI.

These phenotypes are most likely to be the products of single mutations in the coding region of the SI gene. Recently, our group was the first to successfully clone and characterize a cDNA encoding SI from a biopsy sample of a patient with CSID, and to identify a single point mutation that is responsible for the impaired transport behavior of SI in phenotype II (50). This mutation converts a glutamine to a proline in the sucrase subunit of SI at amino acid 1098 (Q1098P) and leads to an accumulation of SI in the *cis*-Golgi and ERGIC. As such, this observation has important implications for current concepts of membrane and protein transport, as it suggests that the Q1098P mutation generates a recognition site for a protein involved in a hypothetical quality control mechanism operating beyond the endoplasmic reticulum; such an event has not been described so far. The Q1098P substitution, therefore, has been investigated in more detail and we were able to show that it is not only functional in intestinal epithelial cells but also produces a similar phenotype when expressed in nonpolarized COS-1 cells (29). It is apparent, therefore, that the Q1098P mutation *per se* is responsible for the generation of the SI phenotype II, and that the onset of this CSID phenotype does not involve cellular factors specifically expressed in the small intestine.

One important observation was the folding state of the mutant SI protein. Here, protease sensitivity assays using trypsin show that the mutant SI is not as stable as its wild-type counterpart and is degraded within a relatively short period. The interesting aspect of these folding experiments is that both the sucrase and the isomaltase subunits are degraded. Malfolding of the sucrase subunit as a result of the mutation Q1098P is expected, along with a different pattern of trypsin sensitivity as compared with wild-type sucrase. Unexpected, however, was the susceptibility of isomaltase

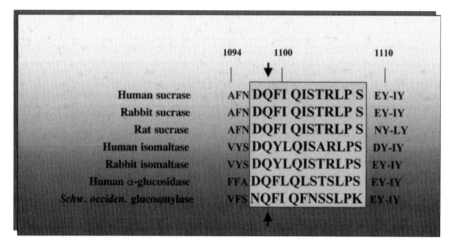

FIG. 4. Identification of the mutation responsible for retention of pro-sucrase-isomaltase (pro-SI) in the *cis*-Golgi apparatus in phenotype II of congenital SI deficiency. The full-length cDNA of pro-SI was isolated by reverse transcriptase polymerase chain reaction from a biopsy sample of a patient with congenital sucrase-isomaltase deficiency (CSID) phenotype II. The cDNA was completely sequenced in both directions and a single mutation, A to C, at nucleotide 3298 in the coding region of sucrase was identified. This mutation leads to a substitution of a glutamine (Q) residue by a proline (P) at amino acid 1098 (Q1098P) (*arrow*). The mutation is contained in a region that shares striking similarities among sucrase and isomaltase from various species, lysosomal α-glucosidase and the yeast *Schwannionmyces occidentalis* glucoamylase. The sequence similarities around the mutation are aligned and shown in the box.

to trypsin in this phenotype, suggesting a different folding pattern from the wild-type isomaltase. This implies that the association between sucrase and isomaltase takes place very early in the endoplasmic reticulum, where the subunits possibly assist each other to fold properly and in this way function as ''intramolecular chaperones'' (16). In mutant SI, these protective associations might be absent, resulting in exposed protease-sensitive sites.

One of the features of the Q1098P mutation is its presence in a region that shares striking homologies between human, rat, and rabbit sucrase and isomaltase variants, as well as human lysosomal α-glucosidase and *Schwannionmyces occidentalis* glucoamylase (Fig. 4) (28). The fact that all these proteins, which may have evolved from a common ancestral gene, are transported along the secretory pathway to their final destinations implies a key role for the region containing the Q1098P in the sorting of these proteins from the endoplasmic reticulum, and a common function of this or structurally similar regions in other proteins along the secretory pathway. Indeed, we were able to show that the Q1098P mutation of sucrase elicits a similar effect when introduced at the corresponding amino acid position 244 in lysosomal α-glucosidase (29). The mutated lysosomal α-glucosidase precursor does not undergo maturation in the Golgi apparatus, is not cleaved into mature enzyme, and is not transported through the Golgi cisternae. It is therefore conceivable that the Q1098P mutation has introduced a retention signal for the *cis*-Golgi or, alternatively, the mutation has led to a structural alteration that functions as a recognition site for a quality control machinery operating in the intermediate compartment or *cis*-Golgi. The components of this hypothetical machinery have to be unraveled.

FUTURE PERSPECTIVES

A fairly substantial knowledge has accumulated on various aspects of the structure, biosynthesis, sorting, gene expression, and regulation of the function of the intestinal disaccharidases SI and LPH. This basic information is of primary importance in elucidating the mechanisms that control the gene expression of these proteins in carbohydrate absorption disorders, for example in adult-type hypolactasia, congenital lactase deficiency, and CSID. In the latter two disorders, post-translational mechanisms appear to be responsible for their onset (30,31). For adult-type hypolactasia, it is still premature to state with certainty which molecular mechanisms are implicated. A consensus has emerged that LPH activity is controlled at the transcriptional level. Despite ample progress in localization of upstream regions and identification of transcription factors implicated in the onset of hypolactasia, much information is still required to solve the puzzle of LPH deficiency. Major attention should be paid to *trans*-acting elements, which have been almost neglected. For this, transgenes should be made that contain constructs of the entire LPH cDNA decorated with randomly selected *trans*-located introns from individuals with high and low lactose-digesting capacity. The potential role of particular post-translational events in the regulation of LPH activity should also be explored (6). Our preliminary data show that LPH contains an endocytic signal in its cytoplasmic tail that is repressed in ''normal'' LPH by the strong apical signal located in the ectodomain. This signal is located in close proximity to the membrane; it shows minimal flexibility or accessibility for interaction with clathrin-coated pits and becomes effective only when the apical signal of LPH is deleted. It would be interesting to screen representative sequences of the cytosolic tails of the LPH gene from individuals with high and low lactose-digesting capacity.

For SI, it is clear that further identification of the mutations responsible for the five phenotypes identified so far is required. This would provide important clues to the factors involved in the post-translational control of the SI activity, and would serve as a model for elucidating mechanisms of protein transport and polarized sorting. Putative components of the sorting machinery that interact with apical sorting signals (e.g., *N*- and *O*-linked glycans) have also to be identified.

In comparison with the extensive data on SI and LPH, substantially less is known about similar aspects of other disaccharidases such as trehalase and maltase-glucoamylase. Striking structural and functional similarities are found between maltase-glucoamylase and SI (51). It is puzzling why two enzyme complexes with such elaborate structures are present to perform virtually the same function. It would be interesting to see whether the expression patterns of these proteins were subject to mechanisms similar to SI or LPH. Furthermore, it will also be important to determine whether maltase-glucoamylase has an auxiliary function not shared by SI and whether it is implicated in novel and presently unsuspected digestive pathways. Correlation of the expression and function patterns of SI and maltase-glucoamylase in carbohydrate disorders would provide important clues in this respect.

ACKNOWLEDGMENTS

The original work from our laboratory cited in this review was supported by grants from the Swiss National Science Foundation, Bern, Switzerland, the German Ministry for Education and Research (BMBF), and the German Research Foundation, Bonn, Germany. I am indebted to Dr. Ralf Jacob for his assistance in the preparation of the manuscript.

REFERENCES

1. Naim HY, Sterchi EE, Lentze MJ. Biosynthesis and maturation of lactase–phlorizin hydrolase in the human small intestinal epithelial cells. *Biochem J* 1987; 241: 427–34.
2. Naim HY, Sterchi EE, Lentze MJ. Biosynthesis of the human sucrase-isomaltase complex. Differential *O*-glycosylation of the sucrase subunit correlates with its position within the enzyme complex. *J Biol Chem* 1988; 263: 7242–53.
3. Hauri HP, Sterchi EE, Bienz D, Fransen JA, Marxer A. Expression and intracellular transport of microvillus membrane hydrolases in human intestinal epithelial cells. *J Cell Biol* 1985; 101: 838–51.
4. Colombo V, Lorenz-Meyer H, Semenza G. Small intestinal phlorizin hydrolase: the "beta-glycosidase complex." *Biochim Biophys Acta* 1973; 327: 412–24.
5. Mantei N, Villa M, Enzler T, *et al.* Complete primary structure of human and rabbit lactase–phlorizin hydrolase: implications for biosynthesis, membrane anchoring and evolution of the enzyme. *EMBO J* 1988; 7: 2705–13.
6. Naim HY, Lentze MJ. Impact of *O*-glycosylation on the function of human intestinal lactase–phlorizin hydrolase. Characterization of glycoforms varying in enzyme activity and localization of *O*-glycoside addition. *J Biol Chem* 1992; 267: 25494–504.
7. Naim HY, Lacey SW, Sambrook JF, Gething MJ. Expression of a full-length cDNA coding for human intestinal lactase–phlorizin hydrolase reveals an uncleaved, enzymatically active, and transport-competent protein. *J Biol Chem* 1991; 266: 12313–20.
8. Jacob R, Radebach I, Wuthrich M, Grunberg J, Sterchi EE, Naim HY. Maturation of human intestinal lactase–phlorizin hydrolase: generation of the brush border form of the enzyme involves at least two proteolytic cleavage steps. *Eur J Biochem* 1996; 236: 789–95.
9. Wuthrich M, Grunberg J, Hahn D, *et al.* Proteolytic processing of human lactase–phlorizin hydrolase is a two-step event: identification of the cleavage sites. *Arch Biochem Biophys* 1996; 336: 27–34.
10. Jacob R, Brewer C, Fransen JA, Naim HY. Transport, function, and sorting of lactase–phlorizin hydrolase in Madin-Darby canine kidney cells. *J Biol Chem* 1994; 269: 2712–21.
11. Boll W, Wagner P, Mantei N. Structure of the chromosomal gene and cDNAs coding for lactase–phlorizin hydrolase in humans with adult-type hypolactasia or persistence of lactase. *Am J Hum Genet* 1991; 48: 889–902.
12. Wacker H, Keller P, Falchetto R, Legler G, Semenza G. Location of the two catalytic sites in intestinal lactase–phlorizin hydrolase. Comparison with sucrase-isomaltase and with other glycosidases, the membrane anchor of lactase–phlorizin hydrolase. *J Biol Chem* 1992; 267: 18744–52.
13. Danielsen EM, Skovbjerg H, Noren O, Sjostrom H. Biosynthesis of intestinal microvillar proteins. Intracellular processing of lactase–phlorizin hydrolase. *Biochem Biophys Res Commun* 1984; 122: 82–90.
14. Buller HA, Montgomery RK, Sasak WV, Grand RJ. Biosynthesis, glycosylation, and intracellular transport of intestinal lactase–phlorizin hydrolase in rat. *J Biol Chem* 1987; 262: 17206–11.
15. Naim HY, Naim H. Dimerization of lactase–phlorizin hydrolase occurs in the endoplasmic reticulum,

involves the putative membrane spanning domain and is required for an efficient transport of the enzyme to the cell surface. *Eur J Cell Biol* 1996; 70: 198–208.

16. Naim HY, Jacob R, Naim H, Sambrook JF, Gething MJ. The pro region of human intestinal lactase–phlorizin hydrolase. *J Biol Chem* 1994; 269: 26933–43.
17. Casanova JE, Apodaca G, Mostov KE. An autonomous signal for basolateral sorting in the cytoplasmic domain of the polymeric immunoglobulin receptor. *Cell* 1991; 66: 65–75.
18. Lisanti MP, Le Bivic A, Saltiel AR, Rodriguez-Boulan E. Preferred apical distribution of glycosyl-phosphatidylinositol (GPI) anchored proteins: a highly conserved feature of the polarized epithelial cell phenotype. *J Membr Biol* 1990; 113: 155–67.
19. Simons K, Ikonen E. Functional rafts in cell membranes. *Nature* 1997; 387: 569–72.
20. Fiedler K, Simons K. The role of N-glycans in the secretory pathway. *Cell* 1995; 81: 309–12.
21. Yeaman C, Le Gall AH, Baldwin AN, Monlauzeur L, Le Bivic A, Rodriguez-Boulan E. The *O*-glycosylated stalk domain is required for apical sorting of neurotrophin receptors in polarized MDCK cells. *J Cell Biol* 1997; 139: 929–40.
22. Jacob R, Preuss U, Panzer P, *et al.* Hierarchy of sorting signals in chimeras of intestinal lactase–phlorizin hydrolase and the influenza virus hemagglutinin. *J Biol Chem* 1999; 274: 8061–7.
23. Naim HY. Processing and transport of human small intestinal lactase–phlorizin hydrolase (LPH). Role of N-linked oligosaccharide modification. *FEBS Lett* 1994; 342: 302–7.
24. Alfalah M, Jacob R, Preuss U, Zimmer KP, Naim H, Naim HY. *O*-linked glycans mediate apical sorting of human intestinal sucrase-isomaltase through association with lipid. *Curr Biol* 1999; 9: 593–6.
25. Panzer P, Preuss U, Joberty G, Naim HY. Protein domains implicated in intracellular transport and sorting of lactase–phlorizin hydrolase. *J Biol Chem* 1998; 273: 13861–9.
26. Hauri HP, Quaroni A, Isselbacher KJ. Biogenesis of intestinal plasma membrane: posttranslational route and cleavage of sucrase-isomaltase. *Proc Natl Acad Sci USA* 1979; 76: 5183–6.
27. Hunziker W, Spiess M, Semenza G, Lodish HF. The sucrase-isomaltase complex: primary structure, membrane-orientation, and evolution of a stalked, intrinsic brush border protein. *Cell* 1986; 46: 227–34.
28. Naim HY, Niermann T, Kleinhans U, Hollenberg CP, Strasser AW. Striking structural and functional similarities suggest that intestinal sucrase-isomaltase, human lysosomal alpha-glucosidase and *Schwannionmyces occidentalis* glucoamylase are derived from a common ancestral gene. *FEBS Lett* 1991; 294: 109–12.
28a. Naim HY, Joberty G, Alfalah M, Jacob R. Temporal association of the N- and O-linked glycosylation events and their implication in the polarized sorting of intestinal brush border sucrase-isomaltase, aminopeptidase N, and dipeptidyl peptidase IV. *J Biol Chem* 1999; 274: 17961–7.
29. Moolenaar CE, Ouwendijk J, Wittpoth M, *et al.* A mutation in a highly conserved region in brush-border sucrase-isomaltase and lysosomal alpha-glucosidase results in Golgi retention. *J Cell Sci* 1997; 110: 557–67.
30. Fransen JA, Hauri HP, Ginsel LA, Naim HY. Naturally occurring mutations in intestinal sucrase-isomaltase provide evidence for the existence of an intracellular sorting signal in the isomaltase subunit. *J Cell Biol* 1991; 115: 45–57.
31. Naim HY, Roth J, Sterchi EE, *et al.* Sucrase-isomaltase deficiency in humans. Different mutations disrupt intracellular transport, processing, and function of an intestinal brush border enzyme. *J Clin Invest* 1988; 82: 667–79.
32. Fiedler K, Simons K. Characterization of VIP36, an animal lectin homologous to leguminous lectins. *J Cell Sci* 1996; 109: 271–6.
33. Traber PG, Silberg DG. Intestine-specific gene transcription. *Annu Rev Physiol* 1996; 58: 275–97.
34. Olsen WA, Lloyd M, Korsmo H, He YZ. Regulation of sucrase and lactase in Caco-2 cells: relationship to nuclear factors SIF-1 and NF-LPH-1. *Am J Physiol* 1996; 271: G707–13.
35. Rings EH, de Boer PA, Moorman AF, *et al.* Lactase gene expression during early development of rat small intestine. *Gastroenterology* 1992; 103: 1154–61.
36. Troelsen JT, Olsen J, Mitchelmore C, Hansen GH, Sjostrom H, Noren O. Two intestinal specific nuclear factors binding to the lactase–phlorizin hydrolase and sucrase-isomaltase promoters are functionally related oligomeric molecules. *FEBS Lett* 1994; 342: 297–301.
37. Yeh KY, Yeh M, Holt PR. Intestinal lactase expression and epithelial cell transit in hormone-treated suckling rats. *Am J Physiol* 1991; 260: G379–84.
38. Markowitz AJ, Wu GD, Bader A, Cui Z, Chen L, Traber PG. Regulation of lineage-specific transcription of the sucrase-isomaltase gene in transgenic mice and cell lines. *Am J Physiol* 1995; 269: G925–39.

39. Troelsen JT, Olsen J, Noren O, Sjöström H. A novel intestinal trans-factor (NF-LPH1) interacts with the lactase–phlorizin hydrolase promoter and co-varies with the enzymatic activity. *J Biol Chem* 1992; 267: 20407–11.

40. Wu GD, Chen L, Forslund K, Traber PG. Hepatocyte nuclear factor-1 alpha (HNF-1 alpha) and HNF-1 beta regulate transcription via two elements in an intestine-specific promoter. *J Biol Chem* 1994; 269: 17080–5.

41. Hecht A, Torbey CF, Korsmo HA, Olsen WA. Regulation of sucrase and lactase in developing rats: role of nuclear factors that bind to two gene regulatory elements. *Gastroenterology* 1997; 112: 803–12.

42. Kretchmer N. Expression of lactase during development [Editorial]. *Am J Hum Genet* 1989; 45: 487–8.

43. Buller HA, Kothe MJ, Goldman DA, *et al.* Coordinate expression of lactase–phlorizin hydrolase mRNA and enzyme levels in rat intestine during development [published erratum appears in *J Biol Chem* 1990; 265(22): 13410]. *J Biol Chem* 1990; 265: 6978–83.

44. Fajardo O, Naim HY, Lacey SW. The polymorphic expression of lactase in adults is regulated at the messenger RNA level. *Gastroenterology* 1994; 106: 1233–41.

45. Harvey CB, Wang Y, Hughes LA, *et al.* Studies on the expression of intestinal lactase in different individuals. *Gut* 1995; 36: 28–33.

46. Krasinski SD, Estrada G, Yeh KY, *et al.* Transcriptional regulation of intestinal hydrolase biosynthesis during postnatal development in rats. *Am J Physiol* 1994; 267: G584–94.

47. Troelsen JT, Mitchelmore C, Spodsberg N, Jensen AM, Noren O, Sjöström H. Regulation of lactase–phlorizin hydrolase gene expression by the caudal-related homeodomain protein Cdx-2. *Biochem J* 1997; 322: 833–8.

48. Lifshitz F. Congenital lactase deficiency. *J Pediatr* 1966; 69: 229–37.

49. Treem WR. Congenital sucrase-isomaltase deficiency. *J Pediatr Gastroenterol Nutr* 1995; 21: 1–14.

50. Ouwendijk J, Moolenaar CE, Peters WJ, *et al.* Congenital sucrase-isomaltase deficiency. Identification of a glutamine to proline substitution that leads to a transport block of sucrase-isomaltase in a pre-Golgi compartment. *J Clin Invest* 1996; 97: 633–41.

51. Nichols BL, Eldering J, Avery S, Hahn D, Quaroni A, Sterchi E. Human small intestinal maltase-glucoamylase cDNA cloning. Homology to sucrase-isomaltase. *J Biol Chem* 1998; 273: 3076–81.

DISCUSSION

Dr. Lyonnet: You have very elegant tools to study series of highly glycosylated proteins in the intestine. Have you had the opportunity to test those proteins in children with generalized glycosylation deficiency, and eventually to relate your findings to the intestinal phenotype of those patients?

Dr. Naim: Some groups are doing this work and evidence indicates that sucrase-isomaltase is normally transported. I personally looked at one biopsy done in Paris, and found that the biosynthesis of sucrase-isomaltase was perfectly normal. So, the deficiency there is at some other level in the endoplasmic reticulum involving the enzymes that contribute to the mannoses.

Dr. Lentze: It is fascinating how much this field has progressed since we started many years ago. In the type 2 sucrase-isomaltase deficiency, where you found your point mutation, was that type of enzyme enzymatically active or not?

Dr. Naim: No, it was not enzymatically active.

Dr. Lentze: So, besides the fact that this protein was missorted, it was also inactive. Thus, two properties were influenced by the mutation?

Dr. Naim: Exactly. It is a proline mutation, so it is glutamine to proline. Therefore, although some microdomains will be affected, it is probably more than that. In the studies we performed in the past, we always applied the method of epitope mapping with a panel of epitope-specific monoclonal antibodies and found that some antibodies reacted with the sucrase-isomaltase and some did not. Now in this very case of phenotype II, we had three of four antibodies that reacted properly with sucrase-isomaltase, one that did not. We do not know exactly where the epitope of that antibody is, but I assume it must be somewhere in the region that has been affected by the mutation. Because of that, some folding problems probably may have affected the enzyme activity itself at some active site near the end.

The other problem is the missorting, which means a block in the *cis*-Golgi apparatus. The nice thing about this phenotype is that when looking at the biosynthesis of this transfected, mutated protein in COS-1 cells at reduced temperatures (from 37°C to ~22°C), you find transport of the molecule to the cell surface. It seems that recycling of the molecule occurs back and forth between the Golgi and the endoplasmic reticulum until it has acquired sufficient folding for it to leave the *cis*-Golgi and proceed further to the cell surface. A quality control mechanism probably operates beyond the endoplasmic reticulum involving this region, or maybe this mutation has generated a retention signal that is recognized by a yet to be identified protein. We are trying to define this putative quality control mechanism beyond the endoplasmic reticulum.

Dr. Lentze: My second question is related to lactase. The precursor is a big 96-kd molecule, which is probably what had been called the ''missing piece.'' Is it necessary for sorting or not?

Dr. Naim: It is not.

Dr. Lentze: Then, why has nature provided something that is not necessary?

Dr. Naim: It is necessary, but not for sorting. It is required for some other function. It is not required for activity, as I have shown, because the whole molecule is as active as the cleaved molecule, so it is not a sort of a zymogen that is being cleaved to activate lactase. The fragment appears to be required to assist in folding of the LPH-β region. We call it an ''intramolecular chaperone.'' These fragments are found in many proteins.

Dr. Delvin: Going back to the isomaltase and the α-glucosidase story, a single point mutation would mislead the cell with respect to trafficking of the protein to the brush border membrane and trafficking to the lysosomes. That means that this single mutation will affect both trafficking processes. As a corollary to this, are any other lysosomal hydrolases, which should have a somewhat similar signal for trafficking, also affected by that single mutation, or does that motif not exist in other hydrolases for lysosomes?

Dr. Naim: It would be great to be able to demonstrate that for other proteins. Cell biologists would love to have this type of mutation, because then they could start to put some hypotheses forward relating to the cellular aspects of certain phenomena. Of course, we would like to have other proteins that generate a similar phenotype by introducing this type of mutation, but I do not know of any other examples of lysosomal proteins that have a similar region. The other protein I showed is a yeast protein, the *Schwanniomyces occidentalis* glucoamylase, and it is useful to do the same type of experiment with that protein, because the yeast cell is eukaryotic and we know that transport pathways are common between mammalian and yeast cells. If this quality control mechanism behind the endoplasmic reticulum is generalized, than we ought to find it in the yeast cell as well.

Dr. Büller: You referred to phenotype IV missorting to the basal lateral membrane. That is exciting, because it provides a role for *O*-glycosylation. Is that generalizable or was it just found in the phenotype IV in that particular patient group?

Dr. Naim: These experiments on *O*-glycosylation in the sorting of sucrase-isomaltase were done with reagents that block *O*-glycosylation. So, we are blocking *O*-glycosylation not only in the stalk region of sucrase-isomaltase, but in all the other potential *O*-glycosylation sites. This tells us that *O*-glycans are involved, which can be generalized for sucrase-isomaltase, but not for lactase. *O*-glycans are not involved in lactase sorting. Now that we know that *O*-glycans are involved in sucrase sorting, we have a better chance of narrowing down the region where we have to search for the mutation.

Dr. Büller: Could you explain why and how adult low lactase occurs?

Dr. Naim: I would suspect both translation and processing. We looked at the biosynthesis and processing of lactase in adult-type hyperlactasia some years ago and found differences in the molecular forms and in the turnover of the molecule, although only in a few cases (1).

Dr. E. Wright: With the Q1098P mutation—the proline in sucrase-isomaltase—have you tried in the CHO cells to look at other mutants at that position to see whether it is the loss of the glutamine or the gain of the proline that causes the trafficking? The other part of this question: How do you think that the ectodomain of the protein actually regulates trafficking?

Dr. Naim: In answer to the first question, we have done some experiments where we mutated the proline, putting in alanine and other amino acids from different groups, and no effect was seen; the trafficking was perfect. As to the second question, in the ectodomain I believe that the signal should not be located at the distal part of the molecule; it must be somewhere structurally near the membrane to interact with these types of protein.

Dr. Roy: On the basis of kinetic studies looking at glucose transport, it was found that the feeding of glucose in the form of sucrose was more efficient. Have you looked at the localization of these proteins—the glucose transporters and the sucrase-isomaltase—with regard to proximity or the way they are inserted into the membrane to explain these kinetic studies?

Dr. Naim: No, we have not looked at that. We know the distribution of the sucrase-isomaltase along the gut, because those studies have been done, but nothing in respect to what you asked.

Dr. Mäki: Do you know whether the same gene is involved in congenital lactase deficiency as in adult hypolactasia?

Dr. Naim: I do not think this is known as yet, but I believe it should be the same gene.

Dr. Büller: But, we know that these people with congenital lactase deficiency do not make the protein, do they?

Dr. Naim: No, we do not know with certainty whether or not they make the protein.

REFERENCE

1. Sterchi EE, Mills PR, Fransen JA, *et al.* Biogenesis of intestinal lactase–phlorizin hydrolase in adults with lactose intolerance. Evidence for reduced biosynthesis and slowed-down maturation in enterocytes. *J Clin Invest* 1990; 86; 1329–37.

Gastrointestinal Functions, edited by Edgard E. Delvin and Michael J. Lentze. Nestlé Nutrition Workshop Series, Pediatric Program, Vol. 46, Nestec Ltd., Vevey/Lippincott Williams & Wilkins, Philadelphia © 2001.

Testing Intestinal Function

Possibilities Offered by $^{13}CO_2$ Breath Tests and Stable Isotopes

Y. Ghoos, B. Geypens, and P. Rutgeerts

Department of Pathophysiology, Catholic University of Leuven, Leuven, Belgium

The $^{13}CO_2$ breath test is a reliable, noninvasive method of studying the principal gastrointestinal functions, including the assimilation of food ingredients. Stable isotopes offer the possibility of monitoring various metabolic events as well.

THE PRINCIPLE OF THE $^{13}CO_2$ BREATH TEST

Breath tests have in common the fact the subject is given a substrate in which ^{12}C atoms normally present in the functional group are replaced by the stable isotope ^{13}C. This functional group is cleaved enzymatically under specific circumstances, during either transit through the gastrointestinal tract, absorption, or further metabolism of the absorbed substrate. After cleavage, the labeled subgroups undergo a metabolic process that ends with the expiration of labeled CO_2. It is necessary that the speed-determining (rate-limiting) factor of the whole physiologic process is directly related to the genesis of $^{13}CO_2$. The $^{13}CO_2$ mixes with the body pool of CO_2/HCO_3^- and is expired. In this way, the exhalation of $^{13}CO_2$ reflects the function to be investigated. The process is shown schematically in Fig. 1.

For $^{13}CO_2$ measurement to be used to demonstrate a well-defined gastrointestinal function, an enzyme activity, or bacterial metabolism, the ^{13}C substrate has to be chosen in such a way that the enzyme or function is the rate-limiting step in $^{13}CO_2$ production. When the excretion of the tracer in the breath is expressed as percent dose per hour or as cumulative percent dose excreted over a defined time period, a dynamic analysis of the variable examined is obtained over time.

The $^{13}CO_2$ breath tests are excellent investigative methods, as their scientific basis is sound and well conceived, the results have been validated in an unequivocal way, and their application is accepted by a growing number of scientists.

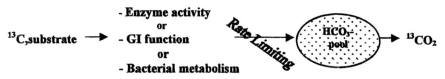

FIG. 1. Schematic diagram of the principle of the $^{13}CO_2$ breath test.

$^{13}CO_2$ BREATH TESTS AS CLINICAL DIAGNOSTIC TOOLS

Originally, breath tests were designed as diagnostic tools for use in gastrointestinal and hepatology clinics. Fig. 2 shows the breath tests used in clinical practice in the Digestion-Absorption Laboratory of the University Hospital Gasthuisberg, Leuven.

Substrates Used in $^{13}CO_2$ Breath Tests

Hepatic function:

- Demethylating and oxidative capacity: [^{13}C]aminopyrine (1)
- Hepatic mass: [^{13}C]galactose (2)
- Mitochondrial activity: [^{13}C]ketoisocaproic acid (3)

Transit measurement:

- Gastric emptying: [^{13}C]octanoic acid and [^{13}C]glycine (4,5)
- Orocecal transit: lactose-[^{13}C]ureide (6,7)
- Small intestinal transit: by mathematical deduction (8)

Helicobacter pylori in stomach:

- [^{13}C]urea (9)

Digestive, absorptive, and fermentative functions:

- Carbohydrates: [^{13}C]naturally enriched compounds, starch, lactose (10–12)
- Lipids: [^{13}C]mixed triglyceride (13,14)

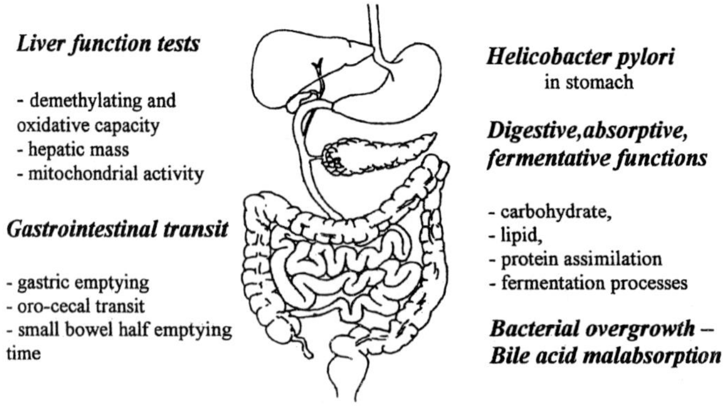

Liver function tests

- demethylating and
oxidative capacity
- hepatic mass
- mitochondrial activity

Gastrointestinal transit

- gastric emptying
- oro-cecal transit
- small bowel half emptying
time

Helicobacter pylori
in stomach

*Digestive, absorptive,
fermentative functions*

- carbohydrate,
- lipid,
- protein assimilation
- fermentation processes

*Bacterial overgrowth –
Bile acid malabsorption*

FIG. 2. Clinical uses of breath tests.

- Proteins: [^{13}C],[^{15}N]egg white proteins (15)
- Fermentation process: lactose-[^{15}N]ureide (16); [^{15}N],[^{2}H]proteins (17)

Bacterial overgrowth or bile acid malabsorption:

- The only [^{14}C]substrate in use (i.e., glycocholic acid + 3 days fecal collection + [^{3}H] polyethyleneglycol transit marker correction) (18–20)

Mathematical Expression of the Functions

An elegant method has been developed to express the meaning of gastrointestinal events by a mathematical formula (21,22). This is discussed later in the chapter.

Good Reasons for Performing $^{13}CO_2$ Breath Tests

A wide range of gastrointestinal techniques are used to investigate gastrointestinal function in clinical practice. These techniques classically are composed of intubation and perfusion to study pancreatic exocrine excretion (23), biopsy to determine brush border enzyme activity (24), and aspiration of intestinal juice to culture for bacterial overgrowth (25). These techniques are complemented by radiography for morphologic examination of the small intestine and colon (26), by radioscintigraphy to demonstrate gastrointestinal segmental transit (27), and by endoscopy with biopsy (28). Less invasive techniques are being developed, such as endoechography (29) and nuclear magnetic resonance imaging (30). Investigation methods based on the analysis of feces and urine for intestinal absorptive capacity are still in daily diagnostic use in hospitals.

Although these techniques are considered reference methods in clinical investigation, they may have some serious shortcomings. For example, intubation, perfusion, aspiration, and biopsy are static methods (i.e., they provide values obtained under nonphysiologic conditions). Methods based on imaging can display dynamic information, and further developments in these techniques may improve clinical investigation in gastroenterology. There remains, however, a need for noninvasive methods providing the same information as the classic methods, but which are simpler and cheaper to perform. $^{13}CO_2$ breath tests may meet these requirements.

If asked, patients request tests that can be executed in a simple way and whenever possible at home (i.e., with minimal absence from family life or work). Doctors ask for tests that can be done repetitively without major discomfort or radiation hazard for the patient, and without time-consuming involvement of equipment and personnel. Public health asks for tests with minimal hospital costs and which do not cause a problem of waste disposal. These advantages are all offered by $^{13}CO_2$ breath tests.

The isotope ratio mass spectrometry technique in current use allows breath $^{13}CO_2$ to be measured in centralized units. Breath samples are sent to the unit and results are available the next day after overnight measurement. It is not claimed that $^{13}CO_2$ breath tests can yet replace the classic tests; at present, they must be considered strictly as important adjuncts to the overall plan of clinical investigation. Thus, it is mandatory that the interpretation of the results should only be made after detailed discussion with the clinician requesting the test.

Special attention must be paid to the execution of the $^{13}CO_2$ breath tests. These tests appear very simple to perform, and some investigators have tried to make them even simpler by reducing the sample numbers or by changing the other test conditions (e.g., meals, sampling time, calculation of results). These modifications can lead to a false interpretation of the test results and make them unsuitable for interlaboratory comparison. The standardized conditions under which these tests are performed, the way the samples are analyzed, and the fact that the calculations can be expressed in relation to an international standard represent a unique advantage over other methods of clinical investigation. An attempt has been made to ensure standardization by the European concerted action BIOMED PL93-1239 project (31). The best way to safeguard uniformity in test design is to do breath tests in specialized clinical units, along the lines of those performing other investigations involving highly technical analytic procedures such as radioscintigraphy. A centralized unit has the additional advantage that breath tests can be performed on several patients at the same time. Samples can be sorted by clinical presentation and the analysis performed overnight.

ADVANTAGES OF $^{13}CO_2$ BREATH TESTS

Three clinical or experimental situations occur in which $^{13}CO_2$ breath tests have a real advantage over classic tests.

1. Combinations of tests. With the combined use of [^{13}C] and [^{14}C] labeling, it is possible to measure two gastrointestinal functions simultaneously. This makes it possible to demonstrate the influence of one function on the other, for example the rate of lipid digestion following the rate of gastric emptying (32). The use of carbon-13 as the sole label to measure gastric emptying as well as orocecal transit time in a single test is under current investigation (see later).
2. Patients can serve as their own controls. For example, to demonstrate a dose-response relation of a prokinetic drug on gastric emptying or orocecal transit (33), or to investigate the digestibility of pretreated food (34). Under these conditions, interindividual variations such as differences in CO_2 production, gastric emptying, and so on, which can influence the test results, are excluded.
3. When several tests are used to monitor different functions in the same patient. In cases such as cystic fibrosis, breath tests could be used to assess the absorption of carbohydrates, lipids, and proteins and to monitor liver function and gastrointestinal transit. In this way, it may also be possible to optimize pulmonary function. The breath tests can be complemented by other functional tests based on the use of stable isotopes, including the measurement of energy expenditure. Once suitable instruction has been given, all these tests can be done at home without discomfort to the patient.

$^{13}CO_2$ BREATH TESTS IN NUTRITIONAL AND PHARMACEUTICAL RESEARCH

Lipids

The test molecule of choice is the 1,3 distearyl-2,[^{13}C]octanoyl glycerol, also called "mixed triglyceride" ([^{13}C]MTG) (13,14). The marker is incorporated in the lipid phase of the meal, which is taken in the morning. The test lasts 6 hours and every 30 minutes a breath sample is obtained. After 4 hours, a light meal is allowed. This does not affect the test results.

Figure 3 shows the mean $^{13}CO_2$ excretion curves in normal individuals and in patients with pancreatic insufficiency receiving different pharmacologic treatments. The curves are the averaged results from five subjects (unpublished observations). Curve 1 shows $^{13}CO_2$ excretion in normal individuals after a [^{13}C]-labeled breakfast (chocolate paste incorporating [^{13}C]MTG). Curve 4 shows $^{13}CO_2$ excretion when patients with pancreatic insufficiency had the same meal. When enzyme replacement therapy is given with the meal, improvement is seen in lipid absorption (curve 3). Maximal recovery of the tracer is obtained when gastric acid secretion is simultaneously inhibited by an Na^+/H^+-adenosine triphosphatase (ATPase) blocker (curve 2), as it is well known that pancreatic lipase is only active at nearly neutral pH. If the environment in the proximal small bowel is acid, enzyme supplementation is relatively ineffective at improving lipid digestion unless the acidity is suppressed.

This test can also be used to study the effect of lipids in relation to:

- Solubilization of lipid in a meal, caloric load, and so on
- Small intestinal conditions that influence lipid assimilation (e.g., transit)
- Inhibition of fat uptake (e.g., the efficiency of lipid assimilation in obesity)

In young children, the [^{13}C]MTG breath test is very useful for monitoring lipid absorption in relation to the composition of formula food and gastric motility. This test is of particular interest in patients with cystic fibrosis. As it can be performed at home, it avoids frequent visits to hospital. It is an elegant method of monitoring the effect of food composition or doses of enzyme supplements on lipid absorption without having to perform stool collections (35–37).

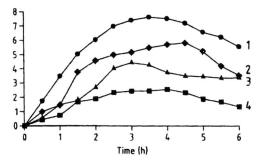

FIG. 3. [^{13}C] mixed triglyceride breath test to demonstrate duodenal lipase activity.

Carbohydrates

To measure the degree and rate of carbohydrate absorption, advantage is taken of the fact that carbohydrates originating from maize or cane are [^{13}C]-enriched naturally by 0.02% (10). This apparently low percentage of enrichment is nevertheless sufficient to allow measurement of [^{13}C] enrichment in the breath with high accuracy.

The carbohydrate most abundantly present in human food is starch. One of the factors that plays a major role in starch assimilation is the physicochemical nature of the test molecule. Its chemical nature is determined by its amylose or amylopectin structure; its physical nature is influenced by pretreatment, specially by heat pretreatment. Heat treatment (gelatinization) has positive effects on the assimilation of starch. Gelatinized starch is more rapidly digested and absorbed than crystalline starch. Branched starch (amylopectin) is much better assimilated than starch with linear configuration (amylose) (38).

In patients with pancreatic insufficiency, starch is less well absorbed than in normal individuals (12). To eliminate the effect of impaired glucose metabolism, correction for glucose oxidation is necessary, as endocrine pancreatic function may also be disturbed. Thus, it is necessary to compare measurements of $^{13}CO_2$ excretion in normal controls and in patients after ingestion of a test meal containing [^{13}C]glucose. Even when these corrections are applied, measurement of starch digestion and absorption remains a test of relatively low sensitivity in demonstrating exocrine pancreatic insufficiency.

The $^{13}CO_2$ breath tests are well suited for monitoring inhibition of starch hydrolysis by acarbose, an inhibitor of brush border alpha-glucosidase (39). The resulting $^{13}CO_2$ excretion curve resembles the malabsorption that occurs in pancreatic failure. Similar changes in $^{13}CO_2$ excretion curves have been obtained in cases where lipid or protein absorption have been inhibited.

Carbohydrates and Fermentation in the Colon: H_2 Excretion in Breath

Malabsorption of carbohydrates in the small intestine results in an increased influx of undigested material in the colon. Bacteria in the colonic lumen metabolize the carbohydrate moiety to short chain fatty acids and gases (40). The most prominent gas is hydrogen, which partly leaves the body in the breath. This phenomenon has been used to demonstrate bacterial overgrowth in the small intestine (41), to measure orocecal transit time (42), and most often to measure carbohydrate malabsorption (43). The combination of $^{13}CO_2$ and H_2 breath tests has the additional advantage that they demonstrate the fate of carbohydrates in foods, such as lactose (11), fructose (44), or carbohydrate-related food additives (45). In daily practice for the diagnosis of lactose absorption or lactose intolerance, both $^{13}CO_2$ and H_2 are measured. The same test procedure is applied to demonstrate sucrose malabsorption.

The metabolic fate of food additives (e.g., sorbitol or xylitol) or of prebiotics (e.g., inulin, polyfructoses) can also be monitored in this way.

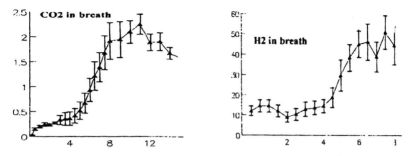

FIG. 4. Evolution of $^{13}CO_2$ and H_2 in breath after the intake of ^{13}C-inulin.

Figure 4 shows how, by measuring $^{13}CO_2$ after the intake of labeled inulin, information can be obtained on energy salvage from nonabsorbable carbohydrates (46). The similar H_2 (right panel) and $^{13}CO_2$ excretion suggests that the $^{13}CO_2$ output is most probably derived from the oxidative metabolism of short chain fatty acids originating from anaerobic bacterial metabolism in the colon.

It has been argued that malabsorption of carbohydrates might be quantified by measuring breath H_2 output after a standardized intake of inulin or lactulose. This method has been abandoned, however, as quantitative measurement of the cumulative excretion of hydrogen over a long period of time is imprecise.

Proteins

Proteins are very important food constituents. Previously, intensive studies have been undertaken to explore the dynamics of various amino acids in the body using stable isotopes. However, few reports have been made on the absorption of proteins or on their metabolic fate in the colon in cases of protein malabsorption. The reason for this is mainly that no reliable substrate was available for monitoring the gastrointestinal events that take place when proteins are taken orally. Our group has described a technique by which it has become possible to incorporate [^{2}H], [^{13}C], or [^{15}N] amino acids, or combinations of these, into eggs in a reproducible way (47). In an extensive study (48), Evenepoel investigated different aspects of the fate of ingested proteins in the gastrointestinal tract. In an initial series of experiments, the gastric phase was studied in relationship to protein digestion. Fig. 5 shows how gastric emptying precedes protein digestion in normal individuals. Protein assimilation follows the delivery of the gastric chyme to the duodenum. Simultaneous measurement of both intestinal functions became possible by using a combination of [^{14}C] and [^{13}C] tracers (48).

In a second experiment, we investigated the influence of the gastric phase and the role of acidity on protein digestion. Predigestion of proteins begins in the stomach under the influence of gastric acid, pepsinogen being converted to pepsin. In clinical practice, it is common for acid secretion in the stomach to be suppressed by H_2 blockers. How does this influence protein digestion? Our experiments show that

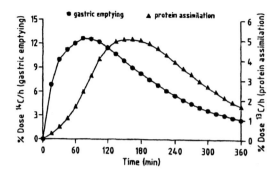

FIG. 5.   Rate of protein digestion following the rate of gastric emptying.

proton pump inhibition does not cause any change in gastric emptying. However, the rate of protein absorption is delayed by approximately 30% when gastric pre-digestion does not take place normally (49).

Food pretreatment also has a marked influence on the rate of protein absorption. Raw egg white leaves the stomach very rapidly, but the digestive phase of raw egg is seriously disturbed: after 6 hours of observation, only one third had been assimilated in comparison with cooked egg. In summary, after ingestion of raw egg, gastric emptying takes half the time it does with cooked egg, but assimilation is three times slower (34).

The application of this technique in ileostomy patients also allows the differentiation between endogenous and exogenous ileal effluents (34).

The most important aspect of our studies on the fate of proteins in the gastrointestinal tract has been the validation of a $^{13}CO_2$ breath test to demonstrate the absorption of proteins. Average values for $^{13}CO_2$ excretion in the breath of normal individuals have been obtained. The amount of the tracer recovered in the breath is markedly diminished in patients with exocrine pancreatic insufficiency. Serum concentrations of [^{13}C]leucine have also been determined. As expected, in the normal individual, the increase of [^{13}C]leucine in the serum following a protein meal precedes the excretion of $^{13}CO_2$ in the breath. In patients with pancreatic insufficiency, serum values are significantly lower than in normal controls. Differences between $^{13}CO_2$ excretion in the breath of normal individuals and in patients have been validated by intestinal perfusion studies and the quantitative recovery of trypsin activity after hormonal stimulation of the pancreas (15). The breath test is promising in monitoring the assimilation of protein from food and in demonstrating the effect of enzyme replacement therapy in cases of exocrine pancreatic insufficiency.

Until now, proteins have been labeled with [^{13}C]leucine only. Additional labeling with [^{15}N]leucine and [ring-$^2H_4$]tyrosine has been shown to be important in detecting protein malabsorption by measuring [^{15}N] losses in the stool (17). This is the only way to differentiate between nitrogen losses originating from exogenous and endogenous sources, not taking into account the recirculating nitrogen pool. The recovery of the [^{2}H$_4$] marker as ring-labeled phenolic compounds in the urine is a reliable way of measuring the degree of fermentation of proteinaceous compounds in the colon (17). Knowledge of this variable might be of value in controlling the formation of toxic compounds in the colon following dietary intake of proteins (50).

To summarize, the technique of multiple labeling of egg white proteins has made it possible to measure the digestion and absorption of proteins in the small intestine, their degree of fermentation in the large bowel, and their loss in the stools.

GASTROINTESTINAL TRANSIT: GASTRIC EMPTYING AND OROCECAL TRANSIT

The rate at which food passes through the gastrointestinal tract is important in determining the nutritional value of food and the extent to which food components are subject to bacterial fermentation in the colon. Whatever the type of food, transit is always subject to complicated feedback mechanisms, either by control of target receptor cells or by direct neural or hormonal regulators. The process starts before food has been taken, as smell, taste, color, consistency, environment, and feelings of satiety have important effects on gut activity and function—the cephalic phase of food assimilation. The influence of these factors is reflected in gastric emptying and orocecal transit time.

Gastric Emptying

Gastric emptying determines the rate at which food is delivered to the duodenum. It is a codeterminant of food acceptability and food assimilation. Breath tests for gastric emptying can be represented in their most simple form by the data shown in Fig. 6. This figure shows gastric emptying in an individual after the intake of a liquid meal (curve 1), a solid meal with same energy content as the liquid meal (curve 2), and a solid meal with twice the energy density (curve 3). This method has multiple applications for food and pharmaceutical research (33,51–53). In com-

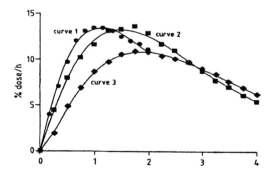

FIG. 6. Typical $^{13}CO_2$ excretion pattern, showing the rate of gastric emptying.

bination with other breath tests, it is an elegant way of showing how the digestion of lipid, carbohydrate, and protein is influenced by gastric emptying when food conditions are altered (by varying their composition, viscosity, consistency, energy density, and so on).

Orocecal Transit

Orocecal transit time (OCTT) is the time needed for food to pass from the mouth to the cecum. It defines the moment when assimilation of food ingredients by the host ceases and the breakdown process by bacteria in the colon begins. Orocecal transit time is determined by the use of a molecule, lactose ureide, in which the urea moiety is labeled with ^{13}C. When also marked with a [^{15}N] tracer, the molecule is very well suited to monitoring the fermentation of N compounds in the colon. The rationale for the use of this molecule is that it is not absorbed in the small intestine, but is well fermented by bacteria in the colon. The method has been evaluated using radioscintigraphy (6). This $^{13}CO_2$ breath test offers many advantages in exploring pharmacologic modulation of the principal gastrointestinal functions of the proximal intestine (54).

Figure 7 shows how gastric and small intestinal transit can be measured in a single experiment (i.e., gastric emptying and orocecal transit time) by measuring the output of $^{13}CO_2$ in the breath (55). The development of appropriate mathematical methods (see later) made it possible to apply this technique of combined breath tests over a wide range of experimental conditions.

In the curve in Fig 7, only the [^{13}C] label is shown and no data are given on the fate of the [^{15}N] tracer from lactose-[^{15}N]ureide. This molecule is very suitable for monitoring the fate of bacterial N metabolites in the colon. Fig. 8 shows clearly the effect of providing a nonabsorbable carbohydrate (lactulose) with a meal: short chain fatty acids are generated from the carbohydrates by bacterial fermentation, which

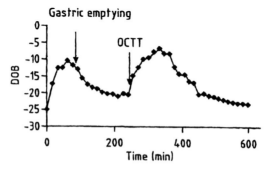

FIG. 7.   Measurement of gastric emptying and orocecal transit time (OCTT) in a single experiment.

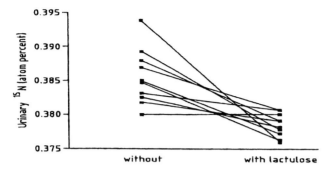

FIG. 8. Monitoring the removal of bacterial N compounds from the body by urinary lactose-[^{15}N]ureide following supplementation of a meal with lactulose.

in combination with [^{15}N] compounds (ammonia, urea, and so on) are utilized by colonic bacteria for cell division. This results in less ^{15}NH$_3$ being delivered to the liver and, consequently, less [^{15}N]-labeled compounds are found in urine (16). This biological system is the key mechanism in avoiding overload of NH$_3$ in cases of hepatic encephalopathy. Lactose-[^{15}N]ureide can be considered a ''biological endo-scope'' for the study of N compounds in the human large intestine.

^{13}CO$_2$ BREATH TESTS IN PEDIATRICS

A need exists for noninvasive tests to investigate gastrointestinal and nutritional function in pediatric patients. Clinical problems particular to childhood require prompt and accurate methods of investigation, which are reliable and ethically acceptable. They should serve both for diagnostic purposes and also for assessing the effects of treatment. The use of ^{13}C offers the possibility of applying ^{13}CO$_2$ breath tests in infants and children, because their noninvasive nature makes them ideally suited for these patients. Another advantage of these noninvasive tests is that they can be performed in the ambulatory patient or at the bedside. It is not necessary for infants to be transported or to stay in hospital.

Methods of performing breath tests in children are currently being investigated in the Department of Pediatrics, Gastroenterology and Nutrition at the Catholic University of Leuven under the supervision of Professor Dr. G. Veereman-Wauters in collaboration with Dr. M. Van Den Driessche. In the pediatric population, the test meal is of particular importance. Children and infants need meals that taste good, look nice, and can be adapted to all age groups. Standardization of the methodology and the test meal is a key factor for success. Most of the breath tests described above have been adapted for use in children, even in preterm infants, and others are subject to ongoing research (5,35,37,55–60).

MATHEMATICAL ANALYSIS OF RESULTS, OBTAINED BY $^{13}CO_2$ BREATH TESTS

Mathematics are the most common way to express results obtained by instrumental analysis. In science mathematics fulfill the same role as words in philology, as expressed by the French philosopher Boileau (1638–1711):

"Ce qui se conçoit bien, s'énonce clairement et les mots pour le dire arrivent aisément."

Relating this statement to breath tests, one could say:

"A well conceived breath test provides those results which can easily be represented by a mathematical formula."

The $^{13}CO_2$ breath tests lend themselves particularly well to mathematical expression as they show a dynamic event over the course of time. A $[^{13}C]$-labeled substrate undergoes a series of steps before the labeled carbon isotope is excreted in breath as $^{13}CO_2$. In breath tests, the function or enzyme activity under investigation is the rate-limiting step, and any variable derived from the breath test curve will reflect the condition of this rate-limiting step. In breath tests for measuring gastrointestinal transit, it is important to obtain precise data describing the process under study alone, unaffected by the influence of any other steps in the complete process undergone by the marker molecule. In general, the problem is to isolate or separate the step of interest from all the other events. This has been done successfully in the case of gastric emptying (21). The unraveling of the rate-limiting step by mathematical analysis is still ongoing. A process of consecutive steps in which an entity undergoes an event resulting from a previous event in cascade may be described mathematically as a convolution. In a convolution, any part of the end result at a well-defined time needs that same amount of time to run through the two consecutive steps that make up the process. The total process is the sum of all the parts needing this total time, divided in any possible way over the separate steps. The action of isolating one of two events from the total is the reciprocal of convolution, called the "deconvolution." Deconvolution can be performed numerically. Separate events can be expressed as mathematical functions, so that the total process can also be expressed mathematically (61,62). This opens the way for the demonstration of physiologic or biochemical processes by unequivocal mathematical equations (8,21,54,63).

USE OF BREATH TESTS IN THE SEARCH FOR FUNCTIONAL FOODS

Many ways are found in which the methods described above could be used in food technology. These include monitoring food modifications to improve (or to inhibit) digestibility and absorption of food components; changing food composition to enhance energy uptake, protein quality, glycemic index, lipid profile, and so on; and testing foods that have been modified to improve their acceptability (the cephalic phase) by altering their consistency, smell, viscosity, and so forth.

New food technology can be directed toward the development of functional foods in relation to substrate utilization (64). One of the possibilities for making food functional is to add or increase the concentration of a component with beneficial biological effects. These effects can be directed toward a function (e.g., immunologic or antioxidant) or toward a specific organ. The gastrointestinal tract is the main target organ for the development of functional foods (65). In gastroenterology, special attention is paid to the colon as the target organ for functional foods: the food then becomes a *colonic food* (i.e., a food ingredient not absorbed in the small intestine that reaches the colon and has health-enhancing properties). The human colon is an ecosystem, maintaining an equilibrium between harmful and beneficial bacteria, and between carbohydrates and proteins as substrates for bacterial fermentation (40). These balances are interlinked: excessive fermentation of proteins can yield toxic compounds (even co-carcinogens), whereas fermentation of carbohydrates by beneficial bacteria generates metabolites that are beneficial for the host. The former group includes ammonia, amines, mercaptanes, and phenolic compounds, whereas beneficial metabolites mainly consist of the short chain fatty acids, among which butyric acid constitutes an important metabolic fuel for colonic cells.

Colonic food that selectively promotes the growth of beneficial bacterial strains is called a *prebiotic food*. Polysaccharoses, specially polyfructoses (inulin), are considered to be prebiotics. Prebiotics are likely to have distinct advantages: stimulation of lactobacilli and bifidobacteria, production of short chain fatty acids, and removal of toxic compounds. Colonic food can also consist of viable bacteria, mainly lactobacillus strains; this is called *probiotic* food (66).

To investigate the potential of functional food, it is necessary to exert control over the main gastrointestinal functions. However, the gastrointestinal tract is a closed system with many different functions and it is inaccessible to direct investigation without disturbing normal physiologic events. $^{13}CO_2$ breath tests and the use of stable isotopes could be of great help in solving these problems. They allow measurement of the digestive and absorptive capacity of the small intestine, to demonstrate gastric emptying and small intestinal transit and to monitor metabolites formed by bacterial fermentation in the colon. These *in vivo* investigations can be completed by careful analysis of the feces for losses of food components, variations in bacterial population, and incorporation of tracers by bacteria. The proposed methods are noninvasive for the individual and risk free. They can be repeated as many times as necessary and, by centralizing the analytic unit, interlaboratory research is easily set up. Clinical investigation protocols can be established for the study of functional food in chronically ill patients with diseases confined to the gastrointestinal tract, especially the colon, such as constipation, ulcerative colitis, colon cancer, Crohn's ileitis, and gastrointestinal fistulas. Patients with diseases that do not depend primarily on colonic events may also benefit from a healthy gastrointestinal environment, particularly patients with uremia.

GENERAL CONCLUSIONS

Our digestion-absorption laboratory in Leuven uses $^{13}CO_2$ breath tests to monitor a wide range of gastrointestinal and hepatic functions. In collaboration with clinicians, these tests are proven to be useful in medical practice. They are also well suited to applications in nutritional and pharmaceutical research. Combined with the administration of molecules labeled with stable isotopes, $^{13}CO_2$ breath tests are a promising development in studies of general metabolism.

The mathematical expression of the results of breath tests is a new area for development and application. Mathematics is a welcome way for physiologists to demonstrate how scientific procedures can give reliable results.

REFERENCES

1. Mion F, Queneau PE, Rousseau M, Brazier JL, Paliard P, Minaire Y. Aminopyrine breath test: development of a ^{13}C breath test for quantitative assessment of liver function in humans. *Hepatogastroenterology* 1995; 42: 931–8.
2. Berry GT, Nissim I, Mazur AT, *et al. In vivo* oxidation of ^{13}C galactose in patients with galactose-1-phosphate uridyltransferase deficiency. *Biochem Mol Med* 1995; 56: 158–65.
3. Lauterburg BH, Grattagliano I, Gmur R, Stalder M, Hildebrand P. Noninvasive assessment of the effect of xenobiotics on mitochondrial function in human beings: studies with acetylsalicylic acid and ethanol with the use of the carbon 13–labeled ketoisocaproate breath test. *J Lab Clin Med* 1995; 125: 378–83.
4. Maes BD, Ghoos YF, Geypens BJ, *et al.* Combined carbon 13–glycine/carbon-14-octanoic acid breath test to monitor gastric emptying rates of liquids and solids. *J Nucl Med* 1994; 35: 824–31.
5. Veereman-Wauters G, Ghoos Y, van der Schoor S, *et al.* The ^{13}C-octanoic acid breath test: a noninvasive technique to assess gastric emptying in preterm infants. *J Pediatr Gastroenterol Nutr* 1996; 23: 111–17.
6. Heine W, Berthold H, Klein P. A novel stable isotope breath test: ^{13}C-labeled glycosyl ureides used as noninvasive markers of intestinal transit time. *Am J Gastroenterol* 1995; 90: 93–8.
7. Geypens B, Bennink R, Peeters M, *et al.* Validation of the lactose-(^{13}C)ureide breath test for determination of orocecal transit time. *J Nucl Med* 1999; 40: 1451–5.
8. Geypens B, Maes B, Ghoos Y, Luypaerts A, Rutgeerts P. Correlation of ileal emptying calculated from simultaneous application of two breath tests. *Gastroenterology* 1998; (suppl 114): G3114.
9. Perri F, Ghoos YF, Maes BD, *et al.* Gastric emptying and *Helicobacter pylori* infection in duodenal ulcer disease. *Dig Dis Sci* 1996; 41: 462–8.
10. Ghoos Y, Hiele M, Rutgeerts P, Vantrappen G. Use of naturally ^{13}C-enriched substrates for the study of carbohydrates and protein assimilation by means of $^{13}CO_2$-breath tests. In: Baillie TA, Jones JR, eds. *Synthesis and application of isotopically labelled compounds.* Amsterdam: Elsevier, 1988: 693–8.
11. Hiele M, Ghoos Y, Rutgeerts P, Vantrappen G, Carchon H, Eggermont E. $^{13}CO_2$ breath test using naturally ^{13}C-enriched lactose for detection of lactase deficiency in patients with gastrointestinal symptoms. *J Lab Clin Med* 1988; 112: 193–200.
12. Hiele M, Ghoos Y, Rutgeerts P, Vantrappen G. Starch digestion in normal subjects and patients with pancreatic disease, using a $^{13}CO_2$ breath test. *Gastroenterology* 1989; 96: 503–9.
13. Ghoos YF, Vantrappen GR, Rutgeerts PJ, Schurmans PC. A mixed-triglyceride breath test for intraluminal fat digestive activity. *Digestion* 1981; 22: 239–47.
14. Vantrappen GR, Rutgeerts PJ, Ghoos YF, Hiele MI. Mixed triglyceride breath test: a noninvasive test of pancreatic lipase activity in the duodenum. *Gastroenterology* 1989; 96: 1126–34.
15. Evenepoel P, Geypens P, Geboes K, Rutgeerts P, Ghoos Y. ^{13}C-egg white breath test: a non-invasive test of pancreatic trypsin activity in the small intestine. *Gut* 2000; 46: 52–7.
16. Geypens B, Evenepoel P, Peeters M, Luypaerts A, Rutgeerts P, Ghoos Y. Direct demonstration of the effect of lactulose on colonic bacterial metabolism by application of lactose-($^{13}C,^{15}N$)-ureide breath test. *Gastroenterology* 1998; (suppl 114): L0196.
17. Evenepoel P, Geypens P, Geboes K, Rutgeerts P, Ghoos Y. Amount and rate of egg protein escaping assimilation in the small intestine of humans. *Am J Physiol* 1999; 277: G935–43.
18. Vantrappen G, Janssens J, Hellemans J, Ghoos Y. The interdigestive motor complex of normal subjects and patients with bacterial overgrowth of the small intestine. *J Clin Invest* 1977; 59: 1158–61.
19. Rutgeerts P, Ghoos Y, Vantrappen G, Eyssen H. Ileal dysfunction and bacterial overgrowth in patients with Crohn's disease. *Eur J Clin Invest* 1981; 11: 199–206.

20. Hellemans J, Joosten E, Ghoos Y, *et al.* Positive $^{14}CO_2$ bile acid breath test in the elderly people. *Age Ageing* 1984; 13: 138–43.
21. Maes BD, Mys G, Geypens BJ, Evenepoel P, Ghoos YF, Rutgeerts PJ. Gastric emptying flow curves separated from carbon-labeled octanoic acid breath test results. *Am J Physiol* 1998; 275: G169–75.
22. Geypens B, Luypaerts A, Maes B, Ghoos Y, Rutgeerts P. Double convolution of breath tests to assess the pharmacological modulation by cisapride of proximal gastrointestinal tract. *Gastroenterology* 1999; (suppl 116): G4332.
23. Go VLW, Hofmann A, Summerskill WHJ. Simultaneous measurements of total pancreatic, biliary, and gastric outputs in man using a perfusion technique. *Gastroenterology* 1970; 48: 321–8.
24. Dalqvist A, Hammond J, Crane R, Dunphy J, Littman A. Intestinal lactase deficiency and lactose intolerance in adults: preliminary report. *Gastroenterology* 1963; 45: 488–91.
25. Hamilton I, Wormsley B, Cobden I, Cooke E, Shoesmith J, Axon A. Simultaneous culture of saliva and jejunal aspirates in the investigation of small bowel bacterial overgrowth. *Gut* 1982; 23: 847–50.
26. Cohen M, Barhm A. Enteroscopy and enteroclysis: the combined procedure. *Am J Gastroenterol* 1989; 84: 1413–15.
27. Caride V, Prokop E, Troncale F, Buddoura W, Winchenbach K, McCallum R. Scintigraphic determination of small intestinal transit time: comparison with the hydrogen breath technique. *Gastroenterology* 1984; 86: 714–20.
28. Kreuning J, Bosman F, Kuiper G, Wal A, Lindeman J. An endoscopic and histopathological study of 50 volunteers. *J Clin Pathol* 1978; 36: 69–77.
29. Bolondi L, Caletti G, Casanova P, Villanacci V, Grigioni W, Labo G. Problems and variations in the interpretation of ultrasound feature of normal upper and lower GI tract wall. *Scand J Gastroenterol* 1986; 123: 16–26.
30. Oliveira R, Baffa O, Troncon LA, Miranda J, Cambrea C. Evaluation of a biomagnetic technique for measurement of orocaecal transit time. *Eur J Gastroenterol Hepatol* 1996; 8: 491–5.
31. Ghoos Y, Coward A, co-ordinators. Clinical application of stable isotopes, BIOMED PL93-1239 project. *Gut* 1998; 43 (suppl 3) S1–S30.
32. Maes BD, Ghoos YF, Geypens BJ, Hiele MI, Rutgeerts PJ. Relation between gastric emptying rate and rate of intraluminal lipolysis. *Gut* 1996; 38: 23–7.
33. Maes B, Ghoos Y, Geypens B, Hiele M, Rutgeerts P. Influence of octreotide on gastric emptying of solids and liquids in normal healthy volunteers. *Aliment Pharmacol Ther* 1995; 9: 11–18.
34. Evenepoel P, Geypens B, Luypaerts A, *et al.* Digestibility of cooked and raw egg protein in humans as assessed by stable isotope techniques. *J Nutr* 1998; 128: 1716–22.
35. De Boeck K, Delbeke I, Eggermont E, Veereman-Wauters G, Ghoos Y. Lipid digestion in cystic fibrosis: comparison of conventional and high-lipase enzyme therapy using the mixed triglyceride breath test. *J Pediatr Gastroenterol Nutr* 1998; 26: 408–18.
36. Lorentz D, Grössle R, Ghoos Y, *et al.* Veränderungen der ^{13}C-Triglyzerid Resorption im Dündarm nach ileoanalem Pouch. In: Schumpelick V, Schippers E, eds. *Pouch, Grundlagen, Funktion, Technik, Ergebniss.* Berlin: Springer Verlag, 1998: 485–91.
37. Van Den Driessche M, Van Malderen M, Geypens B, Ghoos Y, Veereman-Wauters G. Lactose [^{13}C]ureide breath test: A new, noninvasive technique to determine orocecal transit time in children. *J Pediatr Gastroenterol Nutr* 2000; 31: 433–8.
38. Hiele M, Ghoos Y, Rutgeerts P, Vantrappen G, de Buyser K. $^{13}CO_2$ breath test to measure the hydrolysis of various starch formulations in healthy subjects. *Gut* 1990; 31: 175–8.
39. Hiele M, Ghoos Y, Rutgeerts P, Vantrappen G. Effects of acarbose on starch hydrolysis. Study in healthy subjects, ileostomy patients and *in vitro*. *Dig Dis Sci* 1992; 37: 1057–64.
40. Cummings J, MacFarlane G. A review: the control and consequences of bacterial fermentation in the human colon. *J Appl Bacteriol* 1991; 70: 443–59.
41. Kerlin P, Wong L. Breath hydrogen testing in bacterial overgrowth of the small intestine. *Gastroenterology* 1988; 95: 982–8.
42. Gorard D, Libby G, Farthing F. Effect of tricyclic antidepressant on small bowel motility in health and diarrhea-predominant irritable bowel syndrome. *Dig Dis Sci* 1995; 40: 86–95.
43. Levitt M, Hirsch P, Fetzer C, Sheahan M, Levin A. H_2 excretion after ingestion of complex carbohydrates. *Gastroenterology* 1987; 85: 589–95.
44. Hoekstra JH, van den Aker JH, Kneepkens CM, *et al.* Evaluation of $^{13}CO_2$ breath test for the detection of fructose malabsorption. *J Lab Clin Med* 1996; 127: 303–9.
45. Hiele M, Ghoos Y, Rutgeerts P, Vantrappen G. Metabolism of erythritol in humans: comparison with glucose and lactitol. *Br J Nutr* 1993; 69: 169–76.

46. Hiele M. *Assimilation and malabsorption of nutritional carbohydrates in humans* [Doctoral thesis]. University of Leuven: Acco Editions, 1990.

47. Evenepoel P, Hiele M, Luypaerts A, *et al*. Production of egg proteins, enriched with L-leucine-^{13}C, for the study of protein assimilation in humans using breath test technique. *J Nutr* 1997; 127: 327–31.

48. Evenepoel P. *The study of protein assimilation and fermentation using stable isotope techniques* [Doctoral thesis]. Leuven: Acco Editions, 1997.

49. Evenepoel P, Claus D, Geypens B, *et al*. Evidence for impaired assimilation and increased colonic fermentation of protein, related to gastric acid suppression therapy. *Aliment Pharmacol Ther* 1998; 12: 1011–19.

50. Geypens B, Claus D, Evenepoel P, *et al*. Influence of dietary protein supplements on the formation of bacterial metabolites in the colon. *Gut* 1997; 41: 70–6.

51. Maes B, Hiele M, Geypens B, *et al*. Pharmacological modulation of gastric emptying rate of solids as measured by the carbon labelled octanoic acid breath test: influence of erythromycin and propantheline. *Gut* 1994; 35: 333–7.

52. Maes B, Ghoos Y, Geypens B, Hiele M, Rutgeerts P. Relationship between gastric emptying rate and caloric intake in children compared to adults. *Gut* 1995; 36: 183–8.

53. Maes B, Hiele M, Geypens B, Ghoos Y, Rutgeerts P. Gastric emptying of the liquid, solid and oil phase of a meal in normal volunteers and patients with Billroth II gastrojejunostomy. *Eur J Clin Invest* 1998; 28: 197–204.

54. Geypens B. *Use of lactose ureide labelled with stable isotopes in the study of small intestinal transit and colonic metabolism* [Doctoral thesis]. Leuven: University Press, 1999.

55. Van Den Driessche M, Geypens B, Ghoos Y, Veereman-Wauters G. A new technique to assess gastric emptying and orocecal transit time simultaneously. *JPGN* 1997; 25: 483.

56. van Aalst K, Veereman-Wauters G, van de Schoor S, *et al*. [13]C mengtriglyceride ademtest: een kindvriendelijke methode voor het bepalen van de lipase activiteit. *Tijdschr Gastroenterologie* 1996; 8: 19–29.

57. Van Den Driessche M, Veereman-Wauters G, Devlieger H, Ghoos Y. Comparison of the ^{13}C,octanoic acid breath test with the dilution technique to assess gastric emptying in preterm infants. *J Pediatr Gastroenterol Nutr (submitted)*.

58. Van Den Driessche M, Ghoos Y, Veereman-Wauters G. Gastric emptying in formula fed and breast fed infants measured with the ^{13}C-octanoic acid breath test. *J Pediatr Gastroenterol Nutr* 1999; 29: 46–51.

59. Van Den Driessche M, Van Malderen N, Geypens B, Ghoos Y, Veereman-Wauters G. The lactose-^{13}C ureide breath test to determine orocecal transit time: not applicable in very young children and in newborns. *Gastroenterology* 1999; (suppl 116): G0436.

60. Van Den Driessche M, Hoffman I, Ghoos Y, Veereman-Wauters G. Diagnostic application of [13]CO_2 breath tests in pediatrics. *Gastroenterology* 1999; 116: A107.

61. Jacquez J. System identification and the inverse problem. In: *Compartmental analysis in biology and medicine. Kinetics of distribution of tracer-labeled materials*. Amsterdam: Elsevier, 1972: 102–20.

62. Bracewell RN. Convolution. In: *The Fourier transform and its applications*. Tokyo: McGraw-Hill, 1978: 24–37.

63. Geypens B, Luypaerts A, Maes B, Rutgeerts P, Ghoos Y. Deconvolution of octanoic acid breath test results to produce gastric emptying curves, correlating well with scintigraphy. *Gastroenterology* 1999; 116: G4331.

64. Saris W, Asp N, Björk I, *et al*. Functional food science and substrate metabolism. *Br J Nutr* 1998; 80 (suppl 1): S47–75.

65. Salminen S, Bouley C, Boutron-Ruault M-C, *et al*. Functional food science and gastrointestinal physiology and function. *Br J Nutr* 1998; 80 (suppl 1): S147–71.

66. Roberfroid M. *Non digestible oligosaccharides and prebiotics: two new concepts in nutrition*. Proceedings of First Orafti Research Conference, 1995: 3–16.

DISCUSSION

Dr. Zoppi: You said that it is impossible to distinguish between endogenous and exogenous nitrogen losses. Do you mean that typical metabolic balance studies with stool samples over 3 days are no longer useful?

Dr. Ghoos: If protein is not labeled, such studies are not useful.

Dr. Van-Dael: In your methodology for gastric emptying and orocecal transit time, you need to be sure that the marker is completely equilibrated with the food added to it. Are you 100% sure that octanoic acid is completely equilibrated with the formula, and that on acidification, a phase separation does not occur between the curd and the watery whey phase? If that happened, it would be possible for the lipid fraction to enter the small intestinal system in association with one of these two phases but not the other.

Dr. Ghoos: I am not completely sure, but we studied this using radioscintigraphy. We analyzed each step that occurs between eating the food and expiration of CO_2 in the breath, and we ended up with an almost 100% coincidence between the breath test and radioscintigraphy results. This work was published in the *American Journal of Physiology* (1).

Dr. Mansbach: You said that the treatment of the fat before ingestion has an effect on gastric lipase or on the gastric phase of digestion. Could you elaborate on that?

Dr. Ghoos: I can only deal with this in an indirect way. If triglycerides are mixed in saturated butter fat (i.e., as a solid meal when taken), then practically no labeled CO_2 is in breath until 2 hours after intake of the meal. But, if the same label is incorporated in chocopaste, which is a viscous semiliquid that can be smeared on bread, then labeled CO_2 appears in as short a time as 1 hour.

Dr. Roy: Could you discuss the technique for assessing bacterial overgrowth? Do you rely on early rise versus late rise in the CO_2 in breath, or do you have any markers associated with your stable isotope?

Dr. Ghoos: I have been looking for a breath test for bacterial overgrowth for more than 20 years, but in fact there is none. Using a breath test, discrimination cannot be done between bacterial overgrowth and accelerated small intestinal transit. If you really want to look for bacterial overgrowth, then a tube must be inserted. That is the only way to be sure.

Dr. Lentze: In the early studies on the lactose-ureide test for determining orocecal transit time it was found that when volunteers were given unlabeled lactose-ureide in high dose on day 1 and then given the labeled compound on day 2, the apparent transit time was faster than when the subjects were not preloaded. Has that puzzle been solved?

Dr. Ghoos: Normal flora does not have the capacity to split urea immediately from the lactose molecule. This means that to do the test for orocecal transit time, bacterial enzymatic activity must be activated the day before, so we now give one dose of 500 mg of the unlabeled lactose-ureide the evening before the test (2).

Dr. Koletzko: Would you just comment on the reproducibility or the intraindividual variation of this new test of transit time and protein digestion? Even used as a liver function test, we found reproducibility rather disappointing both in healthy children and in children with liver disease.

Dr. Ghoos: For gastric emptying, the coefficient of variation is 19%, and we are happy with that as it is less than for radioscintigraphy. For orocecal transit time, it is of the same order. Unfortunately, not many studies of orocecal transit time have been done by radioscintigraphy: it is difficult to determine the exact time that the chyme enters the colon using that technique.

Dr. Alpers: CO_2 in the breath is many steps removed from protein digestion and will probably be very dependent on the particular amino acid labeled. You intimated that you have, or are going to have, data in the blood immediately afterward. Do you have those data, is the amino acid still intact, and does that correlate differently or better with the CO_2 excretion? (3).

Dr. Ghoos: With respect to [^{13}C]leucine, in normal individuals, a steep rise in ^{13}C occurs in the serum and about 14 minutes after that the CO_2 excretion peaks. In patients with malabsorption, that steep rise of the ^{13}C does not occur, but it increases more slowly to a plateau value, and the CO_2 peak is less than the plateau value. In patients with pancreatic deficiency, a relatively larger rise is seen in ^{13}C leucine in the blood than would be expected from the expiration of ^{13}C CO_2 in breath. That is the first enigma. The second enigma in malabsorption is that after 6 hours, when the chyme would normallyalready be in the colon, the plateau of ^{13}C in the blood is still present, although CO_2 excretion is practically normal; in fact, the plateau of ^{13}C leucine is higher than found in normal individuals (4). We do not at present understand the reason for these two enigmas. I realize a lot of work remains to be done on the metabolism of these labeled amino acids. Until now, we have been discussing only ^{13}C leucine, but what happens to nitrogen? A very fine review by Reeds in the *Annual Review of Nutrition* relates to the recycling of nitrogen in the gut (5). Anybody interested in nitrogen metabolism in the gut should read it.

Dr. Alpers: But your preliminary results are consistent with the idea that if a large amount of amino acid is taken in that is not needed for protein synthesis, then a lot of it will be transaminated, and so the difference between what is found in the blood and what comes out as CO_2 may be very dependent on the nutritional status of the patient.

Dr. Ghoos: You are right. When investigating the catabolic state of an individual, we cannot use CO_2 and blood analyses alone; we need to combine those tests with other biological markers.

Dr. Seidman: Your data suggested that raw egg proteins are less well digested than cooked egg. What is the mechanism? Have you applied this to other proteins? For example, the proteins in milk are routinely consumed raw.

Dr. Ghoos: Until now, we have not studied milk proteins. As to the mechanism of reduced digestion, consider what happens when you try to pick up a cooked egg and a raw egg in your hand. I think the enzymes in the duodenum have the same problem as you have with your hands.

Dr. Seidman: I think that is too simplistic! Could there be some other explanation than digestion? Is it possible that the subjects who took the raw protein did not tolerate it, and vomited the protein?

Dr. Ghoos: I do not think so. But we are dealing with human beings. And as I mentioned at the start, executing breath tests is not always straightforward. Certainly in cases of malabsorption or intolerance of carbohydrates, abdominal complaints could be provoked, so you need to remain nearby the patient.

REFERENCES

1. Maes B, Mys G, Geypens B, *et al.* Gastric emptying flow curves separated from carbon-labeled octanoic acid breath test results. *Am J Physiol* 1998; 275: G169–75.
2. Geypens B, Bennink R, Peeters M, *et al.* Validation of the lactose-(^{13}C)ureide breath test for determination of orocecal transit time. *J Nucl Med* 1999; 40: 1451–55.
3. Cohn JA, Friedman KJ, Noone PG, *et al.* Relation between mutations of the cystic fibrosis gene and idiopathic pancreatitis. *N Engl J Med* 1998; 339: 653–8.
4. Evenepoel P, Geypens P, Geboes K, Rutgeerts P, Ghoos Y. ^{13}C-egg white breath test: a non-invasive test of pancreatic trypsin activity in the small intestine. *Gut* 2000; 46: 52–7.
5. Fuller MF, Reeds PJ. Nitrogen cycling in the gut. *Annu Rev Nutr* 1998; 18: 385–411.

Gastrointestinal Functions, edited by Edgard E. Delvin and
Michael J. Lentze. Nestlé Nutrition Workshop Series, Pediatric
Program, Vol. 46, Nestec Ltd., Vevey/Lippincott Williams &
Wilkins, Philadelphia © 2001.

Esophageal Dysfunction

Yvan Vandenplas

*Department of Pediatrics, Academy Hospital and Faculty of Medicine, Vrije Universiteit
Brussel, Brussels, Belgium*

The function of the esophagus, the first organ of the digestive tube, appears very simple: it is an anteroposteriorly flattened hollow tube organ that transports material from the mouth into the stomach. However, this requires a very complex swallowing mechanism, lubrication of the swallowed material with saliva and other esophageal secretions, transport into the stomach by peristaltic waves, and prevention of retrograde transport from stomach to mouth. The esophagus is located in the thoracic cavity and enters the abdominal cavity through an opening in the diaphragm. Although short, the intra-abdominal length of the esophagus is important, because the intra-abdominal pressure will cause compression of this part of the esophagus, preventing reflux.

Gastroesophageal reflux (GER), regurgitation, and vomiting are considered to be the most typical, although nonspecific, manifestations of esophageal dysfunction. However, by protecting against excessive postprandial gastric dilatation, GER could also be a feature of normal esophageal function. When GER occurs, nature will try to move any refluxed material that is noxious to the esophageal mucosa out of the esophagus as quickly as possible, both in a downward direction, forcing the refluxed material back into the stomach, and in an upward direction, causing regurgitation and vomiting.

Attempts have been made, although with contradictory conclusions (1,2), to evaluate whether the clinical history or a specific questionnaire may be helpful in selecting infants and children with pathologic GER, as has been considered possible in adults (3).

THE MOUTH: MASTICATION AND SALIVA SECRETION

Mastication is poorly developed in infants. Its importance increases when the food becomes more solid. The major function of mastication is to prepare food mechanically for later transport and the initiation of digestion. No information is available on the influence of mastication on GER, but mastication stimulates the parasympathetic nerves that regulate salivary, gastric, and pancreatic secretion. Chewing gum has been suggested as a treatment for pathologic GER (4).

Saliva has different functions. The larger the volume of saliva, the more the food is lubricated, and the easier esophageal transport becomes. In adults, the volume secreted daily is 1,000 to 1,500 ml. Saliva is principally composed of water (99.5%), but also contains enzymes and salts, especially bicarbonate. Saliva secretion is decreased during sleep; normal adults swallow 600 times during 24 hours, but only 50 times during sleep.

Acetylcholine stimulates the salivary glands (5). Cisapride, a prokinetic drug stimulating acetylcholine release in the myenteric plexus, results in a 45% increase in salivary volume secreted in basal conditions, a 32% increase during mastication, a 53% increase during mechanical stimulation, and a 51% increase during chemical stimulation (5). Cisapride also changes the composition of saliva, increasing the bicarbonate and nonbicarbonate buffers, and the protein, glucoconjugate, and epidermal growth factor (EGF) content (5,6). Inorganic phosphate is increased in the saliva of patients with esophagitis (7). GER stimulates salivary secretion, so-called waterbrash, although this esophagosalivary reflex is mainly effective only in prolonged episodes of GER (4).

Saliva secretion is determined by mastication, by the state of alertness, and by GER itself. Saliva is important in our understanding of the pathophysiology of GER as it stimulates swallowing, thus increasing primary esophageal peristalsis, and its volume and alkaline composition also help to clear the esophagus of refluxed material. However, the role of saliva should not be overestimated: a 90% reduction in saliva secretion in experimental rat models did not increase the development of esophagitis (8).

ANATOMIC STRUCTURE OF THE ESOPHAGUS

As with all other parts of the alimentary tract, the esophagus consists of four layers; however, because of its special function, structural differences exist between the esophagus and the rest of the gastrointestinal tract. The upper esophagus has a stratified squamous epithelium of the nonkeratinizing type, which continues from the pharynx into the esophagus. This type of epithelium protects against any rough material that may be swallowed, but does not protect against acid reflux. The dense connective tissue of the submucosa layer, together with the muscularis mucosa, forms numerous longitudinal mucosal folds that result in an irregular luminal in cross section. The elasticity of the connective tissue of the submucous layer allows these folds to be smoothed out when food is swallowed. In contrast with the remainder of the gastrointestinal tract, the outer and inner layers of the muscularis propria in the upper third of the esophagus are composed of striated muscle. It is only in the lower third that the smooth muscle becomes arranged into an outer longitudinal and an inner circular layer, with a myenteric nerve plexus in between. Many spiral or oblique bundles are found in the inner layer. The longitudinal muscularis bundles of the outer layer are irregularly arranged. The extensive system of neural elements in the muscularis externa is known as the "myenteric plexus of Auerbach." In the submucosa, the neural elements form the submucous plexus of Meissner, which appears at approximately 13 weeks of fetal life. Both plexuses are part of intrinsic neural mechanisms. Extrinsic vagal and sympathetic fibers are also present.

The upper and lower esophageal sphincters are not distinct anatomic structures. The lower esophageal sphincter is an extension of the circular muscle of the esophageal body. In some animals (e.g., the dog and the cat) that spend a great part of their life horizontal, the lower esophageal sphincter is an anatomically discrete sphincter. In humans, the musculature of the sphincter differs from that of the esophageal body, with more impressive length-tension characteristics. The lower esophageal sphincter and the gastric fundus are held in place by a prominent phrenoesophageal membrane—a tough fibroelastic layer attached to the thoracic and abdominal diaphragm and the esophagus within the hiatus. At the junction of the esophagus with the cardia of the stomach is found an abrupt transition from stratified squamous to simple columnar epithelium. Macroscopically, the boundary line between the smooth white mucous membrane of the esophagus and the pink surface of the gastric mucosa appears as a jagged (Z) line.

Connective tissue diseases (e.g., mixed connective tissue disease and scleroderma) often involve the esophagus (9). In patients with familial amyloidosis, it is now thought unlikely that amyloid deposits in the mucosal wall cause increased esophageal stiffness; rather, an autonomic, predominantly vagal, denervation probably best explains the disturbed esophageal function in this disease (10). Similarly, a correlation is seen between esophageal dysmotility and cardiovascular autonomic dysfunction (11). Gastroesophageal dysfunction is a major cause of morbidity and mortality in patients with familial dysautonomia (12).

SWALLOWING

Swallowing is a complex, integrated, continuous act involving somatic and visceral afferent and efferent nerves and their associated striated and smooth muscle (Fig. 1). For simplicity, it can be divided in two distinct phases, oropharyngeal and esophageal. Although the fetus has the ability to swallow by the age of 11 weeks, an effective sucking-swallowing mechanism does not appear before 35 weeks. Nonnutritive sucking develops first; it is characterized by its rapidity, exceeding two sucks per second, which is approximately twice that seen in nutritive sucking. As the change to diversified feeding gradually occurs, the sucking reflexes are repressed, although they can later be reinstalled, as in experienced beer drinkers.

In older children and adults, the initiation of deglutition is under conscious control. However, swallowing also often occurs automatically. Afferent impulses arising from contact between the bolus and the anterior pillars of the pharynx, the base of the tongue, and the soft palate take subsequent events out of conscious control by initiating the swallowing reflex. Dynamic ultrasound techniques can detect tongue incoordination and are especially useful in the objective imaging and identification of tongue thrust in orthodontic patients (13).

Following a swallow, the upper esophageal sphincter relaxes, respiration is inhibited, and the glottis closes as the larynx is drawn forward and upward. The nasopharynx is closed by a combination of elevation of the soft palate and contraction of the

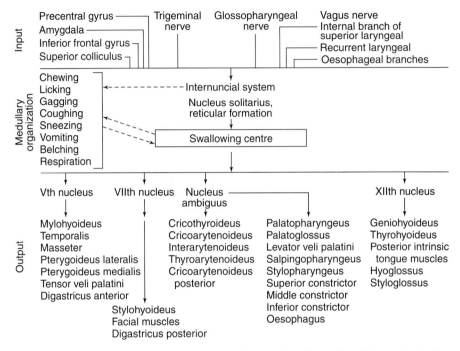

FIG. 1. The complex neuromuscular pattern of swallowing. (Reproduced by permission.)

superior pharyngeal constrictor. The epiglottis tips down, deflecting the bolus laterally and posteriorly away from the larynx. The pharyngeal constrictors contract sequentially, propelling the bolus into the esophagus. The muscles of the esophagus relax and respiration resumes as the upper esophageal sphincter contracts to separate the bolus and the esophagus from the pharynx and the airway. The complex neuromuscular reaction pattern of swallowing involves more than 25 muscle groups (Table 1), controlled by the swallowing center in the brain stem. Although the initiation of swallowing is under voluntary control, it appears impossible to swallow if the pharyngeal afferents are blocked by a local anesthetic. Activation of the swallowing center influences the activities of other centers, most notably the respiratory center, as evidenced by a physiologic apneic pause of 0.5 to 3.5 seconds that accompanies every swallow. Apnea occurs also during belching and vomiting. All these phenomena occur with increased frequency in infants with pathologic GER. This may contribute to the irregular, immature breathing pattern in such infants.

The second or esophageal phase of swallowing, which involves the smooth muscle of the esophageal wall, depends on both central coordination and local intramural neural arcs.

Given the complexity of the swallowing mechanism, it is surprising that dysfunction of this phase does not occur more often; an exception is children with certain neurologic disorders such as cerebral palsy. The large reduction in the swallowing

TABLE 1. *Factors influencing the incidence and noxious effect of gastroesophageal reflux (GER)*

Defense mechanism		Adverse factors
Good	Esophageal clearance (gravity ?)	Delayed
High	Mucosal resistance	Low
High	Lower esophageal sphincter pressure	Low
Long	Abdominal esophagus	Short (hiatus hernia)
Normal	Sphincter position	Dislocated
Acute	Esophagogastric angle	Obtuse
Small	Gastric volume	Large
Normal	Gastric emptying	Delayed
Low	Gastric acid output	High
Low	Pepsin/trypsin/bile salts	High
Low	Intra-abdominal pressure	High
Low	Gastroesophageal reflux	High

rate during sleep can result in delayed esophageal clearance of refluxed material; this would be expected to cause more difficulty for infants than for adults, as they spend more time asleep.

Specific Swallowing Disorders

The *Opitz GBBB syndrome* is characterized by craniofacial and genitourinary abnormalities, swallowing difficulties, esophageal dysfunction, hypotonia, and moderate development delay (14). Frequently, poor deglutition is one of the most striking phenomena. Patients with *globus sensation* have frequent abnormalities such as nonspecific esophageal motor disorders, pharyngoesophageal sphincter dysfunction, pharyngeal stasis, achalasia, and laryngeal penetration or aspiration (15). In esophageal dysfunction, contractions can be of low amplitude, incomplete, or uncoordinated.

OROESOPHAGEAL DYSKINESIA

Weight gain during the first year of life is compromised in many infants. Some investigators call these unexplained feeding disorders ''nonorganic failure to thrive,'' or NOFTT (16,17). The cause of NOFTT is likely to be heterogeneous. Every pediatrician knows infants without any malformations or neurologic deficits but with clearly abnormal sucking, swallowing, and feeding behavior, similar to infants with the Pierre-Robin syndrome. These infants have sucking and swallowing anomalies and esophageal dyskinesia, suggesting that the causative abnormality may be located in the brain stem (18). In most cases, they present with slow feeding (>45 minutes to complete a feed), poor intake, refusal to drink, unexplained and inconsolable crying, and regurgitation and vomiting. During feeding, there may be (micro)aspiration, nasal reflux, and apparent life-threatening events (ALTE). Many infants present with retrognathia and a deep and ogival palate. Early recognition is associated with improved prognosis, even if the cause remains undetermined (19–21). Esophageal peristalsis in children with the Pierre-Robin syndrome is abnormal. Hypertonia of the lower esophageal sphincter or achalasia (insufficient relaxation) has been described in neurovegetative anomalies such as the Pierre-Robin syndrome, ALTE, or hypervagotonia (22,23). Antroduodenal dysmotility has been suggested as the reason why infants with GER tend to refuse feeds. Stress influences the tone of the vagal nerve and may exacerbate symptoms of GER.

ESOPHAGEAL SECRETION

The esophageal glands are irregularly distributed and small, containing only mucous cells. These glands can be detected most often just distal to the upper esophageal sphincter and just proximal to the lower esophageal sphincter. They lubricate the bolus during its passage from the pharynx to the stomach. The bicarbonate-secreting capacity of the human esophagus is small and intrinsic esophageal bicarbonate is unlikely to play an important role in mucosal defense (24). Unlike cisapride, neither omeprazole nor ranitidine affects esophageal bicarbonate secretion (24).

ESOPHAGEAL PERISTALSIS

Swallowing induces a contraction wave that begins at the superior constrictor muscle of the pharynx and sweeps through the striated and smooth muscle to the cardia without interruption. This primary peristaltic contraction pushes a solid bolus down the esophagus into the stomach, taking about 12 seconds in a normal adult. Gravity results in fluids taken in the upright position reaching the cardia before the arrival of the primary peristaltic wave. In the head-down position, fluids are propelled by the esophageal contraction wave. In the resting state between two swallows, the esophagus is closed at both ends by the upper and lower esophageal sphincters. Both the upper sphincter and the lower sphincter relax secondary to deglutition. Transient relaxations of the upper esophageal sphincter occur, and when these occur simultaneously with a transient relaxation of the lower esophageal sphincter, a ''common cavity phenomenon'' is created, resulting in a direct connection between the external world and the stomach. The pressure of the upper esophageal sphincter disappears during sleep, whereas in stress situations and in straining it increases. The activity of the upper esophageal sphincter differs in relation to the kind of material present in the esophagus. It relaxes completely when there is air in the esophagus, as in belching; however, when ingested material or acid refluxes into the esophagus, it normally constricts. Although unproved, it is possible, in patients with chronic aspiration disorders, that the upper esophageal sphincter relaxes instead of contricts secondary to GER.

Secondary peristalsis, which is caused by GER, starts at the highest level in the esophagus reached by the refluxed material. It contributes to clearance of any remnants of the refluxed material that were not cleared by the primary peristaltic wave.

Secondary peristalsis can be produced experimentally by inflation and deflation of an esophageal balloon. Prokinetic agents such as cisapride do not appear to be associated with a greater number or an increased amplitude of secondary peristaltic contractions (25). However, the larger the volume of material refluxed, the greater the amplitude of the secondary waves (25).

Except for their afferent origin, secondary waves are comparable to primary waves. When a subject takes a series of swallows, such as when drinking a glass of water, the upper esophageal sphincter opens and closes at each swallow, whereas the lower esophageal sphincter opens when the first peristaltic wave enters the sphincter, and only closes when the last contraction has passed by. Secondary peristalsis can be inhibited with a swallow. Tertiary peristaltic waves are contractions occurring in the lower smooth muscle segment. These contractions occur spontaneously without any relationship to swallowing or reflux. They do not depend on extrinsic innervation. They can accomplish in quadrupedal animals what gravidity or gravitation does in humans (i.e., clearance of the lower end of the esophagus).

Pain delays esophageal clearance. In adults, normal esophageal transit time takes about 12 seconds, but it takes 25 to 102 seconds if the subject's hand is plunged in iced water. Hot substances increase the speed and amplitude of contractions; cold swallows have the opposite effect.

ESOPHAGEAL INNERVATION AND RECEPTORS

Medullary circuits composed of premotor neurons of the nucleus tractus solitarii are intrinsically capable of generating a rhythmic esophageal motor output, but are subject to powerful modulation by peripheral sensory feedback (26). The role of the vagal nerve endings is still poorly understood. Because all kinds of respiratory symptoms (e.g., wheezing) appear to be related to GER suggests that the vagal nerve endings present in the esophagus and the airways develop simultaneous hyperreactivity secondary to GER.

Three kinds of receptors must be present in the esophagus—mechanical, chemical, and temperature sensitive—although these have not all been convincingly identified anatomically. Under pathologic conditions, receptors become nociceptive, resulting in an increased sensitivity; they then respond with a sensation of pain to physiologic stimuli that normally do not cause pain. In Barrett's esophagus, mucosal sensitivity is decreased (27).

The nociceptors inform the patient about the existence of tissue damage. Two types of afferent neurons have been described: unmyelineated C fibers, responsible for deep burning pain; and delta A fibers, responsible for sharp abrupt pain. Repeated noxious stimuli or one very strong stimulus can sensitize both types of fiber so that typical non-noxious stimuli become very painful. This can result in relatively small esophageal distension secondary to belching, minimal regurgitation, or even the passage of a swallowed food bolus being experienced as very painful. The sensation of pain is transported to the brain by calcitonin gene-related peptide (CGRP) and substance P. Substance P has been studied most extensively; it causes smooth muscle contraction and vasodilatation, with a secondary increase in mucosal permeability. Substance P is released in cases of tissue damage (e.g., with esophagitis), inducing a vicious circle: the more the tissue damage, the more substance P is released and the greater the noxious effect of the refluxed material. Substance P also causes histamine release from the mast cells in the alveoli and, thus, contributes to bronchospasm. The accompanying visceral hyperpalgesia will result in disordered motility, again causing more reflux. All this suggests that pain induced by acid reflux is more likely to be caused by motility phenomena than by the chemical composition of the refluxed material, so treatment should focus on motility.

In the ferret, at least three types of esophageal afferent fibers exist, namely mucosal, tension, and tension/mucosal fibers (28). Vagal efferent neurons respond to gastroesophageal mechanical inputs, and also receive convergent inputs from esophageal acid-sensitive and gastrointestinal bradykinin- and capsaicin-sensitive afferents. Sudden rapid stretch of the mechanoreceptors in the proximal esophagus can trigger the hiccup reflex in normal subjects (29). Only rapid distensions above a determined volume threshold will predictably induce hiccups in a particular subject (29).

ESOPHAGEAL CLEARANCE

Esophageal clearance is influenced by at least three factors: esophageal peristaltic waves, gravity, and saliva (30,31). Esophageal clearance mechanisms are well developed by at least 31 weeks' postmenstrual age (32). Clearance of acid from the esophagus and decreased pressure of the lower esophageal sphincter are the major mechanisms involved in the development of esophagitis (33). The pH of saliva varies from neutral to alkaline. Swallowed saliva contributes to the neutralization of the refluxed acid. Moreover, the bolus effect of swallowed saliva will help in clearing the esophagus of the refluxed material. It seems logical to suppose that gravity also helps to clear the esophagus. The efficacy of positional treatment may be partially related to gravity. The esophagus tends to function normally in healthy controls when they swallow water without gravitational assistance (34). On the other hand, more abnormal contractions (simultaneous, retrograde, and nontransmitted) occur in the upright position than in the supine position (26% and 12%, respectively; $p = .013$) (34). GER most commonly occurs in the seated position, followed by the supine position; it is least common in the prone position.

ESOPHAGEAL MUCOSAL RESISTANCE

The esophageal mucosa has established protective mechanisms that operate within the pre-epithelial, epithelial, and postepithelial compartments. As refluxed acid and pepsin always act from the luminal side of the mucosa, protective factors such as EGF, operating as a part of the pre-epithelial defense, are essential for maintaining the integrity of the esophageal mucosa (35). The resistance of the mucosa to the noxious effects of the refluxed material (e.g., acid, pepsin, chymotrypsin or trypsin, bile) differs from person to person, and is genetically determined. Prostaglandin E_2 and nitric oxide (NO) are said to be protective (in low concentrations) and detrimental (in high concentrations) for esophageal mucosal integrity (36).

Prostaglandins

Prostaglandin E_2 (PGE_2) is the major arachidonic acid metabolite secreted (37). Esophageal perfusion with saline stimulates the secretion of PGE_2, whereas perfusion with acid decreases it. HCl or pepsin infusion causes a further increase in PGE_2 secretion in comparison with saline infusion (6,37,38). PGE_2 decreases the duration of esophageal contractions in healthy volunteers (39). An increase in the rate of salivary PGE_2 excretion during mastication or after mechanical or chemical stimulation suggests that it may have a potential therapeutic effect (6,35). Aspirin renders the esophageal mucosa more permeable to acid and pepsin (40). Prostaglandins are only secreted in the presence of esophageal inflammation (37). These effects, in part, are pH dependent and might be partially reversed by PGE_2 cotherapy (40). The decline in luminal PGE_2 release in healed reflux esophagitis indicates that the increased secretion occurring in active esophageal disease may reflect the mucosal damage induced by HCl or pepsin (40). Inhibition of the rate of luminal release of PGE_2 under the influence of HCl and pepsin may play a role in the development or progression of mucosal damage (41).

Non-steroidal anti-inflammatory drugs (NSAIDs) inhibit the synthesis of prostglandins. As NSAIDs are also reported to have positive effects in animal models of reflux esophagitis, it has been proposed that prostglandins have a deleterious effect in esophagitis (42). This hypothesis could explain the relationship between inflammation and dysmotility (42). However, in the rabbit, PGE_2 has no effect on esophageal mucosal repair (43), although HGF (human growth factor), insulin-like growth factor 1 (IGF-I), and EGF (stimulation), and transforming growth factor β_1 (TGF-β_1) (inhibition) have major effects (43). A study examining PGE_2, $PGF_{2\alpha}$, PGI_2, and thromboxane B_2 (TXB_2) content in esophageal mucosal biopsies from healthy controls and patients with esophagitis showed a difference only for PGI_2 (44). The presence of a murine calcium-sensitive chloride channel in esophageal mucosa suggests the presence of exocrine secretory cells and of transepithelial ion transport (45).

The information presented above can be summarized as follows: PGE_2 (and NO) are protective in low concentrations, whereas in high concentrations they can be harmful (36); in addition, the release of prostaglandins differs in relation to the prostaglandin subtype and according to the composition of the refluxed material (38).

Sex Differences

Severe GER disease (e.g., Barrett's esophagitis) has a male predominance. However, this difference is not found in young infants presenting with uncomplicated reflux disease. Although it was hypothesized that this sex difference is genetically or hormonally mediated, it is likely that lifestyle is a more important determinant.

THE LOWER ESOPHAGEAL SPHINCTER

The lower esophageal sphincter is a functional barrier and represents a zone where the intraluminal pressure is greater than in the stomach and esophagus. In adults, this high pressure zone has a length of 3 to 6 cm and a pressure of approximately 20 mm Hg, ranging between 10 and 40 mm Hg. In infants, its length is only a few millimeters. The lower esophageal sphincter relaxes 2.5 seconds after the initiation of a swallow, well before the arrival of the bolus, and remains open for 10 to 12 seconds, until the bolus has passed through the region. As a rule, increased abdominal pressure is associated with increased sphincter pressure. However, gastric distension not associated with an increased intragastric pressure is accompanied by a fall in lower esophageal sphincter pressure or by inappropriate transient lower esophageal sphincter relaxations (TLESRs), which can last for 10 to 17 seconds. It is believed that these responses are mediated by vagal reflexes. Stimulation of mechanoreceptors in the gastric fundus, or stretching of the gastric fundus, initiates vagosympathetically mediated reflexes resulting in TLESRs.

The lower esophageal sphincter pressure is one of the most classically reported and relevant defense mechanisms against GER, although only 20% of all reflux episodes are associated with decreased resting pressure (33). The lower esophageal sphincter pressure decreases postprandially, both in normal individuals and in patients with GER. Gastric contractions, gastric alkalinization, and protein meals increase the lower esophageal sphincter pressure, as do gastrin, motilin, and substance P. Cord blood gastrin levels are much higher than adult levels, whereas during the first days and weeks of life, gastrin levels are decreased in comparison with adult levels. The role of gastrin in infant regurgitation has not been determined.

Progesterone, atropine (at least in cats), cholecystokinin, glucagon, vasoactive intestinal peptide (VIP), NO, dopamine, secretin, estrogen, mint, and chocolate decrease the pressure of the lower esophageal sphincter. L-arginine, the endogenous source of NO, prolongs TLESRs (46). The type of meal influences the number of reflux episodes and the severity of heartburn, which are increased by red wine and chilli peppers and decreased by fat and chocolate (47). Circulating glucagon and cholecystokinin, which are increased in renal insufficiency, regulate hunger and satiety.

Esophageal balloon dilatation, the presence of fat in the duodenum, nicotine, and alcohol also decrease the lower esophageal sphincter pressure. VIP and NO both induce TLESRs (48). NO also delays gastric emptying (49) and is increased in infants with pyloric stenosis (50), again suggesting that TLESRs are a protective mechanism against gastric overdistension. NO controls several esophageal neuromuscular functions, including relaxation of the lower esophageal sphincter (36), but NO levels were found to be the same in biopsies of normal and inflamed esophageal mucosa (51). On the other hand, nitric oxide synthetase (and cyclooxygenase-2) are involved in the neoplastic progression of Barrett's esophagus (52).

Most reflux episodes occur in relation to TLESRs. TLESRs are also the predominant mechanism of GER in healthy preterm infants (32). TLESRs occur more often in the seated position than in the supine position. Reflux episodes can also occur during periods of prolonged lower esophageal sphincter hypotonia or with pressure drifts, especially in patients with severe esophagitis (53).

Gastric distension and partial or incomplete swallowing induce TLESRs, which are also the normal mechanism for burping and belching. The larger the meal, the more TLESRs occur. Equally, the greater the gastric secretory volume and the higher the intragastric osmolarity, the more TLESRs occur. So TSLERs can be considered protective against overfeeding by enhancing the ''up-clearing'' of the feeds. And it can also be hypothesized that part of the efficacy of proton pump inhibitors and H_2 receptor antagonists is related to a decrease in gastric secretory volume independent of its pH. During sleep, normally no such transient relaxations of the lower esophageal sphincter occur.

All physiologic GER episodes are related to TLESRs, but in patients with severe reflux esophagitis, only 66% of the GER episodes occur in relation to a TLESR. In ''chalasia'' chronic relaxation of the lower esophageal sphincter occurs. In ''achalasia,'' a complete absence of TLESRs is seen. GER is related to reduced lower esophageal sphincter pressure, although not particularly in the resting state. Thus, it is not TLESRs that are pathologic *per se*, but the absence of a control mechanism over this phenomenon. Regurgitation can be considered a natural defense mechanism against overfeeding: when the stomach becomes too distended, TLESRs are induced more frequently, allowing food to flow back into the esophagus.

The major mechanism involved in pathologic GER are TLESRs. However, it is not clear if a decreased resting lower esophageal sphincter pressure should be considered a cause of or a result of GER. It may well be both.

ACHALASIA

Achalasia, which is a complex motor disorder of the entire esophagus, with primary and secondary motility abnormalities of the esophageal body (54), is characterized by a hypertonicity of the sphincter with lack of or incomplete relaxation (55). Achalasia is also associated with extra-esophageal autonomic nervous system dysfunction involving cardiovascular function and the regulation of mesenteric arterial blood flow (56). A lack of NO synthetase in the lower esophageal sphincter, cardia, and gastric fundus is involved in the pathophysiology of cardiac achalasia in children (57). In patients with achalasia, esophageal tonic activity is impaired (58).

INTRA-ABDOMINAL ESOPHAGUS (HIATUS HERNIA)

The crural diaphragm bolsters the lower esophageal sphincter during inspiration, straining, and so on. The intra-abdominal part of the esophagus is very short during the first weeks of life. No data exist on the prevalence of hiatus hernia in children; in adults more than 50 years of age, however, the incidence is reported to be more than 50%. Only 9% of the adults with a hiatus hernia have complaints suggestive of GER pathology. However, 75% of adults with reflux esophagitis also have a hiatus hernia.

The incidence of reflux symptoms in a population with hiatus hernia is low, however, on the other hand, a high incidence of hiatus hernia occurs in adults with reflux symptoms. The reason for this seems to be that the length of the intra-abdominal esophagus is shortened or nonexistent in patients with a hiatus hernia. Thus, the lower esophageal sphincter region is located in the thorax, where it is exposed to a negative pressure and cannot function as a high pressure zone. As a result, gastric contents are aspirated back into the esophagus because of the pressure differences between the abdomen (positive pressure) and the thoracic cavity (negative pressure during inspiration). During the first year of life, the intra-abdominal esophagus is physiologically very short, which contributes to the increased incidence of regurgitation in this age group.

ANGLE OF INDENTATION

Normally, an acute angle is found between the greater curvature of the stomach and the esophagus. In some patients (e.g., those with a hiatus hernia), this angle is obtuse and favors GER episodes. The function of this acute angle is comparable with the function of a valve. It has been hypothesized that the angle is more obtuse in young infants, and only becomes acute after the age of 1 year.

GASTRIC VOLUME; GASTRIC EMPTYING

It is logical to relate gastric volume to the incidence of GER; if the stomach is empty, no material is available to reflux into the esophagus. Gastric electrical abnormalities underlying delayed gastric emptying have been documented in children with severe GER (59). To accommodate the intake of food or liquid, gastric reservoir functions—adaptive and receptive relaxations—are important reflexes (60). *Adaptive relaxation* is a reflex in which the fundus of the stomach dilates in response to small increases in intragastric pressure when food enters the stomach. *Receptive relaxation* is a reflex in which the gastric fundus dilates when food passes down the esophagus. Nitric oxide is involved in both pathways (60). Stretch of the gastric wall activates the mechanoreceptors in the gastric mucosa, inducing the release of NO which causes relaxation of the circular muscle and, thus, of the fundus. Receptive relaxation is mediated by vagal motor fibers. In contrast to the pressure-induced adaptive relaxation, ganglionic nicotinic transmission is essential in the vagally mediated receptive relaxation (60). Phasic relaxations of the lower esophageal sphincter are induced through afferent vagal pathways by stimulation of mechanoreceptors in the fundus of the stomach (61). Children with central nervous system disorders who vomit often have abnormal GER as abnormal gastric motility (62).

In neurologically normal children, gastric dysrhythmias can also play a major role in the pathogenic components of GER (63).

Approximately 50% of adults with GER pathology have delayed gastric emptying. Children with untreated delayed gastric emptying have a doubling of reflux frequency (64). However, preoperative selection of these patients seems extremely difficult (65). The role of the vagal nerve endings in the esophagus could be involved in the mechanism: the esophageal nerve endings are very rapidly ''irritated'' once GER occurs, which increases the local tissue prostaglandin levels, whereas the irritated vagal nerve endings also cause pylorospasm. The NO donor nitroglycerin inhibits pyloric motility, alters the organization but not the number of antral pressure waves, and slows gastric emptying (50). Patients with GER and chronic respiratory disease or GER and failure to thrive present with delayed gastric emptying. The frequency of postprandial GER is related to meal size; gastric bolus feeding causes a greater intragastric pressure increase and more TLESRs. Increasing feed osmolality and volume slows gastric emptying and increases postprandial GER.

Mechanoreceptors are present in the fundus, near to the gastric part of the cardiac region. When these are stimulated because of gastric distension, they induce TLESRs.

GASTRIC ACID OUTPUT

''The more acid is produced, the more acid the gastroesophageal reflux'' seems logical (33). Large variation is seen in the secretion of gastric acid during a 24-hour period, and this is regulated by the vagus nerve (66). The volume secreted may be more relevant than the pH; thus, proton pump inhibitors are very potent in the treatment of esophagitis despite the nocturnal breakthrough of acid secretion.

PEPSIN, TRYPSIN, AND BILE SALTS

The noxious effect of pepsin on the esophageal mucosa is greater than that of acid (67). The effect of bile salts is influenced by the pH of the refluxed material: at acid pH, it is conjugated bile salts that are noxious, whereas at neutral pH it is deconjugated bile salts and trypsin that are noxious (68). Bile salts increase the permeability of the esophageal mucosa to acid (69). For this reason, ''mixed'' reflux (as occurs in regurgitation) may be more noxious to the mucosa than pure acid GER. Both endogenous and exogenous cholecystokinin decrease the lower esophageal sphincter pressure and increase the number of TLESRs (67). Cholestyramine increases gall bladder emptying and the number of TLESRs (67).

INTRA-ABDOMINAL PRESSURE

Intra-abdominal pressure is probably an important, although as yet little studied, mechanism favoring GER. In adults, 17% of the GER episodes are related to transient

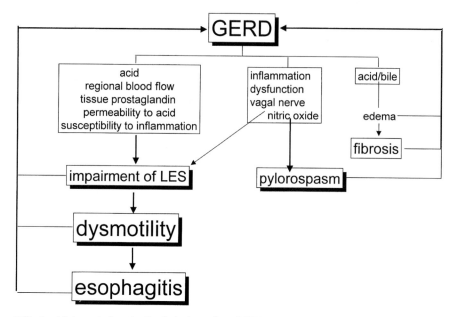

FIG. 2. Vicious circles of reflux inducing reflux. GERD, gastroesophageal reflux disease; LES, lower esophageal sphincter.

increases in intra-abdominal pressure. The role of increased intra-abdominal pressure in children, as with constipation or a tight diaper, has not been evaluated.

GER CAUSING GER

An important mechanism favoring GER is GER itself, because of its effect on the esophageal mucosa, which causes a vicious cycle (Fig. 2): GER contains acid; as a result of the contact of the acid with the esophageal mucosa, regional blood flow increases, which also increases the local tissue content of PGE_2; prostaglandins increase the permeability of the mucosa to acid, which enhances the susceptibility of the mucosa to inflammation; inflammation of the mucosa of the lower part of the esophagus causes impairment of the lower esophageal sphincter (favoring GER), dysmotility of the lower esophageal sphincter (favoring GER), and finally esophagitis; NO aggravates the problem by delaying gastric emptying (49).

Contact of acid with the esophageal mucosa causes irritation, dysfunction, and inflammation of the local vagal nerve endings, impairing the lower esophageal sphincter and causing pylorospasm. Both phenomena favor GER. If the refluxed materials also contain bile, local edema and fibrosis presents in the mucosa.

CONCLUSIONS

Some individuals may be particularly susceptible to the development of pathologic GER for one or a combination of the following reasons: lack of mucus and bicarbonate secretion by surface epithelial cells; lack of defensive enhancement by prostaglandin release; lack of an effective mucous cap after injury; and an apparent failure to heal erosions rapidly by epithelial restitution. A possible mechanism of GER is as follows. The initiating phenomenon may be delayed gastric emptying (e.g., because of overfeeding, overweight, or increased intra-abdominal pressure). Gastric distension then stimulates mechanoreceptors in the gastric wall near the cardia, which has vasovagal effects, resulting in abnormal neural control of the lower esophageal sphincter by the central nervous system. As a consequence, lower esophageal sphincter motility becomes defective, and TLESRs increase. This finally results in defective basal lower esophageal sphincter tone, favoring GER. In the presence of a hiatus hernia, GER will be further facilitated. Ineffective acid clearance (inadequate neutralization of the pH by saliva and inefficient volume clearance by poor motility) enhances the noxious effect of the refluxed material. Finally, poor mucosal resistance, which is partially genetically determined, contributes to the development of reflux esophagitis.

REFERENCES

1. Orenstein SR, Shalaby TM, Cohn J. Reflux symptoms on 100 normal infants: diagnostic validity of the infant gastroesophageal reflux questionnaire. *Clin Pediatr* 1996; 35: 607–14.
2. Heine RG, Jaquiery A, Lubitz L, Cameron DJ, Catto-Smith AG. Role of gastro-oesophageal reflux in infant irritability. *Arch Dis Child* 1995; 71: 121–5.
3. Carlsson R, Dent J, Bolling-Sternevald E, *et al.* The usefulness of a structured questionnaire in the assessment of symptomatic gastroesophageal reflux disease. *Scand J Gastroenterol* 1998; 33: 1023–9.
4. von Schonfeld J, Hector M, Evans DF, Wingate DL. Oesophageal acid and salivary excretion: is chewing gum a treatment option for gastro-oesophageal reflux? *Digestion* 1997; 58: 111–14.
5. Goldin GF, Marcinkiewicz M, Zbroch T, *et al.* Esophagoprotective potential of cisapride. An additional benefit for gastroesophageal reflux disease. *Dig Dis Sci* 1997; 42: 1362–9.
6. Namiot Z, Yu ZJ, Piascik R, *et al.* Modulatory effect of esophageal intraluminal mechanical and chemical stressors on salivary prostaglandin E_2 in humans. *Am J Med Sci* 1997; 31: 90–8.
7. Bouchoucha M, Callais F, Renard P, *et al.* Relationship between acid neutralization capacity of saliva and gastro-oesophageal reflux. *Arch Physiol Biochem* 1997; 105: 19–26.
8. Aldazabal P, Lopez de Torre B, Uriarte S, *et al.* Saliva in experimental gastroesophageal reflux. *Cir Pediatr* 1998; 11: 19–24.
9. Lock G, Strozter M, Straub RH, *et al.* Air oesophagram: a frequent, but not a specific sign of oesophageal involvement in connective tissue disease. *Br J Rheumatol* 1998; 37: 1011–14.
10. Bjerle P, EK B, Linderholm H, Steen L. Oesophageal dysfunction in familial amyloidosis with polyneuropathy. *Clin Physiol* 1993; 13: 57–69.
11. Jermendy G, Fornet B, Koltai MZ, Pogatsa G. Correlation between oesophageal dysmotility and cardiovascular autonomic dysfunction in diabetic patients without gastrointestinal symptoms of autonomic neuropathy. *Diabetes Res* 1991; 16: 193–7.
12. Krausz Y, Maayan C, Faber J, *et al.* Scintigraphic evaluation of esophageal transit and gastric emptying in familial dysautonomia. *Eur J Radiol* 1994; 18: 52–6.
13. Fuhrmann R, Diedrich P. Video-supported dynamic B-mode sonography of tongue function during swallowing. *Fortschr Kieferorthop* 1993; 54: 17–26.
14. Urioste M, Arroyo I, Villa A, *et al.* Distal deletion of chromosome 13 in a child with the ''Opitz'' GBBB syndrome. *Am J Genet* 1995; 59: 114–22.
15. Schima W, Pokieser P, Schober E, *et al.* Globus sensation: value of static radiography combined with videofluoroscopy of the pharynx and oesophagus. *Clin Radiol* 1996; 51: 177–85.
16. English PC. Failure to thrive without organic reason. *Pediatr Ann* 1978; 7: 774–81.
17. Burklow KA, Phelps AN, Schultz JR, McConnel K, Rudolph C. Classifying complex pediatric feeding disorders. *J Pediatr Gastroenterol Nutr* 1998; 27: 143–7.
18. Abadie V, Chéron G, Couly G. Le syndrome néonatal de dysfonctionnement du tronc cérébral. *Arch Pediatr* 1993; 50: 347–52.

19. Hampton D. Resolving the feeding difficulties associated with non-organic failure to thrive. *Child Care Health Dev* 1996; 22: 261–71.

20. Moores J. Non-organic failure to thrive—dietetic practice in a community setting. *Child Care Health Dev* 1996; 22: 251–9.

21. Black MM, Dubowitz H, Hutcheson J, *et al.* A randomized clinical trial of home intervention for children with failure to thrive. *Pediatrics* 1995; 95: 807–14.

22. Goutet JM, Baudon JJ, Vasquez MP, *et al.* La dykinesie oesophagienne du syndrome de Pierre Robin est-elle la conséquence de l' immaturité physiologique ou du reflux gastro-oesophagien? [Abstract]. *Arch Pediatr* 1998; 2: 236(A).

23. Katzka DA, Sidhu M, Castell DO. Hypertensive lower esophageal sphincter pressure: an apparent paradox that is not unusual. *Am J Gastroenterol* 1995; 90: 280–4.

24. Mertz-Nielsen A, Hillingso J, Bukhave K, Rask-Madsen J. Reappraisal of bicarbonate secretion by the human oesophagus. *Gut* 1997; 40: 582–6.

25. Holloway RH, Penagini R, Schoeman MN, Dent J. Effect of cisapride on secondary peristalsis in patients with gastroesophageal reflux disease. *Am J Gastroenterol* 1999; 94: 799–803.

26. Lu W, Zhang M, Neuman RS, Bieger D. Fictive oesophageal peristalsis evoked activation of muscarinic acetylcholine receptors in rat nucleus tractus solitarii. *Neurogastroenterol Motil* 1997; 9: 247–56.

27. Niemantsverdriet EC, Timmer R, Breumelhof R, Smout AJ. The roles of excessive gastro-oesophageal reflux, disordered oesophageal motility and decreased mucosal sensitivity in the pathogenesis of Barrett's oesophagus. *Eur J Gastroenterol Hepatol* 1997; 9: 515–19.

28. Page AJ, Blackshaw LA. An *in vitro* study of the properties of vagal afferent fibres innervating the ferret oesophagus and stomach. *J Physiol (Lond)* 1998; 512: 907–16.

29. Fass R, Higa L, Kodner A, Mayer EA. Stimulus and site specific induction of hiccups in the oesophagus of normal subjects. *Gut* 1997; 41: 590–3.

30. Helm JF. Determinants of esophageal acid clearance in normal subjects. *Gastroenterology* 1987; 85: 607–12.

31. Kahrilas PJ. Effect of peristaltic dysfunction on esophageal volume clearing. *Gastroenterology* 1988; 94: 73–80.

32. Omari TI, Barbett C, Snel A, *et al.* Mechanisms of gastroesophageal reflux in healthy premature infants. *J Pediatr* 1998; 133: 650–4.

33. Cadiot G, Bruhat A, Rigaud D, *et al.* Multivariate analysis of pathophysiological factors in reflux oesophagitis. *Gut* 1997; 40: 167–74.

34. Allen ML, Zamani S, Dimarino AJ. The effect of gravity on oesophageal peristalsis in humans. *Neurogastroenterol Motil* 1997; 9: 71–6.

35. Marcinkiewicz M, Grabwska SZ, Czyzewska E. Role of epidermal growth factor (EGF) in oesophageal mucosal integrity. *Curr Med Res Opin* 1998; 14: 145–53.

36. Zicari A, Corrado G, Cavaliere M, *et al.* Increased levels of prostaglandins and nitric oxide in esophageal mucosa of children with reflux esophagitis. *J Pediatr Gastroenterol Nutr* 1998; 26: 194–9.

37. Jimenez P, Lanas A, Piazuelo E, Bioque G, Esteva F. Prostaglandin E_2 is the major arachidonic acid metabolite secreted by esophageal mucosal cells in rabbits. *Inflammation* 1997; 21: 419–29.

38. Sarosiek J, Yu Z, Namiot Z, *et al.* Impact of acid and pepsin on human esophageal prostaglandins. *Am J Gastroenterol* 1994; 89: 588–94.

39. Holtmann G, Kolbel CB, Ewers M, Giese A, Mayer P. Effect of prostaglandin E_2 analog nocloprost on motility and acid clearance of the tubular esophagus in man. *Med Klin* 1993; 88: S2–4.

40. Lanas AI, Sousa FL, Ortego J, *et al.* Aspirin renders the oesophageal mucosa more permeable to acid and pepsin. *Eur J Gastroenterol Hepatol* 1995; 7: 1065–72.

41. Marcinkiewicz M, Sarosiek J, Edmunds M, *et al.* Monophasic luminal release of prostaglandin E_2 in patients with reflux esophagitis under the impact of acid and acid/pepsin solutions. Its potential pathogenic significance. *J Clin Gastroenterol* 1995; 21: 268–74.

42. Morgan G. Deleterious effects of prostaglandin E_2 in reflux oesophagitis. *Med Hypotheses* 1996; 46: 42–4.

43. Jimenez P, Lanas A, Piazuelo E, Esteva F. Effect of growth factors and prostaglandin E_2 on restitution and proliferation of rabbit esophageal epithelial cells. *Dig Dis Sci* 1998; 43: 2309–16.

44. Tihanyi K, Rozsa I, Banai J, Dobo I, Bajtai A. Tissue concentrations and correlations of prostaglandins in healthy and inflamed human esophageal and jejunal mucosa. *J Gastroenterol* 1996; 31: 149–52.

45. Gruber AD, Gandhi R, Pauli B. The murine calcium-sensitive chloride channel (mCaCC) is widely expressed in secretory epithelia and in other select tissues. *Histochem Cell Biol* 199; 110: 43–9.

46. Luiking YC, Weusten BL, Portincasa P, *et al.* Effects of long-term oral L-arginine on esophageal motility and gallbladder dynamics in healthy humans. *Am J Physiol* 1998; 274: G984–91.
47. Rodriguez S, Miner P, Robinson M, *et al.* Meal type affects heartburn severity. *Dig Dis Sci* 1998; 43: 485–90.
48. Hirsch DP, Holloway RH, Tytgat GN, Boeckxstaens GE. Involvement of nitric oxide in human transient lower esophageal sphincter relaxations and esophageal primary peristalsis. *Gastroenterology* 1998; 115: 1374–80.
49. Sun WM, Doran S, Jones KL, *et al.* Effects of nitroglycerin on liquid gastric emptying and antropyloroduodenal motility. *Am J Physiol* 1998; 275: G1173–8.
50. Vanderwinden JM, Mailleaux P, Schiffmann SN, Verhaeghen JJ, De Laet MH. Nitric oxide synthase activity in infantile hypertrophic pyloric stenosis. *N Engl J Med* 1992; 327: 511–15.
51. Gupta SK, Fitzgerald JF, Chong SK, Croffie JM, Garcia JG. Expression of inducible nitric oxide synthase (iNOS) mRNA in inflamed esophageal and colonic mucosa in a pediatric population. *Am J Gastroenterol* 1998; 93: 795–8.
52. Wilson KT, Fu S, Ramanujam KS, Meltzer SJ. Increased expression of inducible nitric oxide synthase and cyclooxygenase-2 in Barrett's esophagus and associated adenocarcinomas. *Cancer Res* 1998; 58: 2929–34.
53. Dent J, Holloway RH, Toouli J. Mechanism of lower esophageal sphincter incompetence in patients with symptomatic gastro-esophageal reflux. *Gut* 1988; 29: 1020–8.
54. Kalicinski P, Dluski E, Drewniak T, Kaminski W. Esophageal manometric studies in children with achalasia before and after operative treatment. *Pediatr Surg Int* 1997; 12: 571–5.
55. Tovar KA, Prieto G, Molina M, Arana J. Esophageal function in achalasia: preoperative and postoperative manometric studies. *J Pediatr Surg* 1998; 33: 834–8.
56. von Herbay A, Heyer T, Olk W, *et al.* Autonomic dysfunction in patients with achalasia of the oesophagus. *Neurogastroenterol Motil* 1998; 10: 387–93.
57. Lui H, Vanderwinden JM, Ji P, De Laet MH. Nitric oxide synthase distribution in the enteric nervous system of children with cardiac achalasia. *Chin Med J (Engl)* 1997; 110: 358–61.
58. Gonzalez M, Mearin F, Vasconez C, Armengol JR, Malagelada JR. Oesophageal tone in patients with achalasia. *Gut* 1997; 41: 291–6.
59. Cucchaira S, Salvia G, Borelli O. Gastric electrical dysrhythmias and delayed gastric emptying in gastroesophageal reflux disease. *Am J Gastroenterol* 1997; 92: 1103–8.
60. Arakawa T, Uno H, Fukuda T, *et al.* New aspects of gastric adaptive relaxation, reflex after food intake for more food: involvement of capsaicin-sensitive sensory nerves and nitric oxide. *J Smooth Muscle Res* 1997; 33: 81–8.
61. Martin CJ, Patrikios J, Dent J. Abolition of gas reflux and transient lower esophageal sphincter relaxation by vagal blockade in the dog. *Gastroenterology* 1986; 91: 890–6.
62. Ravelli AM, Milla PJ. Vomiting and gastroesophageal motor activity in children with disorders of the central nervous system. *J Pediatr Gastroenterol Nutr* 1998; 26: 56–63.
63. Cucchiara S, Salvia G, Borrelli O, *et al.* Gastric electrical dysrhythmias and delayed gastric emptying in gastroesophageal reflux disease. *Am J Gastroenterol* 1997; 92: 1103–8.
64. Bustorff Silva J, Fonkalsrud EW, Perez CA, *et al.* Gastric emptying procedures decrease the risk of postoperative recurrent reflux in children with delayed gastric emptying. *J Pediatr Surg* 1999; 34: 79–82.
65. Johnson DG, Reid BS, Meyers RL, *et al.* Are scintiscans accurate in the selection of reflux patients for pyloroplasty? *J Pediatr Surg* 1998; 33: 573–9.
66. Mistry FP, Sreenivasa D, Narawane NM, Abraham P, Bhatia SJ. Vagal dysfunction following endoscopic variceal sclerotherapy. *Indian J Gastroenterol* 1998; 17: 22–3.
68. Harmon JW. Effects of acid and bile salts on the rabbit esophageal mucosa. *Dig Dis Sci* 1981; 26: 65–72.
67. Clave P, Gonzalez A, Moreno A, *et al.* Endogenous cholecystokinin enhances postprandial gastroesophageal reflux in humans through extrasphincteric receptors. *Gastroenterology* 1998; 115: 597–604.
69. Safaie-Shirazi S. Effect of bile salts on the ionic permeability of the esophageal mucosa and their role in the production of esophagitis. *Gastroenterology* 1975; 69: 728–33.

DISCUSSION

Dr. Zoppi: In atrophic gastritis, is GER enhanced or diminished?

Dr. Vandenplas: I do not think we have any answers regarding the incidence of reflux.

What is probably different is the pH of the refluxed material. This has been seen in adults with *Helicobacter pylori* gastritis and atrophic gastritis: if the *H. pylori* is eradicated and the atrophy disappears, more esophagitis occurs. I think a relationship probably exists between acid secretion and esophagitis.

Dr. Infante: In my experience, we often see infants with symptoms that you describe as nonorganic failure to thrive. What kind of treatment do you think is indicated for these infants?

Dr. Vandenplas: We do not have any medical treatment at this moment for most of these children. Of course, an anatomic problem such as retrognathia has to be corrected surgically. For those in whom the problem is mainly functional, it seems to disappear after a while, usually about a year. These children may need tube feeding but later on they are able to eat normally. The mechanism is not yet understood, as far as I know.

Dr. Milla: I enjoyed your ideas about nociception in the esophagus. I think we all have patients with reflux who we treat with large doses of proton pump inhibitors because the primary complaint is pain. Yet, they steadfastly refuse to stop complaining of the pain. Do you have any insight into how we might deal with that? Should we be looking at their nociception pathways rather than their reflux and esophageal mucosa?

Dr. Vandenplas: We are going to start to try to do that. This is a provocative approach, but it should be explored. We all know of regurgitating babies without esophagitis who cry for hours, and it may be that this shows that the volume they regurgitate is painful for them. This is purely speculative.

Dr. Büller: We have taught for centuries that babies who regurgitate or vomit should be kept upright and held in that position for a long time. If I interpret your work correctly, you seem to be suggesting that we should not do that. We should put them down immediately because in the upright position transient lower esophageal sphincter relaxation is increased. Is that a fair conclusion?

Dr. Vandenplas: I do not think we have the answer to that. People hold infants upright after feeding because that decreases regurgitation, and milk is less frequently ejected from the mouth. But whether that has the same effect lower in the esophagus, I do not know. From the physiologic data, it seems likely that more transient relaxations occur in the upright position.

Dr. Büller: As a clinician, what would you advise me to do?

Dr. Vandenplas: It depends. If talking about a regurgitating baby, the regurgitation must be taken away. If referring to severe GER—a condition that occurs in a very small number of all regurgitating babies—then in these children it may be that they feel happier when they are lying down after a feed than being held upright. Mothers sometimes do tell you that. But systematic investigation is needed to provide an answer to this question.

Dr. Jirapinyo: I once did a study on gastric emptying in infants and was surprised to find that in some infants 20 or 30 minutes after the feed, the gastric volume increased to more than 100% of the milk that was taken in. We found that some infants had 130% of their intake in their stomachs at that time. So, I think the volume of secretions—probably from saliva but also from the stomach—may be a problem and cause pain to the infant, and also cause reflux.

Dr. Vandenplas: I agree that this may be one of the possible mechanisms of reflux. Gastric secretion is something we do not consider often enough in infants and children. However, if that viewpoint is taken, then medications (e.g., proton pump inhibitors) would be effective, because they greatly decrease the secretory volume. It would be too easy if only one mechanism was causing reflux or pain in the infant! Likely, a variety of mechanisms are operating, including combinations of the different factors that I discussed. Probably, we will end up with different therapeutic approaches, because the pathophysiologic mechanism may be very different from patient to patient.

Dr. Naim: My question is regarding sleep patterns in children in relationship to the risk of GER. As you mentioned, infants who show patterns of reduced swallowing and increased sleeping may be at higher risk of GER than others in that age group. It is a normal physiologic process for infants and children to sleep for relatively long periods, but if this normal sleep pattern increases the risk of esophagitis, how are we going to prevent or reduce the risk of GER in this age group?

Dr. Vandenplas: It is of course a normal part of life that infants sleep a lot, and it is normal that they sleep in the horizontal position. I would like to be provocative again. We all know that more cases of sudden infant death occur in the prone sleeping position than in the supine position. That is why it is now recommended that infants sleep supine. The arousal threshold in the prone sleeping position is much higher than in supine sleeping position, which means that infants sleeping prone tend to sleep more deeply. If that is translated to reflux, much more reflux occurs in the supine position than in prone position; because of the reflux, apneas and arousals ensue and no sudden infant death occurs. I believe these factors are related, although I am not saying the relationship is causal. However, it does offer another way of looking at the problem. We do not see much severe esophagitis in those young infants; all we see most of the time is a little redness in the distal esophagus. What that means is unclear.

Dr. Black: Your statement about the inverse relationship between reflux and sudden infant death syndrome is fairly provocative. Some physicians and pediatricians regularly prescribe antireflux formulas for infants. Are you suggesting that this may not be a good thing to do? If not, we should be very careful about what we prescribe and what we produce as manufacturers.

Dr. Vandenplas: I would not like to go that far. One important mistake is found in what you said: I do not consider those formulas to be antireflux formulas, but antiregurgitation formulas. They reduce the symptom of regurgitation but they have no influence on reflux whatsoever. The studies that have been done show that in nearly one third of patients reflux does improve; in one third, no difference is seen, and in one third the reflux worsens (1,2); thus, overall, no change is seen. If such infants do need help, however, then the most physiologic way to do so is probably with dietary treatment, which is better than medication. But the primary recommendation for regurgitating babies is to convince the parents that everything is OK.

Dr. Brandtzaeg: I just wonder if you would update me on Barrett's esophagus. A discussion has occurred to whether these are hypogastric glands, ectopic glands, metaplastic glands, or whatever. Also, what is the relationship to reflux—do these hypoplastic glands affect the tendency to reflux? What is the chicken and what the egg in these cases?

Dr. Vandenplas: The only thing I can say about this is that the only patients in whom I still see Barrett's esophagitis are neurologically impaired children. Those are the ones with the most severe reflux that has been present for the longest time. From a pediatric point of view, I think it is clear a relationship exists between the severity and duration of reflux, and whether the reflux has been treated, and the incidence of Barrett's esophagitis. It is very rare in children and rather outside my area of interest, so I cannot say anything about the different kinds of glands.

Dr. Brandtzaeg: It is not so rare in adults. I am curious about the nature of these glands.

Dr. Vandenplas: I think Dr. Wright may have the answer.

Dr. N. Wright: Three hypotheses relate to the histogenesis of Barrett's mucosa. The first one is that the cardiac mucosa extends into the esophagus. The second one is that stem cells at the bases of the esophageal rete pegs have the ability to differentiate into glandular epithelium. The third one is that they actually rise from the ducts of the esophageal glands, because when looking at the three-dimensional structure, particularly of regenerating mucosa after omeprazole, the squamous epithelium can be seen in juxtaposition to the esophageal glands. Barrett's esophagus epithelium is not necessarily unstable until it undergoes metaplasia, and that metaplasia results in so-called specialized mucosa or type 2B, sulphomucin Muc-2, secreting epithelium. That is the epithelium that shows p53 mutations, loss of heterozygocity of APC, and gradually clonal expansion and dysplasia. In a nutshell, that is the histogenesis of Barrett's esophagus.

Dr. Goulet: You pointed out many factors involved in gastric emptying, but what about intrathoracic pressure and the relationship between ventilatory function and esophageal function? In clinical practice, a clear relationship is seen between GER and bronchopulmonary disease. Have you a view on this, and also on the value of investigating upper esophageal sphincter function?

Dr. Vandenplas: Regarding respiratory disease, it has been shown that in chronic bronchopulmonary disease giving oxygen by continuous positive airway pressure (CPAP) to those children decreases GER. So, just by changing pressures in the thorax, the reflux is treated. It has also been shown that in infants with wheezing, the greater the respiratory problem and the more negative the intrathoracic pressure, the higher the intra-abdominal pressure becomes and the more the patient will aspirate what is in the stomach.

Investigation of the upper esophageal sphincter is an area on which we need to focus in the coming years. The lower sphincter has been very well studied, but the upper sphincter probably also plays a major role. For instance, it may be that in children with pathologic apneas related to reflux, the response of the upper esophageal sphincter is different from normal. It is difficult to investigate but it needs to be done.

Dr. Fyderek: Would you give us your opinion on the role of alkaline reflux in gastroesophageal reflex disease, and what is the best method to investigate this?

Dr. Vandenplas: A really a good method is not currently available to investigate alkaline reflux. At least two pH probes are needed and the pH has to be clearly shown rising first in the lower pH probe and then in the higher probe. In theory, this is nice, but when attempting to do it in practice, it is very hard—if not impossible—to demonstrate the phenomenon in a large series of children. I do not know how common it is because it is so difficult to investigate. The question to be answered is whether duodenogastric reflux is an important factor in GER; large amounts of bile are needed in the stomach to neutralize gastric acidity, so even with acid reflux bile can be present in the refluxate. The question of the role of bile reflux is a difficult one, because we have no way of clearly demonstrating the presence of bile in the refluxate, and that is what is of principal interest.

Dr. Fyderek: What about the Biletech method?

Dr. Vandenplas: I have never used it and I do not know many people who have. Those who did use it do not use it any more as far as I know. Maybe that answers your question.

Dr. Mäki: Do we have any solid long-term data on reflux disease in infancy? What do we know about its natural history and the consequence of treatment?

Dr. Vandenplas: I have no idea. The problem is that long-term follow-up studies of 40 to 50 years, at least, are needed. These have not been done and, in practice, it would be very difficult to do so. The only information I have about this is in relationship to North African immigrant families in western Europe. A lot of these families are seen now and, in this population, we hardly ever see esophageal stenosis in childhood as a complication of GER.

In North Africa, however, they still see a lot of it in children of the same genetic background. This is not evidence that early treatment improves later outcome, but it is suggestive.

Dr. Steenhout: I like the concept of an initiating stimulus in the upper part of the esophagus. What might be the role of food at this level? Do you think a food additive or colorant, for example, could trigger the release of a hormone such as substance P, or is this purely a mechanical mechanism?

Dr. Vandenplas: That it is a very good question. We really do not know how relevant factors such as substance P are. Studies clearly show that these factors change in concentration, depending on the circumstances, but what initiates those changes and how important they are in clinical practice is unknown as yet.

Dr. Seidman: A provocative Italian study (3) suggested that regurgitation caused by reflux can be distinguished from regurgitation caused by cow's milk protein allergy in infants with challenge-proved protein allergy on the basis of their pH probe pattern: the infants proved to have allergy had a progressive and prolonged decrease in esophageal pH after a feed, as opposed to the frequent short-term changes in pH in benign reflux. I would appreciate your comments on that study.

Dr. Vandenplas: We were unable to reproduce that. The diagnosis of cow's milk protein allergy is not one that should be made by pH monitoring—challenge tests are needed, which is the only way to diagnose it properly. That reflux should be related to cow's milk protein allergy is logical, because here something is being ingested which is not tolerated and must be gotten rid of. But, on that basis, a lot of short reflux episodes should be expected that provoke vomiting to get rid of what is not being tolerated, rather than prolonged reflux episodes.

REFERENCES

1. Vandenplas Y, Belli D, Cadranel S, *et al.* I. Dietary treatment for regurgitation—recommendations from a working party. *Acta Paediatr* 1998; 87: 462–8.
2. Vandenplas Y. Clinical use of cisapride and its risk-benefit in paediatric patients. *Eur J Gastroenterol Hepatol* 1998; 10: 871–81.
3. Cavataio F, Iacono G, Montalto G, *et al.* Clinical and pH-metric characteristics of gastro-oesophageal reflux secondary to cows' milk protein allergy. *Arch Dis Child* 1996; 75: 51–6.

Gastrointestinal Functions, edited by Edgard E. Delvin and
Michael J. Lentze. Nestlé Nutrition Workshop Series, Pediatric
Program, Vol. 46, Nestec Ltd., Vevey/Lippincott Williams &
Wilkins, Philadelphia © 2001.

Celiac Disease

Markku Mäki

*Institute of Medical Technology, University of Tampere and Department of Pediatrics, Tampere
University Hospital, Tampere, Finland*

CHANGING CLINICAL FEATURES OF CELIAC DISEASE

Celiac disease is caused by ingested gluten. In genetically susceptible individuals, it leads to malabsorption of food and nutrients. Characteristically, it has manifested during infancy. Symptoms and signs of malabsorption became obvious within months after starting a gluten-containing diet, and the child typically had chronic diarrhea or loose stools, vomiting, and a distended abdomen. Failure to thrive was a common presentation. These symptoms are those of the classic form of childhood celiac disease. In adults, diarrhea, weight loss, and weakness used to be the classic signs of celiac disease, and a severe malabsorption syndrome was generally found. Nowadays, however, in many countries celiac disease presenting as a malabsorption syndrome is the exception rather than the rule, and a changing symptom pattern has been experienced in both children and adults (1). Clinical celiac disease represents only the tip of the iceberg (Fig. 1).

As seen today, celiac disease can still present with the traditional symptoms and signs but usually in a very mild form. Symptoms such as indigestion in adults and recurrent abdominal pain in children are common. A typical monosymptomatic form of the disease is isolated iron deficiency, a sign of malabsorption. Despite the presence of the diagnostic mucosal lesion, the disease can even be symptom-free and clinically silent (Fig. 1). Approximately 10% of the healthy relatives of patients with celiac disease also have silent celiac disease (2).

Extraintestinal Manifestations and Associated Diseases

Until the 1960s, celiac disease was recognized as a gastrointestinal disease because the diagnosis was based solely on the finding of gastrointestinal symptoms, and even the laboratory tests measured only intestinal absorption. When the typical small bowel mucosal lesion became the "gold standard" of diagnosis and serologic tests were developed as safe screening tools, it became clear that celiac disease is a complex disorder with manifestations that are not confined to the gastrointestinal tract; in fact, malabsorption is now no longer regarded as essential for the diagnosis.

It is widely accepted that dermatitis herpetiformis is gluten induced and a classic

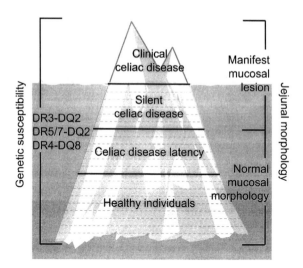

FIG. 1.   The celiac disease iceberg and spectrum of gluten sensitivity. From 1. Mäki M, Collin P. Coeliac disease. *Lancet* 1997; 349: 1755–9; with permission.

example of the extraintestinal manifestation of celiac disease. This disorder affects the skin when gluten is ingested by individuals with a particular genetic background (3,4) (Fig. 2). Other linked disorders include permanent tooth enamel defects (5), epilepsy and cerebral calcification (6), liver involvement (7), malignancies (8,9), osteopenia (10,11), idiopathic ataxia (12), and even autoimmune diseases in general (13). Clearly, indications are that extraintestinal, gluten-induced manifestations can develop in the latent stage of the disease when the mucosa is still morphologically normal (6,12,14–17). The cooking pot in Fig. 2 indicates that celiac disease with the classic flat mucosal lesion is only one of the disease entities splashing out of the pot. Physicians need to remember as well that celiac disease is related to certain specific conditions such as selective IgA deficiency (18) and Down's syndrome (19).

Our current understanding is that celiac disease presents as a clinical disease ranging symptomatically from mild to severe, or with atypical symptoms, or it can present in a silent form with only the gluten-sensitive intestinal mucosal lesion.

LATENT CELIAC DISEASE

By definition, celiac disease is excluded in patients who have normal small bowel mucosal morphology when eating a normal gluten-containing diet. However, gluten sensitivity is no longer restricted to villous atrophy (Fig. 1). Small bowel mucosal damage develops gradually from normal mucosal morphology to overt atrophy with crypt hyperplasia. Individuals with initially normal small bowel villous architecture while eating normal amounts of gluten can still be gluten sensitive—they may have

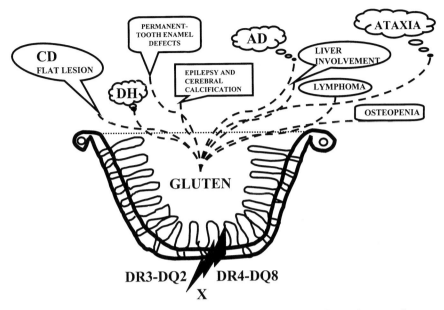

FIG. 2. The gluten cooking pot with splashing disease entities. AD, autoimmune diseases; CD, celiac disease; DH, dermatitis herpetiformis; X, unknown genes.

latent celiac disease. This means that small bowel villous atrophy and crypt hyperplasia develop later (20–23).

Celiac-type gluten sensitivity should also include in its definition the susceptibility genes for celiac disease (Fig. 1), and the term "celiac trait" has been suggested (1). Latent celiac disease can be suspected in individuals who are positive for tissue autoantibodies (i.e., reticulin, endomysial, or tissue transglutaminase antibodies) and in patients with a high density of intraepithelial lymphocytes bearing the γδ T-cell receptor who also carry the susceptibility genes for celiac disease, the DQ2 or DQ8 molecules.

OCCURRENCE

During the early 1980s it seemed that the incidence of celiac disease in children was decreasing. In some countries (e.g., the Netherlands and Denmark), the prevalence in the childhood population was reported to be very low, at between 1 of 5,000 and 1 of 10,000 (24,25). In Finland, the decrease was also observed, but it occurred in young infants and an increasing incidence was found in older children and adolescents (26,27). It has become evident that the disease still exists or now appears later, although the classic forms have disappeared.

At a time when the disease seemed to be disappearing in many European countries, in Sweden the opposite occurred. The incidence of celiac disease in Swedish infants reached 1 of 250, a figure much higher than that in the neighboring countries (28,29).

The differences were thought to reflect different infant feeding practices, especially the amount of ingested gluten (30). Infant feeding recommendations were recently re-evaluated in Sweden; however, before that had been done, the incidence of celiac disease had already begun to decline (31). It is now apparent that large differences are found in the incidence of celiac disease between various European countries (32). However, screening studies have shown that many clinically silent cases of celiac disease lie under the tip of the iceberg (33) (Fig. 1), and the true prevalence of the disease in different populations may be around 1 of 100 (34–37).

Few incidence and prevalence figures are seen from North America, and the diagnosis seems rare there (38). The incidence of celiac disease seems to be dependent on the primary care physicians' knowledge of the disease complex. Today, physicians working in primary care must have a high index of suspicion of the disease and be ready to use serologic screening tests freely (1). Today, these patients are mostly not referred to specialized centers on clinical grounds. A high prevalence of endomysial antibodies in blood donors in the United States (39) and the occurrence of silent celiac disease among insulin-dependent diabetic patients in North America (40–42) indicate that the clinical situation may be similar there to that in Europe.

DIAGNOSIS AND TREATMENT

The diagnostic criteria of celiac disease, as stated by the European Society for Pediatric Gastroenterology and Nutrition (ESPGAN) in 1970, are (a) small bowel mucosal atrophy with improvement or normalization on a gluten-free diet, and (b) a deterioration of the villous morphology during intake of a gluten-containing diet. These criteria were modified in 1990 (43). The findings of characteristic small bowel mucosal atrophy and clinical remission on a gluten-free diet are essential. In symptom-free patients, a second biopsy is needed to show mucosal recovery on a gluten-free diet. The presence of circulating antibodies and their disappearance on a gluten-free diet support the diagnosis. The old ESPGAN criteria, including gluten challenge, can be used when needed—for example, in children younger than 2 years who live in countries where intolerance to protein in cow's milk is common, or in patients for whom the findings from their first biopsy sample was equivocal. Gluten challenge after mucosal healing in children who initially test negative for serum endomysial antibodies is also advisable. In the Nordic countries, a manifest mucosal lesion generally indicates celiac disease, irrespective of whether the patient has symptoms or signs of malabsorption. Small bowel biopsy sampling is essential, and the diagnosis should not be based on symptoms or serologic tests alone (44).

Oral glucose tolerance tests, fecal fat excretion, D-xylose excretion tests, hematologic investigations, and radiologic examination of the small bowel have failed to distinguish patients with suspected malabsorption with mucosal atrophy from those without atrophy, and frequently give misleading results (45). The focus in case finding and screening today is on serologic tests, particularly tests for certain tissue autoantibodies (46). Patients with malabsorption syndrome or other features that raise a strong suspicion of celiac disease do not need screening tests for intestinal mucosal injury; jejunal biopsy should be the first diagnostic test in the workup (1).

Noninvasive screening tests are helpful in patients without malabsorption and with only slight clinical suspicion of celiac disease.

In celiac disease, treatment with a strict, lifelong, gluten-free diet results in complete clinical and histologic recovery. Wheat, rye, and barley prolamins should be withdrawn from the diet, but the issue whether oats can be safely consumed by celiac patients has been debated. Recent studies in adults show no adverse effects of oats on small bowel mucosal integrity (47,48). Our preliminary data suggest that oats can also safely be used in children with celiac disease. Studies are in progress in many centers. Rice, maize, buckwheat, and millet are also nontoxic cereals.

Wheat starch-based, gluten-free flour products meeting the ''old'' *Codex Alimentarius* standard have always been permitted in the treatment of celiac disease and dermatitis herpetiformis in the United Kingdom and the Nordic countries, but discouraged in many countries in southern Europe and in North America. Treatment with these products has not resulted in excess mortality or morbidity in celiac disease patients (46,49).

A problem with naturally gluten-free flours and products is gluten contamination, as these products are not tested and are labeled as ''gluten-free.'' International trade tolerates about 5% extraneous grain in a cereal. When flours that are gluten-free by nature have been tested, gluten contamination is common and often very high. Gliadin was found in millet, rice, maize, soybean, and buckwheat, and values exceeding the new *Codex* proposed allowance (200 ppm gluten) by as much as tenfold were obtained (50). It appears that industrially produced wheat starch-based, gluten-free flours may be more pure than flours that are gluten-free by nature.

AUTOIMMUNE ASPECTS OF CELIAC DISEASE

From both a clinical and a biological point of view, celiac disease can be classified among the autoimmune diseases (1). Celiac disease is triggered by ingested gluten, a single major environmental factor. The disease also has a very narrow, highly specific, HLA class II association, DR3-DQ2, and to a lesser extent DR4-DQ8. These HLA types are also typical for many autoimmune diseases. Common disease associations in celiac disease are insulin-dependent diabetes mellitus, Sjögren's syndrome, and autoimmune thyroiditis. Another typical feature of celiac disease is the presence of autoantibodies directed against the extracellular matrix, the so-called ''reticulin and endomysial tissue structures.'' Also typical for the gluten-induced small bowel mucosal lesion is a high density of intraepithelial $\gamma\delta+$ T lymphocytes.

The pathogenic mechanisms behind the gluten-induced, small bowel mucosal lesion are unknown. Continuing gliadin ingestion seems to be responsible for the self-maintenance of the disease by revealing disease-triggering self-epitopes. Celiac disease is self-perpetuating and irreversible if the environmental trigger, gluten, is not removed; if it is removed, the immunologic response is reduced and mucosal healing is seen. It is not known what would be the outcome in other autoimmune diseases if all the environmental triggers, including viral infections, could be removed early enough, and if the target tissues had a high regenerating capacity as with the small bowel mucosa.

My group has based the autoimmune hypothesis in celiac disease pathogenesis—as formulated in the Proceedings of the Sixth International Symposium on celiac disease held at Trinity College, Dublin in July 1992 (51)—mainly on the high disease specificity of IgA class reticulin antibodies and on the fact that these antibodies are targeted against self-epitopes (2,52–54). Here, we proceed one step forward. We hypothesize that these disease-specific autoantibodies are disease inducing, because, in an *in vitro* crypt–villus axis model, both IgA from serum of untreated patients with celiac disease and antibodies against tissue transglutaminase inhibit the fibroblast-induced transforming growth factor (TGF) β1 mediated differentiation of epithelial cells (55). Nature might, in fact, have meant celiac disease–specific autoantibodies to have a biological function, not merely to be an epiphenomenon—and perhaps even to play a role in protection against disease.

Reticulin and Endomysial Autoantibodies

Serum reticulin antibody tests have been in use since 1971 (46). The antigen has routinely been detected by a standard indirect immunofluorescence method using unfixed cryostat sections of rat kidney, liver, and stomach as antigens, and the R1 type reticulin antibodies were claimed to be specific for celiac disease and dermatitis herpetiformis. However, the sensitivity of this tissue antibody test in detecting untreated celiac disease has been variable and often unsatisfactory. By measuring IgA class R1 type reticulin antibodies, a sensitivity and specificity of 97% and 98%, respectively, were claimed (52), positivity entailing a typical staining pattern in both rat kidney and liver. More recent studies have confirmed this test to be reliable and valuable in assisting in the early recognition of occult celiac disease (56). The IgA class reticulin antibody test has also been used to screen selected groups of at risk patients, with the expected results. Positivity has clearly predicted clinically silent celiac disease among patients with insulin-dependent diabetes mellitus, Sjögren's syndrome, and autoimmune thyroid diseases. The clinician must be aware of selective IgA deficiency, where IgG class reticulin antibodies are again predictive of gluten-sensitive enteropathy (18).

Sera from patients with celiac disease react not only with rodent tissues but also with human and other primate tissues. Hällström (57) showed that all reticulin antibody-positive sera tested gave a moderate to strong immunofluorescent reticular network pattern in human jejunum, liver, lung, spleen, thymus, and pancreas and a weaker reaction in human skin, kidney, and colon. Kárpáti et al. (58) have used jejunum for this purpose and named the test the "jejunal antibody test." Chorzelski et al. (59,60) used monkey esophagus to test for tissue antibodies in patients with celiac disease and dermatitis herpetiformis and named this the "endomysial antibody test." This IgA class tissue antibody test has gained popularity in recent years, as it gives an almost 100% sensitivity and specificity for celiac disease. In our hands, both reticulin and endomysial antibody tests perform adequately and cannot in clinical practice be distinguished from one another (46). Ladinser et al. (61) were first to show that reticulin and endomysial antigens are also present in human umbilical cord vessels. The IgA class human umbilical cord autoantibody test today often replaces the classic endomysial antibody test using monkey esophagus as antigen (62–68). This new autoantibody test correlates well with the classic IgA class R1 type reticulin antibody test.

Tissue Autoantibodies in Individuals with Normal Mucosa

Tissue autoantibodies in celiac disease are gluten induced and work well in clinics. We have also learned that a positive reticulin or endomysial antibody test not only predicts undiagnosed clinically silent celiac disease in symptomless first degree relatives of celiac disease patients, but also identifies a small number of relatives with normal mucosal architecture expressing celiac type HLA haplotypes (A1;B8; DR3) (2). Also, outside celiac disease families, a positive autoantibody test in patients with normal mucosal morphology correlates with positivity for DQA1*0501 and DQB1*0201 alleles (69). A positive IgA class reticulin or endomysial antibody test in individuals with normal mucosa on biopsy should be followed up, as the test evidently reveals latent celiac disease, where mucosal deterioration is seen later (2,21). Positivity for reticulin antibodies in patients with normal jejunal mucosal morphology predicted subsequent villus atrophy in 83% of cases (21). Individuals with low titers of these autoantibodies and a normal mucosal morphology often have no sign of an infiltrative lesion, and counts of intraepithelial lymphocytes have been below 30 lymphocytes per 100 epithelial cells (21,46). We have not diagnosed such individuals as having celiac disease. To do that, we would first need to change the diagnostic criteria for celiac disease. However, clinicians should be aware that gluten sensitivity is not restricted to villous atrophy. The definition of celiac-type gluten sensitivity (celiac trait) should also include the susceptibility genes for celiac disease (1).

Although endomysial antibodies in most studies have been highly efficient in detecting untreated celiac disease and have revealed prevalences of up to 1 of 100 in population-based studies, contradictory reports have been made. According to Rostami et al. (70) endomysial antibody testing has only limited value in screening programs for celiac disease, as many celiac patients were initially negative for these antibodies. Only one third of patients with partial villous atrophy (Marsh IIIa) and none of the first degree relatives with Marsh I-II were endomysial antibody positive. In another study, the same group showed that half of their patients with nonfamilial celiac disease with a Marsh II lesion were DQ2 and DQ8 negative (71).

Searching for the Autoantigen, Tissue Transglutaminase

The antigen recognized by reticulin and endomysial antibodies is highly preserved among both rodents and primates. In humans, the antigen is present in the extracellular matrix of most tissues (57), and the antibodies have been interpreted as being the target organ related IgA class autoantibodies in celiac disease (58). IgA antibodies in sera from patients recognize a common antigen in an amorphous component associated with collagen fibers (72,73). Pursuit of the autoantigen has been in progress for years. In 1973, Pras and Glynn isolated a noncollagenous reticulin component from kidney tissue (74), and subsequent studies suggested that histologic reticulin was not a single entity (75). Interestingly, Unsworth et al. (76) showed specific gliadin binding in a reticulinlike manner to connective tissue fibers of mammalian tissues. We again have identified and purified extracellular matrix, noncollagenous protein molecules in human fetal lung tissue that bound specifically to serum reticulin and endomysial IgA from patients with celiac disease, and we called this complex protein "celiac disease autoantigen protein," CDAP. We further showed the autoantigen to be expressed by human fibroblasts (53,54). Other groups have also lately joined the chase for the autoantigen (77–80).

Recently, Dieterich et al. (81) showed that immunoprecipitation of human fibrosarcoma cell lysates (cell line HT 1080) using the IgA fraction from serum samples of patients with celiac disease resulted in a single protein band with a molecular weight of 85 kd. Immunoprecipitation occurred exclusively with 25 celiac disease serum samples, but with none of the 25 control samples. The 85-kd antigen was cleaved with endoproteinase Asp-N and, after amino-terminal sequence analysis, the three cleavage products tested all yielded sequences that could be assigned to tissue transglutaminase (EC 2.3.2.13). To prove that tissue transglutaminase obtained from the fibrosarcoma cells binds to the endomysial antibody fraction of celiac serum IgA, these investigators performed indirect immunofluorescence with high titer celiac disease serum samples on monkey esophagus with or without prior incubation of those samples with a commercially available tissue transglutaminase extract. Pretreatment with tissue transglutaminase also almost completely abolished endomysial antibody labeling. Dieterich et al. concluded they have identified this enzyme as the unknown endomysial autoantigen (81).

The identification of tissue transglutaminase as the endomysial autoantigen has given us an additional tool for screening. IgA class tissue transglutaminase autoantibodies seem to be highly accurate in detecting untreated celiac disease (82,83). These studies confirm that this enzyme is the target self-antigen for endomysial antibodies. Further, Lock et al. (84) show that both reticulin and endomysial reactivities seen in celiac disease arise because of an immune response to tissue transglutaminase. The possibility, however, remains that further autoantigenic epitopes exist that are not related to tissue transglutaminase (84,85).

Tissue transglutaminase is widely distributed in human organs and belongs to a family of calcium-dependent enzymes catalyzing cross-link formation between glutamine residues and lysine residues in substrate proteins. Gliadin is one of its substrates. Furthermore, deamidation of gliadins by this enzyme creates an epitope that binds efficiently to both DQ2 and DQ8 and is recognized by gut-derived T cells (86,87). This is a new mechanism that may be relevant for loss of tolerance and the initiation of autoimmune disease.

Autoantibodies and Celiac Disease Pathogenesis

The pathogenic mechanisms behind the gluten-induced celiac disease, small bowel lesion are unknown. No attempts have yet been made to prove or disprove whether

celiac disease–specific tissue autoantibodies could have a pathogenic role in inducing the mucosal lesion. This hypothesis, presented earlier (51), is often totally dis-
missed on the grounds that the serum endomysial antibody test is sometimes, or in
certain centers, negative at the time of diagnosis. However, these autoantibodies are
originally synthesized at intestinal level (88–90) and detectable serum antibodies
may appear later on, perhaps decades later. Also, in untreated celiac disease, IgA
deposits are seen in the small bowel mucosa and on subepithelial fibroblasts (91).
It seems that the IgA is trapped in the mucosa. In all, we felt that the hypothesis
was valid and worth testing. By no means, do we infer that gluten sensitivity is
caused exclusively by endomysial antibody production (92). On the other hand, in
myasthenia gravis, for example, muscle weakness and fatigue are caused by autoantibodies binding to the acetylcholine receptors (93). Furthermore, it was recently
shown that autoantibodies can induce arthritis; the disease requires T cells; surprisingly, however, B cells are also needed (94).

The differentiation programs of gut epithelial cells are influenced by reciprocal
permissive and instructive interactions (cross talk) between different cell compartments. In particular, mesenchymal fibroblasts—which in the small intestinal pericryptal area lie immediately beneath the epithelial cell basement membrane, where
they replicate and migrate in parallel and in approximate synchrony with the replicat-
ing and migrating epithelial cells—play a central role in the regulation of epithelial
cell proliferation and differentiation through the growth factors they produce. We,
thus, hypothesized that celiac disease–associated IgA class antibodies interfere with
the fibroblast-epithelial cell cross talk in the crypt–villus axis. We took advantage of
our recently described three-dimensional fibroblast–epithelial cell coculture method,
whereby we showed that the differentiation and organization of intestinal cryptlike
T84 epithelial cells into luminal formations was induced by fibroblasts through TGF-
β_1 (95). We were able to show that celiac disease serum IgA, together with antibodies
against tissue transglutaminase, interferes with the mesenchymal cell–epithelial cell
cross talk in our *in vitro* model, resulting in inhibition of epithelial cell differentiation
and increased proliferation (55). As part of the process leading to villous atrophy and
crypt hyperplasia in celiac disease, the reticulin and endomysial tissue autoantibodies
specific for tissue transglutaminase might also disturb the biological functioning of
TGF-β_1 *in vivo*.

In Fig. 3 a potential role of tissue transglutaminase (reticulin and endomysial)
antibodies is shown. Tissue transglutaminase is involved in the activation of latent
TGF-β by cross-linking the latent TGF-β complex through latent TGF-β binding
protein 1 to the extracellular matrix. Activated TGF-β_1 is needed for epithelial cell
differentiation (95). We have recently shown that celiac disease–associated IgA
class antibodies, such as monoclonal tissue transglutaminase antibodies, indeed have
a biological effect and disturb TGF-β mediated fibroblast-epithelial cell cross talk
(55). The need for tissue transglutaminase in the activation of latent TGF-β might
well be the explanation of how endomysial autoantibodies inhibit epithelial cell
differentiation. If this occurs *in vivo*, it will result in the migration of more immature
crypt epithelial cells to the surface. Nature might have meant local autoantibodies
to work in a protective way in this situation (i.e., ''to get rid of the bug''), which

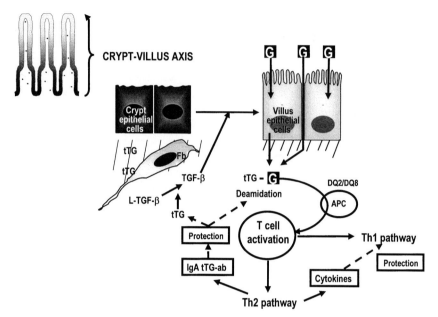

FIG. 3. Gliadin-induced T-cell activation on the small bowel crypt–villus axis in celiac disease. Tissue transglutaminase-activated transforming growth factor (TGF) β is required for epithelial cell differentiation on the normal crypt–villus axis (95). In patients with celiac disease, tissue transglutaminase deamidated gliadin is presented by either the DQ2 or DQ8 molecule to immuno-competent T cells (86,87). Celiac disease–specific IgA has been shown to have a biologic effect (i.e., tissue transglutaminase antibodies inhibit epithelial cell differentiation) (55). It is hypothe-sized that nature has meant a protective role for mucosal tissue autoantibodies. APC, antigen-presenting cell; Fb, fibroblast; G, gluten, gliadin.

in our case is gluten. Continuing gluten ingestion could cause a spillover effect: a vicious circle resulting in morphologic changes, villous atrophy, crypt hyperplasia, and the presence of circulating autoantibodies. If deamidation of gliadin by tissue transglutaminase occurs *in vivo* and is crucial for celiac disease pathogenesis, it is tempting to speculate that local tissue transglutaminase autoantibodies are meant for protection. By inhibiting tissue transglutaminase activity and thus gliadin deami-dation (or overdeaminating gliadin), T cells would not be activated as no modified gliadin would fit to the DQ2 or DQ8 groove. Again, continuing gluten ingestion for years would break this protective effect.

GENETICS, CELLULAR IMMUNITY AND PATHOGENESIS OF CELIAC DISEASE

The tendency for celiac disease to run in families is well recognized (1). The disease prevalence among healthy first degree relatives has varied from 1% to 18%. Twin studies have also shown that the genetic component is clear. Concordance between identical twins is 70%, and may even be higher because individuals found to be discordant have later been shown to be concordant (individuals negative for celiac disease on biopsy sampling who later developed the disease i.e., latent celiac disease).

Celiac disease is associated with the HLA class II extended haplotypes DR3-DQ2 or DR5/7-DQ2 (Fig. 1). The DQ2 molecule, an α/β heterodimer, is situated on the surfaces of cells involved in immune responses and is encoded by the alleles DQA1*0501 and DQB1*02 (96). Approximately 10% of patients with celiac disease have the haplotype DR4-DQ8 (DQA1*03, DQB1*0302). Most patients with celiac disease carry the risk alleles, but this is also the case for DQ2 alone in approximately 20% of the general population. Thus, it is probable that other genes outside the HLA region are involved in celiac disease susceptibility (Figs. 1 and 2). Recently, autosomal genomic screening has provided evidence for linkage of several non-HLA loci to celiac disease (97,98). One of the future targets in celiac disease research is to identify additional susceptibility genes and their function.

Several major hypotheses regarding the nature of the primary host defect in celiac disease have been proposed, but the immunologic theory is the one most widely accepted (1). HLA class II molecules on antigen-presenting cells expose processed peptides to immunocompetent T cells (Fig. 3), thus initiating the disease mechanisms (Fig. 4) (55,86,87,99–102). The major environmental trigger is the ingested gluten, but adenovirus infection has also been suggested to play a role. In addition, gliadin-triggered autoimmune mechanisms might be operative in the pathogenesis of celiac disease (51,89,103).

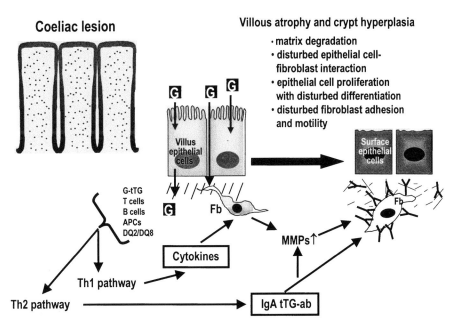

FIG. 4. Pathogenic mechanisms possibly leading to the celiac small bowel lesion. APC, anti-gen-presenting cell; Fb, fibroblast; G, gluten, gliadin; G-tTG, tissue transglutaminase deamidated gliadin; MMP, matrix metalloproteinase.

REFERENCES

1. Mäki M, Collin P. Coeliac disease. *Lancet* 1997; 349: 1755–9.
2. Mäki M, Holm K, Lipsanen V, *et al.* Serological markers and HLA genes among healthy first-degree relatives of patients with coeliac disease. *Lancet* 1991; 338: 1350–3.
3. Reunala T, Kosnai I, Karpati S, Kuitunen P, Török E, Savilahti E. Dermatitis herpetiformis: jejunal findings and skin response to gluten-free diet. *Arch Dis Child* 1984; 59: 517–22.
4. Reunala T, Mäki M. Dermatitis herpetiformis: a genetic disease. *Eur J Dermatol* 1993; 3: 519–26.
5. Aine L, Mäki M, Collin P, Keyriläinen O. Dental enamel defects in celiac disease. *J Oral Pathol Med* 1990; 19: 241–5.
6. Gobbi G, Bouquet F, Greco L, *et al.* Coeliac disease, epilepsy and cerebral calcifications. *Lancet* 1990; 340: 439–43.
7. Volta U, De Franceschi L, Lari F, Molinaro N, Zoli M, Bianchi FB. Coeliac disease hidden by cryptogenic hypertransaminasaemia. *Lancet* 1998; 352: 26–9.
8. Holmes GKT, Prior P, Lane MR, Pope D, Allan RN. Malignancy in coeliac disease—effect of a gluten free diet. *Gut* 1989; 30: 333–8.
9. Collin P, Pukkala E, Reunala T. Malignancy and survival in dermatitis herpetiformis: a comparison with coeliac disease. *Gut* 1996; 38: 528–30.
10. Mazure R, Vazquez H, Gonzalez D, *et al.* Bone mineral affection in asymptomatic adult patients with celiac disease. *Am J Gastroenterol* 1994; 89: 2130–4.
11. Mustalahti K, Collin P, Sievänen H, Salmi J, Mäki M. Osteopenia in patients with clinically silent coeliac disease warrants screening. *Lancet* 1999; 354: 744–5.
12. Hadjivassiliou M, Grunewald RA, Chattopadhyay AK, *et al.* Clinical, radiological, neurophysiological, and neuropathological characteristics of gluten ataxia. *Lancet* 1998; 352: 1582–5.
13. Ventura A, Magazzu G, Greco L, *et al.* Duration of exposure to gluten and risk for autoimmune disorders in patients with celiac disease. *Gastroenterology* 1999; 117: 297–303.
14. Freeman HJ, Chiu BK. Multifocal small bowel lymphoma and latent celiac sprue. *Gastroenterology* 1986; 90: 1992–7.
15. Mäki M, Aine L, Lipsanen V, Koskimies S. Dental enamel defects in first-degree relatives of coeliac disease patients. *Lancet* 1991; 337: 763–4.
16. Savilahti E, Reunala T, Mäki M. Increase of lymphocytes bearing the gamma/delta T-cell receptor in the jejunum of patients with dermatitis herpetiformis. *Gut* 1992; 33: 206–11.
17. Mäki M, Huupponen T, Holm K, Hällström O. Seroconversion of reticulin autoantibodies predicts coeliac disease in insulin-dependent diabetes mellitus. *Gut* 1995; 36: 239–42.
18. Collin P, Mäki M, Keyriläinen O, Hällström O, Reunala T, Pasternack A. Selective IgA-deficiency and coeliac disease. *Scand J Gastroenterol* 1992; 27: 367–71.
19. Carlsson A, Axelsson I, Borulf S, *et al.* Prevalence of IgA-antigliadin antibodies and IgA-antiendomysium antibodies related to celiac disease in children with Down syndrome. *Pediatrics* 1998; 101: 272–5.
20. Mäki M, Holm K, Koskimies S, Hällström O, Visakorpi JK. Normal small bowel biopsy followed by coeliac disease. *Arch Dis Child* 1990; 65: 1137–41.
21. Collin P, Helin H, Mäki M, Hällström O, Karvonen A-L. Follow-up of patients positive in reticulin and gliadin antibody tests with normal small bowel biopsy findings. *Scand J Gastroenterol* 1993; 28: 595–8.
22. Troncone R. Latent coeliac disease in Italy. *Acta Paediatr* 1995; 84: 1252–7.
23. Corazza GR, Andreani ML, Biagi F, Bonvicini F, Bernardi M, Gasbarrini G. Clinical, pathological, and antibody pattern of latent celiac disease: report of three adult cases. *Am J Gastroenterol* 1996; 91: 2203–7.
24. George EK, Mearin ML, van der Velde EA, *et al.* Low incidence of childhood coeliac disease in the Netherlands. *Pediatr Res* 1995; 37: 213–18.
25. Weile B, Krasilnikoff PA. Extremely low incidence rates of coeliac disease in the Danish population of children. *J Clin Epidemiol* 1993; 46: 661–4.
26. Mäki M, Kallonen K, Lähdeaho M-L, Visakorpi JK. Changing pattern of childhood coeliac disease in Finland. *Acta Paediatr Scand* 1988; 77: 408–12.
27. Mäki M, Holm K. Incidence and prevalence of coeliac disease in Tampere. Coeliac disease is not disappearing. *Acta Paediatr Scand* 1990; 79: 980–2.
28. Ascher H, Holm K, Kristiansson B, Mäki M. Different features of coeliac disease in two neighbouring countries. *Arch Dis Child* 1993; 69: 375–80.
29. Weile B, Cavell B, Nivenius K, Krasilnikoff PA. Striking differences in the incidence of childhood

coeliac disease between Denmark and Sweden: a plausible explanation. *J Pediatr Gastroenterol Nutr* 1995; 21: 64–8.

30. Mäki M, Holm K, Ascher H, Greco L. Factors affecting clinical presentation of coeliac disease: role of type and amount of gluten-containing cereals in the diet. In: Auricchio S, Visakorpi JK, eds. Common food intolerances. 1: Epidemiology of coeliac disease. *Dynamic Nutrition Research* 1992; 2: 76–82.

31. Hallert C. The epidemiology of coeliac disease: a continuous enigma. In: Lohiniemi S, Collin P, Mäki M, eds. *Changing features of coeliac disease*. Tampere: The Finnish Coeliac Society, 1998: 83–7.

32. Greco L, Mäki M, Di Donato F, Visakorpi JK. Epidemiology of coeliac disease in Europe and the Mediterranean area. In: Auricchio S, Visakorpi JK, eds. Common food intolerances. 1: Epidemiology of coeliac disease. *Dynamic Nutrition Research* 1992; 2: 25–44.

33. Catassi C, Rätsch IM, Fabiani E, *et al.* Coeliac disease in the year 2000: exploring the iceberg. *Lancet* 1994; 343: 200–3.

34. Johnston SD, Watson RG, McMillan SA, Sloan J, Love AH. Prevalence of coeliac disease in Northern Ireland. *Lancet* 1997; 350: 1370.

35. Korponay-Szabó IR, Kovács J, Czinner A, Gorácz Gy, Vámos A, Szabó T. High prevalence of silent coeliac disease in preschool children screened with IgA/IgG anti-endomysium antibodies. *J Pediatr Gastroenterol Nutr* 1999; 28: 26–30.

36. Meloni G, Dore A, Fanciulli G, Tanda F, Bottazzo GF. Subclinical coeliac disease in schoolchildren from northern Sardinia. *Lancet* 1999; 353: 37.

37. Csizmadia CGDS, Mearin ML, von Blomberg BME, Brand R, Verloove-Vanhorick SP. An iceberg of childhood coeliac disease in the Netherlands. *Lancet* 1999; 353: 813–14.

38. Fasano A. Where have all the American celiacs gone? *Acta Paediatr* 1996; 85 (suppl 412): 20–4.

39. Not T, Horvath K, Hill ID, *et al.* Celiac disease risk in the USA: high prevalence of antiendomysium antibodies in healthy blood donors. *Scand J Gastroenterol* 1998; 33: 494–8.

40. Rossi TM, Albini CH, Kumar VJ. Incidence of celiac disease identified by the presence of serum endomysial antibodies in children with chronic diarrhea, short stature, or insulin-dependent diabetes mellitus. *J Pediatr* 1993; 123: 262–4.

41. Talal AH, Murray JA, Goeken JA, Sivitz WI. Celiac disease in an adult population with insulin-dependent diabetes mellitus: use of endomysial antibody testing. *Am J Gastroenterol* 1997; 92: 1280–4.

42. Fraser-Reynolds KA, Butzner JD, Stephure DK, Trussell RA, Scott R. Use of immunoglobulin A–antiendomysial antibody to screen for celiac disease in North American children with type 1 diabetes. *Diabetes Care* 1998; 21: 1985–9.

43. Walker-Smith JA, Guandalini S, Schmitz J, Shmerling DH, Visakorpi JK. Revised criteria for diagnosis of coeliac disease. *Arch Dis Child* 1990; 65: 909–11.

44. Walker-Smith JA. Discussion of diagnostic criteria for coeliac disease. In: Mäki M, Collin P, Visakorpi JK, eds. *Coeliac disease*. Tampere: University of Tampere, 1997: 191–3.

45. Sanderson MC, Davis LR, Mowat AP, *et al.* Failure of laboratory and radiological studies to predict jejunal mucosal atrophy. *Arch Dis Child* 1975; 50: 526–31.

46. Mäki M. The humoral immune system in coeliac disease. In: Howdle PD, ed. Coeliac disease. *Baillieres Clin Gastroenterol* 1995; 9: 231–49.

47. Janatuinen EK, Pikkarainen PH, Kemppainen TH, *et al.* A comparison of diets with and without oats in adults with celiac disease. *N Engl J Med* 1995; 333: 1033–7.

48. Mäki M, Kaukinen K, Holm K, Collin P. Treatment of coeliac patients with oats and wheat starch. In: Lohiniemi S, Collin P, Mäki M, eds. *Changing features of coeliac disease*. Tampere: The Finnish Coeliac Society, 1998: 93–6.

49. Kaukinen K, Collin P, Holm K, *et al.* Wheat starch-containing gluten-free flour products in the treatment of coeliac disease and dermatitis herpetiformis. *Scand J Gastroenterol* 1999; 34: 163–9.

50. Deutsch H. Food legislation and contamination. In: Lohiniemi S, Collin P, Mäki M, eds. *Changing features of coeliac disease*. Tampere: The Finnish Coeliac Society, 1998: 37–44.

51. Mäki M. Autoantibodies as markers of autoimmunity in coeliac disease pathogenesis. In: Feighery C, O'Farrelly C, eds. *Gastrointestinal immunology and gluten-sensitive disease*. Dublin: Oak Tree Press, 1994: 246–52.

52. Mäki M, Hällström O, Vesikari T, Visakorpi JK. Evaluation of a serum IgA class reticulin antibody test for the detection of childhood celiac disease. *J Pediatr* 1984; 105: 901–5.

53. Mäki M, Hällström O, Marttinen A. Reaction of human non-collagenous polypeptides with coeliac disease autoantibodies. *Lancet* 1991; 338: 724–5.

54. Marttinen A, Mäki M. Purification of fibroblast-derived coeliac disease autoantigen molecules. *Pediatr Res* 1993; 34: 420–3.
55. Halttunen T, Mäki M. Serum immunoglobulin A from patients with celiac disease inhibits human T84 intestinal crypt epithelial cell differentiation. *Gastroenterology* 1999; 116: 566–72.
56. Unsworth DJ, Brown DI. Serological screening suggests that adult coeliac disease is underdiagnosed in the UK and increases the incidence by up to 12%. *Gut* 1994; 35: 61–4.
57. Hällström O. Comparison of IgA-class reticulin and endomysial antibodies in celiac disease and dermatitis herpetiformis. *Gut* 1989; 30: 1225–32.
58. Kárpáti S, Bürgin-Wolff A, Krieg T, *et al.* Binding to human jejunum of serum IgA antibody from children with coeliac disease. *Lancet* 1990; 336: 1335–8.
59. Chorzelski TP, Sulej J, Tschorzewska H, *et al.* IgA class endomysial antibodies in dermatitis herpetiformis and celiac disease. *Ann N Y Acad Sci* 1983; 420: 325–34.
60. Chorzelski TP, Beutner EH, Sulej J, *et al.* IgA-antiendomysial antibody. A new immunological marker of dermatitis herpetiformis and celiac disease. *Br J Dermatol* 1984; 111: 395–402.
61. Ladinser B, Rossipal E, Pittschieler K. Endomysium antibodies in coeliac disease: an improved method. *Gut* 1994; 35: 776–8.
62. Volta U, Molinaro N, de-Franceschi L, Fratangelo D, Bianchi FB. IgA anti-endomysial antibodies on human umbilical cord tissue for celiac disease screening. Save both money and monkeys. *Dig Dis Sci* 1995; 40: 1902–5.
63. Carroccio A, Cavataio F, Iacono G, *et al.* IgA antiendomysial antibodies on the umbilical cord in diagnosing celiac disease. Sensitivity, specificity, and comparative evaluation with the traditional kit. *Scand J Gastroenterol* 1996; 31: 759–63.
64. Yiannakou JY, Dell'Olio D, Saaka M, *et al.* Detection and characterisation of anti-endomysial antibody in coeliac disease using human umbilical cord. *Int Arch Allergy Immunol* 1997; 112: 140–4.
65. Kolho KL, Savilahti E. IgA endomysium antibodies on human umbilical cord: an excellent diagnostic tool for coeliac disease in childhood. *J Pediatr Gastroenterol Nutr* 1997; 24: 563–7.
66. Not T, Citta A, Lucchesi A, Torre G, Martelossi S, Ventura A. Anti-endomysium antibody on human umbilical cord vein tissue: an inexpensive and sensitive diagnostic tool for the screening of coeliac disease. *Eur J Pediatr* 1997; 156: 616–18.
67. Sulkanen S, Halttunen T, Marttinen A, Leivo EL, Laurila K, Mäki M. Autoantibodies in coeliac disease: importance of fibroblasts. *J Pediatr Gastroenterol Nutr* 1998; 27: 206–13.
68. Sulkanen S, Collin P, Laurila K, Mäki M. IgA- and IgG-class antihuman umbilical cord antibody tests in adult coeliac disease. *Scand J Gastroenterol* 1998; 33: 251–4.
69. Iltanen S, Holm K, Partanen J, Laippala P, Mäki M. Increased density of jejunal γδ+ T cells in patients having normal mucosa—marker of operative autoimmune mechanisms? *Autoimmunity* 1999; 29: 179–87.
70. Rostami K, Kerckhaert J, Tiemessen R, von Blomberg BM, Meijer JW, Mulder CJ. Sensitivity of antiendomysium and antigliadin antibodies in untreated celiac disease: disappointing in clinical practice. *Am J Gastroenterol* 1999; 94: 888–94.
71. Crusius JBA, Mulder CJJ, Wahab P, *et al.* HLA-DQ typing of gluten sensitive patients with a Marsh II lesion. *Abstracts of Eighth International Symposium on Celiac Disease*, Castel Sant'Elmo, Naples, Italy, 21–24 April 1999: 108.
72. Kárpáti S, Stolz W, Meurer M, *et al.* Extracellular binding sites of IgA anti-jejunal antibodies on normal small bowel detected by indirect immunoelectron microscopy. *J Invest Dermatol* 1991; 96: 228–33.
73. Kárpáti S, Meurer M, Stolz W, *et al.* Ultrastructural binding sites of endomysium antibodies from sera of patients with dermatitis herpetiformis and coeliac disease. *Gut* 1992; 33: 191–3.
74. Pras M, Glynn LE. Isolation of a non-collagenous reticulin component and its primary characterization. *Br J Exp Pathol* 1973; 54: 449–56.
75. Unsworth DJ, Scott DL, Almond TJ, *et al.* Studies on reticulin. I: Serological and immunohistological investigations of the occurrence of collagen type III, fibronectin, and the non-collagenous glycoprotein of Pras and Glynn in reticulin. *Br J Exp Pathol* 1982; 63: 154–66.
76. Unsworth DJ, Leonard JN, Hobday CM, *et al.* Gliadin binds to reticulin in a lectin-like manner. *Arch Dermatol Res* 1987; 279: 232–5.
77. Kárská K, Tucková L, Steiner L, *et al.* Calreticulin—the potential autoantigen in celiac disease. *Biochem Biophys Res Commun* 1995; 209: 597–605.
78. Whelan A, Willoughby R, Weir D. Human umbilical vein endothelial cells: a new easily available source of endomysial antigens. *Eur J Gastroenterol Hepatol* 1996; 8: 961–6.

79. Börner H, Osman AA, Meergans T, *et al.* Isolation of antigens recognized by coeliac disease autoantibodies and their use in enzyme immunoassay of endomysium and reticulin antibody-positive human sera. *Clin Exp Immunol* 1996; 106: 344–50.

80. Uibo R, Uibo O, Reimand K, Peterson P, Krohn K. Characterization by molecular cloning an antigen reactive with antireticulin antibodies. *Ann NY Acad Sci* 1997; 815: 509–11.

81. Dieterich W, Ehnis T, Bauer M, *et al.* Identification of tissue transglutaminase as the autoantigen of coeliac disease. *Nat Med* 1997; 3: 797–801.

82. Sulkanen S, Halttunen T, Laurila K, *et al.* Tissue transglutaminase autoantibody enzyme-linked immunosorbent assay in detecting celiac disease. *Gastroenterology* 1998; 115: 1322–8.

83. Dieterich W, Laag E, Schöpper H, *et al.* Autoantibodies to tissue transglutaminase as predictors of celiac disease. *Gastroenterology* 1998; 115: 1317–21.

84. Lock RJ, Gilmour JE, Unsworth DJ. Anti-tissue transglutaminase, anti-endomysium and anti-R1-reticulin autoantibodies—the antibody trinity of coeliac disease. *Clin Exp Immunol* 1999; 116: 258–62.

85. Uhlig H, Osman AA, Tanev ID, Viehweg J, Mothes T. Role of tissue transglutaminase in gliadin binding to reticular extracellular matrix and relation to coeliac disease autoantibodies. *Autoimmunity* 1998; 28: 185–95.

86. Molberg O, McAdam SN, Korner R, *et al.* Tissue transglutaminase selectively modifies gliadin peptides that are recognized by gut-derived T cells in coeliac disease. *Nat Med* 1998; 4: 713–17.

87. van de Wal Y, Kooy Y, van Veelen P, *et al.* Selective deamidation by tissue transglutaminase strongly enhances gliadin-specific T cell reactivity. *J Immunol* 1998; 161: 1585–8.

88. Mawhinney H, Lowe AHG. Anti-reticulin antibody in jejunal juice in celiac disease. *Clin Exp Immunol* 1975; 21: 394–8.

89. Picarelli A, Maiuri L, Frate A, Greco M, Auricchio S, Londei M. Production of antiendomysial antibodies after in-vitro gliadin challenge of small intestine biopsy samples from patients with coeliac disease. *Lancet* 1996; 348: 1065–7.

90. Sblattero D, Not T, Marzari R, Bradbury A. Phage antibody library from celiac disease patients. *J Pediatr Gastroenterol Nutr* 1999; 28: 568.

91. Mäki M, Hällström O, Sulkanen S, Marttinen A. Antibodies in coeliac disease. In: Auricchio S, Ferguson A, Troncone R, eds. Mucosal immunity and the gut epithelium: interactions in health and disease. *Dynamic Nutrition Research* 1995; 4: 115–26.

92. Mulder C, Rostami K, Marsh MN. When is a coeliac a coeliac? *Gut* 1998; 42: 594.

93. Vincent A, Willcox N, Hill M, Curnow J, MacLennan C, Beeson D. Determinant spreading and immune responses to acetylcholine receptors in myasthenia gravis. *Immunol Rev* 1998; 164: 157–68.

94. Korganow AS, Ji H, Mangialaio S, *et al.* From systemic T cell self-reactivity to organ-specific autoimmune disease via immunoglobulins. *Immunity* 1999; 10: 451–61.

95. Halttunen T, Marttinen A, Rantala I, Kainulainen H, Mäki M. Fibroblasts and transforming growth factor β induce organization and differentiation of T84 human epithelial cells. *Gastroenterology* 1996; 111: 1252–62.

96. Sollid LM, Thorsby E. HLA susceptibility genes in celiac disease: genetic mapping and role in pathogenesis. *Gastroenterology* 1993; 105: 910–22.

97. Zhong F, McCombs CC, Olson JM, *et al.* An autosomal screen for genes that predispose to celiac disease in the western counties of Ireland. *Nat Genet* 1996; 14: 329–33.

98. Greco L, Corazza G, Babron MC, *et al.* Genome search in celiac disease. *Am J Hum Genet* 1998; 62: 669–75.

99. Lundin KEA, Scott H, Hansen T, *et al.* Gliadin-specific, HLA.DQ(α_1*0501,β_1*0201) restricted T cells isolated from the small intestinal mucosa of celiac disease patients. *J Exp Med* 1993; 178: 187–96.

100. Pender SLF, Ticle SP, Docherty AJP, Howie D, Wathen NC, MacDonald TT. A major role for matrix metalloproteinases in T cell injury in the gut. *J Immunol* 1997; 159: 1583–90.

101. Bajaj-Elliott M, Poulsom R, Pender SL, Wathen NC, MacDonald TT. Interactions between stromal cell-derived keratinocyte growth factor and epithelial transforming growth factor in immune-mediated crypt cell hyperplasia. *J Clin Invest* 1998; 102: 1473–80.

102. Maiuri L, Auricchio S, Coletta S, *et al.* Blockage of T-cell costimulation inhibits T-cell action in celiac disease. *Gastroenterology* 1998; 115: 564–72.

103. Mäki M. Coeliac disease and autoimmunity due to unmasking cryptic epitopes. *Lancet* 1996; 348: 1046–7.

DISCUSSION

Dr. Roy: I think the interpretation of what you call autoantibodies requires caution. Recent studies, particularly in *nod* mice, where the investigators were able to prevent the development of diabetes by desensitization of the animals to glutamic acid decarboxylase, was convincing evidence that, in fact, they may play a pathogenic role. Antibodies may not be merely spectators of an ongoing difficulty. The problem with the transglutaminase is the fact that no real animal model for celiac disease exists.

Dr. Mäki: I agree. The problem is that we have no animal model, so we established this model on the crypt–villus axis where we can look at mesenchyme–epithelial cell cross talk and the genes involved, and we did show that these antibodies have biological effects. Also, a recent paper in *Immunity* described a mouse model where autoantibodies induce autoimmune disease (1).

Dr. Bjarnason: You say no animal model has been bred for celiac disease; if I remember correctly, however, Batt has bred a unique strain of Irish Setter that is clearly gluten sensitive.

Dr. Mäki: We have collaborated with Dr. Batt's laboratory. When you look at these dogs, they are gluten sensitive, but their mucosa is not the same as in celiac disease. They lack the crypt hyperplasia. They are gluten sensitive in a way we see in atopic humans, with infiltration, gliadin antibodies, and so on. These dogs do not have reticulin antibodies or endomysial antibodies. Gluten-sensitive enteropathy in the dogs does not appear to be determined by variation within the major histocompatibility complex (MHC) class II cluster (DQ). This is not a model for celiac disease (2).

Dr. Koletzko: Is there any difference in the pathogenesis between celiac disease with selective IgA deficiency and that in patients who are nondeficient?

Dr. Mäki: I do not know. We are trying to solve the main problem first, and then we will look at the exceptions. Perhaps no big differences exist and maybe IgM takes over. I do not know where these antibodies come from and I am not saying that they provoke the disease.

Dr. Parsons: My question goes back to the epitope in food. How broad are the epitopes that are represented by the HLA-DQ2? Would you modify the gluten in such a way that it does not present those epitopes?

Dr. Mäki: If you modify wheat genetically by removing the gliadin, the baking properties will probably be lost. Maybe we have this already: we call it potato, we call it rice! However, an enormous amount of money is being invested in this in Germany. It now seems that glutinins might not be disease inducing. In the past, when they have been shown to be disease inducing, contamination with gliadin was always found. If it can be shown that they are not disease inducing when they are not contaminated by gliadin, it should be possible to produce "gluten-free" wheat by genetic engineering. This should preserve the baking properties in the absence of disease-inducing gliadin.

Dr. Spolidoro: Autoimmune enteropathy is associated with an atrophic mucosa and also with Crohn's disease. These patients usually do not respond very well to a gluten-free diet—they need to receive immune suppressive drugs. Have you studied tissue transaminase in these patients?

Dr. Mäki: No, I have not.

Dr. Seidman: I can perhaps answer that. The patients with autoimmune enteropathy we have studied are all antiendomysium and antigliadin positive to a high degree; I have not yet studied transglutaminase, but I suspect that will be positive as well.

Dr. Mäki: I believe that the literature reports that they are antiendomysial antibody negative. It is very surprising to hear that they are endomysial antibody positive.

Dr. Goulet: To my knowledge and in our experience, they are negative.

Dr. N. Wright: You referred to the concept of the myofibroblast escalator, whereby epithelial cells move up the crypt in the villi on the back of the myofibroblast. Recent studies by Neal et al. (3,4) have shown that the migration rate of myofibroblast is extremely slow. In the small intestine, they do not get beyond the crypt–villus junction; they move off in the lamina propria and become polypoid. So, it is highly unlikely that myofibroblasts actually carry epithelial cells up the villi.

Dr. Mäki: I did not mean that they go all the way up. I know those studies showing that they only travel halfway. My point was that there should be cross talk.

Dr. N. Wright: In your coculture system, you had the fibroblasts above a membrane, without cell-to-cell contact. Could you identify collagen in the gel after the T84 cells were differentiated?

Dr. Mäki: We have not looked for that. We used rat tendon tail type I collagen when we built up the system. I took the model from Montesano's paper in *Cell* in 1991 (5).

Dr. N. Wright: So, is this process of differentiation RGD dependent? Can you inhibit it with RGD antibodies?

Dr. Mäki: We have not looked at this.

Dr. N. Wright: Well, you should, because epithelial cells and RGD with type I collagen can produce differentiation of things such as HT29 and so on.

Dr. Mäki: In monolayers, HT29 is active, but not in this three-dimensional system. They are not organized into luminal formations, even in the presence of type I collagen and even when given fibroblast support or TGF-β support.

Dr. N. Wright: But HRA19 cell lines will differentiate in type I collagen.

Dr. Lionetti: TGF-β has been mentioned many times. This is a molecule associated with well-differentiated enterocytes; it is an immunosuppressive cytokine. Therefore, one would expect it to be decreased in cases of inflammation. However, this is not the case, because it increases in the lamina propria in inflammatory bowel disease. We have also recently found increased expression of TGF-β in the lamina propria in celiac disease, whereas in normal control mucosa, very little expression is seen in the lamina propria. How does that fit with your work? Do you have any speculations?

Dr. Mäki: We shall have to find out how it fits in. At present, I have no comment.

Dr. Brandtzaeg: It should very easy to test part of your hypothesis experimentally. If your antiendomysial antibodies, which are not species specific, inhibit maturation of TGF-β and thereby inhibit differentiation of epithelial cells, this effect should be reproducible in a mouse by causing an epithelial lesion (e.g., with alcohol) and the regeneration of this epithelium examined after injecting human IgA antibodies. That should be easy to do.

Dr. Endres: One very simple question about treatment: what does gluten-free mean? Is it 200 ppm, or less, provided that we have a reproducible precise method?

Dr. Mäki: A very active polarized discussion is going on in the *Codex* commission and worldwide about this. In Finland, we have been treating patients with celic disease for 40 years with gluten-free diets based on the *Codex* allowance, which means industrial gluten-free flours that are based on starch. They contain very small amounts of gluten. We did biopsies in these patients after 10 years—adults and children—and the mucosa is very healthy—much better than in an Italian study that is often quoted where they used a naturally gluten-free diet (6,7). However, discussion about this is ongoing, although it is now known that industrially purified gluten-free flour may be much more pure than naturally gluten-free flour. For example, soya flour may contain 3,000 ppm of gluten, and similar amounts may be present in rice, maize, buckwheat, and so on—probably because international trade allows grain dockage. Without notification, 5% wheat can be found in corn or rice. This is a political issue. If the next *Codex* specifies 200 ppm, that is fine; it is less than today, and the industry will cope with that.

Dr. Panagiotou-Angelakopoulou: Over recent years, we have seen a dramatic increase in the diagnosis of silent forms of celiac disease. Do you think these patients are at the same risk as those with classic celiac disease for developing malignancy and should, therefore, be placed on a lifelong strict gluten-free diet?

Dr. Mäki: I think they have the same risk, but for malignancy the risk is small. In looking at the new publications, it is very low. The risk is probably greater for other things such as infertility, central and peripheral nervous system disorders, osteopenia, and general quality of health. If I do a biopsy and find it flat, I will treat, whatever the symptoms. But whether population screening would be ethical is another matter. If we found 100,000 patients with celiac disease in the streets of Montreal, should they be treated or not? We do not know if we would be doing more harm than good.

Dr. Seidman: In the infant with classic celiac disease who has positive autoantibodies, is a biopsy essential?

Dr. Mäki: Today, a biopsy is essential because it is required to fulfill our diagnostic criteria. When we have proved over and over, in different settings, that serologic diagnosis works, then we may be able to skip biopsies. We know now that celiac disease is a continuum from normal looking to flat mucosa, but we need more research and proof. Currently, however, we must stick to today's criteria, otherwise we will lose the case.

Dr. Seidman: The comparison I would like to raise is that many years ago cystic fibrosis was diagnosed by jejunal capsule biopsy, on the basis of staining of the mucous glands, and yet we do not now require jejunal biopsies to confirm the sweat test. The predictive value of the transglutaminase test is comparable to, if not superior to, the sweat test.

Dr. Mäki: The predictive value of transglutaminase is very good, but problems still exist, as assays are done with crude liver extracts, which contain a lot of other antigens. From batch to batch, 25% to 75% of the total protein is transglutaminase, which is disappointing. We may do better with human recombinant transglutaminase; we will see.

REFERENCES

1. Korganow AS, Ji H, Mangialaio S, *et al*. From systemic T cell self-reactivity to organ-specific autoimmune disease via immunoglobulins. *Immunity* 1999; 10: 451–61.
2. Polvi A, Garden OA, Houlston RS, *et al*. Genetic susceptibility to gluten sensitive enteropathy in Irish setter dogs is not linked to the major histocompatibility complex. *Tissue Antigens* 1998; 52: 543–9.
3. Neal JV, Potten CS. Description and basic cell kinetics of the murine pericryptal fibroblast sheath. *Gut* 1981; 14: 19–24.
4. Neal JV, Potten CS. Polyploidy in the murine colonic pericryptal fibroblast sheath. *Cell Tissue Kinetics* 1981; 14: 527–36.
5. Montesano R, Matsumoto K, Nakamura T. Identification of a fibroblast-derived epithelial morphogen as hepatocyte growth factor. *Cell* 1991; 67: 901–8.
6. Kaukinen K, Collin P, Holm K, *et al*. Wheat starch-containing gluten-free flour products in the treatment of coeliac disease and dermatitis herpetiformis. A long-term follow-up study. *Scand J Gastroenterol* 1999; 34: 163–9.
7. Catassi C, Rossini M, Rätsch IM, *et al*. Dose dependent effects of protracted ingestion of small amounts of gliadin in coeliac disease children: a clinical and jejunal morphometric study. *Gut* 1999; 34: 1515–9.

Gastrointestinal Functions, edited by Edgard E. Delvin and Michael J. Lentze. Nestlé Nutrition Workshop Series, Pediatric Program, Vol. 46, Nestec Ltd., Vevey/Lippincott Williams & Wilkins, Philadelphia © 2001.

Autoimmune Enteropathy

Olivier Goulet

Department of Pediatrics, University of Paris - Necker; Department of Gastroenterology, Hôpital Necker-Enfants Malades, Paris, France

The definition, presentation, and outcome of the syndrome of intractable diarrhea of infancy (IDI) have changed considerably during the last three decades because of a better understanding of the pathology of the small bowel mucosa and major improvements in nutritional management. IDI was first described by Avery et al. in 1968 (1). Its definition included the following features: diarrhea of more than 2 weeks' duration, age less than 3 months, and three or more negative stool cultures for bacterial pathogens. All cases were managed with intravenous fluids and, despite hospital management, diarrhea was persistent and intractable, with a high mortality rate from infection or malnutrition. Most of the time no specific diagnosis was provided. This syndrome remains a difficult challenge for the pediatrician.

The term ''intractable diarrhea of infancy'' embraces a heterogeneous syndrome with a diverse etiology. ''Intractable diarrhea of infancy with persistent villous atrophy'' alludes to children whose diarrhea starts within the first 2 years of life, is profuse ($\geq$100 ml/kg/d), and persists despite bowel rest. It rapidly becomes life threatening, and long-term total parenteral nutrition (TPN) is required. It is associated with a persistent histologic intestinal lesion and may continue for years despite various therapeutic trials including steroids, cyclosporine A, or both, or tacrolimus. These characteristics clearly differentiate IDI from protracted diarrhea of infancy, which responds to bowel rest or enteral feeding or both and always recovers even after several weeks or months of parenteral or enteral nutrition. The so-called ''protracted diarrhea of infancy'' is either caused by a specific immune deficiency or sensitization to a common food protein (e.g., cow's milk, gluten), or by severe infection of the digestive tract. Three recent studies have shown that IDI is clearly different from protracted diarrhea or severe colitis of infancy, even if the onset is sometimes similar (2–4).

CLASSIFICATION OF INTRACTABLE DIARRHEA OF INFANCY

Within the heterogeneous group of children with IDI, conditions such as autoimmune enteropathy (5) or microvillous atrophy (microvillous inclusion disease) (6) were characterized early on. More recently, an attempt to classify intractable diarrhea according to villous atrophy was proposed on the basis of immunohistologic criteria

275

emphasizing the role of activated T cells in the intestinal mucosa (7). Finally, recent work performed by the European Society of Paediatric Gastroenterology, Hapatology, and Nutrition (ESPGHAN) by collecting cases of IDI and villous atrophy with precisely defined light microscopic characteristics has allowed the categorization of several types of IDI (8). This survey was done to analyze the clinical, histologic, biological, and immunologic features and the outcome of the syndrome of IDI, but excluding microvillous inclusion disease. The main diagnostic criteria for identifying IDI were (a) severe life-threatening diarrhea occurring within the first 24 months of life and requiring TPN, (b) persistent villous atrophy demonstrated in consecutive biopsies, and (c) resistance to several therapeutic trials.

Histologic analysis included the degree of villous atrophy (mild, moderate, severe); crypt size and appearance (hyperplastic or normoplastic), necrotic or branched, and the presence of crypt abscesses; epithelial cell height and appearance (an epithelial cell tuft was defined as focal crowding and disorganization of surface enterocytes); the mononuclear cellularity of the lamina propria; the density of intraepithelial lymphocytes; an increased number of neutrophils and eosinophils, either in the epithelium or in the lamina propria; and the uniform or patchy nature of the enteropathy.

According to clinical and histologic analysis, several groups were identified. The first presented with extradigestive symptoms suggestive of autoimmune enteropathy, including arthritis, diabetes, nephrotic syndrome, dermatitis, anemia, and thrombocytopenia, and tended to have a later onset of diarrhea, which was more profuse than in a group of patients who had only gastrointestinal symptoms and gut autoantibodies. Two other groups included patients who did not have mononuclear cell infiltration of the lamina propria. Some patients were small for gestational age and presented with phenotypic abnormalities corresponding to the previously described "syndromatic diarrhea" (9). Other infants presented with mucosal changes including mild to moderate villous atrophy, epithelial cell tufts, and branching or pseudocystic glands (10). The last group included infants with villous atrophy in which histologic analysis did not result in specific features being recognized.

Histologic analysis seems to be the most important procedure in the diagnosis of IDI. Patients present histologically in two clearly different forms: the first is characterized by mononuclear cell infiltration of the lamina propria and is considered to be associated with activated T cells. The second pattern includes the early onset of severe intractable diarrhea with villous atrophy without mononuclear cell infiltration of the lamina propria but with specific histologic abnormalities involving the epithelium, in which molecular abnormalities of intestinal mucosal development are said to be involved (11).

IMMUNE-MEDIATED INTRACTABLE DIARRHEA OF INFANCY

Clinical Features

The most commonly recognized form of immune-mediated IDI is autoimmune enteropathy. Several observations have led to the concept of autoimmune enteropathy (12–39). The association of severe enteropathy with total villous atrophy and circulating gut autoantibodies was first reported in an adolescent with IgA deficiency

(12). In 1982, Powell et al. reported a familial history involving three generations and 17 boys with various autoimmune disorders, with severe protracted diarrhea in eight who died (13). Unsworth and Walker-Smith suggested the term "autoimmune enteropathy" for severe persistent diarrhea, in the absence of immune deficiency but associated with autoimmune disorders (5). In 1985, Savage et al. (14) described two infants who developed severe secretory diarrhea and an enteropathy in the first few months of life. Their disease was associated with the presence of specific complement-fixing antibodies to small intestinal and colonic epithelium. One patient also had hypothyroidism and diabetes mellitus, with thyroid and islet cell antibodies. Parenteral nutrition was required and one patient died despite treatment with a variety of immunosuppressive drugs. The other patient's diarrhea resolved spontaneously. Subsequently, Mirakian et al. (16) reported a series of 14 infants, aged between 1 month and 1 year, in whom severe protracted diarrhea was accompanied by circulating antibodies to enterocytes and a variety of other probably autoimmune phenomena. Antoantibodies were mainly IgG class. High titers and complement-fixing ability were associated with a poorer prognosis. Half the patients were treated with immunosuppression (prednisolone, azathioprine, or both) and five required TPN.

Such enteropathies seem to include a specific dysfunction of the gut-associated lymphoid tissue with the development of enterocyte autoantibodies in patients in whom enteropathy is not ascribable either to a dietary antigen or to an infectious agent. Nevertheless, they may differ in terms of their age of onset, the severity of the disease, and the presence of other extradigestive symptoms known to be autoimmune.

The onset of the disease is usually early, during the first 2 years of life. Several neonatal cases with a poor prognosis have been reported (17,18). Diarrhea is usually characterized as secretory, but it varies in intensity and type. In our experience, fecal output of 150 ml/kg/d was seen, as well as blood and mucous discharge. Patients with this severe form of clinical expression and a protein-losing enteropathy usually have extensive histologic lesions and the prognosis is poor. The fact that a vast predominance of boys is seen, as well as a family history in several male patients, suggests that some cases may be inherited in an X-linked fashion. Several reports have been made of significant numbers of affected siblings (14–16), first degree relatives (17,19), or other family history (20).

Tests for circulating gut epithelial cell autoantibodies are usually positive. These are primarily IgG, and indirect immunofluorescence has shown that they are directed against components of the brush border or cytoplasm of the enterocytes of normal small bowel mucosa (6,16,25,26).

Histologic Features

Villous atrophy is moderate to severe and always associated with an intestinal mononuclear cell infiltration. This infiltration helps to differentiate immune-mediated enteropathy from other cases of IDI related to an inherited defect of enterocytic differentiation (8). Crypt hyperplasia is variable. A low mitotic rate has been reported (27). In most cases, severe to total villous atrophy is associated with crypt hyperplasia. Total villous atrophy can initially lead to the suspicion of celiac disease. However, in celiac disease, total villous atrophy is associated with a striking increase in the number of intraepithelial lymphocytes (40). In contrast, T-cell infiltration in immune-mediated enteropathy predominates in the lamina propria, with no, or moderate, increase of intraepithelial lymphocytes (8). Immunologic studies have shown an increase in the T-cell receptor (TCR) γδ subset in celiac disease (41); in immune-mediated IDI, the T-cell increase is restricted to the TCR αβ+ subset (8).

In some patients, total villous atrophy is associated with epithelial cell necrosis and crypt abscess formation. The surface epithelium is reduced in height with dedifferentiated and basophilic cells. The number of goblet cells is reduced and, in some cases, no or very few goblet cells could be recognized (42,43). It has been shown in similar cases that mononuclear cell infiltration within the lamina propria includes mainly CD4+ T lymphocytes and macrophages; numerous cells express CD25, whereas HLA-DR expression is increased in crypt epithelium (8). These changes are largely observed in small bowel mucosa, but it also seems important to look for such phenomena in other segments of the digestive tract such as the colon (21) and stomach. When involved, they show the same type of lesions, including epithelial cell necrosis, crypt abscess formation, and mononuclear cell infiltration of the lamina propria. Extensive digestive involvement is usually associated with poor outcome.

T-Cell Activation

In the ESPGHAN study, several cases were characterized by a mononuclear cell infiltrate of the lamina propria and by gut autoantibodies; these may be considered to be associated with activated T cells and epithelial injury, as previously reported (8).

The effect of the enterocyte autoantibodies detected in the serum of most of the patients studied was initially presumed to be deleterious (6,14,16,17,25–27,38). In one study, a high titer of autoantibodies fixing complement was associated with the most severe histologic lesions (16). However, *in situ* detection of autoantibodies observed in one patient (12) was absent in another (27). Moreover, a precise kinetic study performed in one patient showed that the appearance of autoantibodies had followed the appearance of intestinal lesions (25). Treatment with cyclophosphamide caused the disappearance of autoantibodies but only minimal histologic and clinical improvement (26). Finally, autoantibodies were not detected in all patients, and they were also observed in low titer in other enteropathies (16). Together, these data suggest that autoantibodies may be a secondary response to gut epithelial lesions and are more likely to play an aggravating than a primary role in epithelial damage.

Recently, the possible role of intestinal T cells activated by an autoimmune process has been proposed (8). Studies of murine models of graft-versus-host disease (44,45), as well as human fetal organ culture (46), have shown that excessive activation of intestinal T cells can lead to villous atrophy, which may or may not be associated with crypt destruction. The primary role of T lymphocytes attaching to the TCR-αβ in the pathogenesis of autoimmune disease has been demonstrated in several animal models and is strongly suggested to occur in humans (47). The mechanisms by which T cells can induce epithelial damage are unclear (48). T cells may act directly against epithelial cells by exerting cytotoxic activity or through lymphokine secretion. They could also recruit and activate macrophages or favor the production of autoantibodies.

MANAGEMENT AND OUTCOME

The prognosis of autoimmune enteropathy is related to the need for long-term TPN. Because of the clues suggesting that this is an autoimmune disease, or because of associated autoimmune disorders, various immunosuppressive treatments have been attempted. Immunoglobulins (20,22,28), steroids alone (15,30) or with azathioprine or cyclosporine A (14,16,19–22,25,28,29,31–33), cyclophosphamide (14, 17,21,25,26,31), or more recently FK506/tacrolimus (37) have produced clinical improvement and even recovery in several patients. However, other patients' conditions have been only minimally or transiently improved by immunosuppressive regimens, including cyclophosphamide, cyclosporine A, steroids, and antilymphocytic immunoglobulins (31). The various reports suggest that neonatal onset, diarrhea exceeding 150 ml/kg/d, extensive crypt destruction, associated lesions in the colon or the upper digestive tract, severe renal involvement, and perhaps a high titer of circulating enterocyte autoantibodies are associated with a bad prognosis, a poor response to immunosuppressive treatment, and the likelihood of a fatal outcome. It is possible that FK506 treatment will result in a better response (37). We recently performed a fully compatible bone marrow transplant in an infant with IDI, diabetes, and dermatitis. Two months after the procedure, he was weaned from parenteral nutrition with almost normal histology. One year later he is still doing very well without any treatment.

AUTOIMMUNE ENTEROPATHY

In autoimmune enteropathy, the onset of diarrhea is usually several months after birth and associated with extradigestive manifestations such as arthritis, diabetes, dermatitis, thrombocytopenia, and renal disease. Villous atrophy seems to be more pronounced, with severe crypt damage, including necrosis and abscess formation. The high masculine incidence of autoimmune enteropathy suggests an X-linked mode of inheritance (6,13–17,19,25–27,33,38).

Tests for circulating gut epithelial cell autoantibodies are usually positive. Goblet cell autoantibodies have also been detected (42,43). Other associated autoantibodies are mainly directed against the nucleus, the DNA, smooth muscle, or mitochondria. In some cases of autoimmune enteropathy associated with nephropathy, circulating autoantibodies reactive with the renal tissue have also been reported (31,32). No autoantigens specific to autoimmune enteropathy have yet been identified (49). A 75-kd antigen reacting with the autoantibody from two unrelated patients with X-linked autoimmune enteropathy associated with tubulonephropathy has been reported (50). Because this 75-kd antigen is distributed in the intestine and kidney, it was speculated that it could be a common component involved in the development of the tissue damage in both these organs (51). Further studies are needed to confirm this hypothesis. The significance and precise role of gut autoantibodies in the pathogenesis of the disease remain unknown, although the partial response to cyclosporine

A (28,39) and the promising use of FK506 (37) indicate that T cells may be important in the pathogenesis of this disorder.

Finally, in infants with IDI, T-cell infiltration of the lamina propria with or without extradigestive manifestations may correspond to a different degree of expression of the same mechanism that involves activation of intestinal mucosal T cells. Extradigestive symptoms may reflect the presence of shared epitopes between tissues producing cross-reacting autoimmunity. The mechanisms by which activated T cells are responsible for epithelial damage could be through a direct cytotoxic action, lymphokine release, or recruitment and activation of macrophages. It would be worthwhile studying the intestinal T-cell repertoire to investigate the existence of autoreactive intestinal T lymphocytes.

REFERENCES

1. Avery GB, Villacivencio O, Lilly JR, Randolph JG. Intractable diarrhea in early infancy. *Pediatrics* 1968; 41: 712–22.
2. Guarino A, Spagnulo MI, Russo S, *et al.* Etiology and risk factors of severe and protracted diarrhea. *J Pediatr Gastroenterol Nutr* 1995; 20: 173–8.
3. Goulet O, Besnard M, Girardet JP, *et al*, and the French Speaking Group of Hepatology, Gastroenterology and Nutrition. Protracted diarrhoea of infancy—place of parenteral nutrition. *Clin Nutr* 1998; 17: 9(A).
4. Catassi C, Fabiani E, Spagnuolo MI, *et al.* Severe and protracted diarrhea: results of the 3-year SIGEP multicenter survey. *J Pediatr Gastroenterol Nutr* 1999; 29: 63–8.
5. Unsworth DJ, Walker-Smith JA. Auto-immunity in diarrheal disease. *J Pediatr Gastroenterol Nutr* 1985; 4: 375–80.
6. Phillips AD, Jenkins P, Raafat F, Walker-Smith JA. Congenital microvillous atrophy: specific diagnostic features. *Arch Dis Child* 1985; 60: 135–40.
7. Cuenod B, Brousse N, Goulet O, *et al.* Classification of intractable diarrhea in infancy using clinical and immunohistological criteria. *Gastroenterology* 1990; 99: 1037–43.
8. Goulet O, Brousse N, Canioni D, Walker-Smith JA, Schmitz J, Philipps AD. Syndrome of intractable diarrhea with persistent villous atrophy in early childhood: a clinicopatological survey of 47 cases. *J Pediatr Gastroenterol Nutr* 1998; 26: 151–61.
9. Giraut D, Goulet O, Ledeist F, *et al.* Intractable diarrhea syndrome associated with phenotypic abnormalities and immune deficiency. *J Pediatr* 1994; 125: 36–42.
10. Goulet O, Kedinger M, Brousse N, *et al.* Intractable diarrhea of infancy: a new entity with epithelial and basement membrane abnormalities. *J Pediatr* 1995; 127: 212–19.
11. Murch SH. The molecular basis of intractable diarrhoea of infancy. *Bailleres Clin Gastroenterol* 1997; 11: 413–40.
12. McCarthy DM, Katz SI, Gazze L, *et al.* Selective IgA deficiency associated with total villous atrophy of small intestine and an organ-specific anti-epithelial cell antibody. *J Immunol* 1978; 120: 932–8.
13. Powell BR, Buist NRM, Stenzel P. An X-linked syndrome of diarrhea, polyendocrinopathy, and fatal infection in infancy. *J Pediatr* 1982; 100: 731–7.
14. Savage MO, Mirakian R, Wozniak ER, *et al.* Specific autoantibodies to gut epithelium in two infants with severe protracted diarrhea. *J Pediatr Gastroenterol Nutr* 1985; 4: 187–95.
15. Charritat IL, Polonovski C. Entéropathies auto-immunes pédiatriques avec autoanticorps anti cytoplasme entérocytaire. *Ann Pediatr* 1987; 34: 195–203.
16. Mirakian R, Richardson A, Milla PJ, *et al.* Protracted diarrhoea of infancy: evidence in support of an autoimmune variant. *BMJ* 1986; 293: 1132–6.
17. Ellis D, Fisher SE, Smith WI, Jaffe R. Familial occurrence of renal and intestinal disease associated with tissue autoantibodies. *Am J Dis Child* 1982; 136: 323–6.
18. Kanof ME, Rance NE, Hamilton ST, Luk GD, Lake AM. Congenital diarrhea with intestinal inflammation and epithelial immaturity. *J Pediatr Gastroenterol Nutr* 1987; 6: 141–6.
19. Mitton SG, Mirakian R, Larcher VF, Dillon MJ, Walker-Smith JA. Enteropathy and renal involvement in an infant with evidence of widespread autoimmune disturbance. *J Pediatr Gastroenterol Nutr* 1989; 8: 397–400.

20. Satake N, Nakanishi M, Okano, *et al.* A Japanese family of X-linked auto immune enteropathy with haemolytic aneamia and polyendocrinopathy. *Eur J Pediatr* 1993; 152: 313–15.
21. Hill SM, Milla PJ, Bottazzo GF, Mirakian R. Autoimmune enteropathy and colitis: is there a generalised autoimmune gut disorder? *Gut* 1991; 32: 36–42.
22. Lachaux A, Bouvier R, Cozzani E, *et al.* Familial autoimmune enteropathy with circulating antibullous pemphigoid antibodies and chronic autoimmune hepatitis. *J Pediatr* 1994; 125: 858–62.
23. Martini A, Scotta MS, Notarangelo LD, *et al.* Membranous glomerulopathy and chronic small-intestinal enteropathy associated with antibodies directed against renal tubular basement membrane and the cytoplasm of intestinal epithelial cells. *Acta Paediatr Scand* 1983; 72: 931–4.
24. Fischer SE, Smith WI, Rabin BS, *et al.* Secretory component and serum immunoglobulin A deficiencies with intestinal autoantibody formation and autoimmune disease: a family study. *J Pediatr Gastroenterol Nutr* 1982; 1: 35–42.
25. Walker-Smith JA, Unsworth DJ, Hutchins P, *et al.* Autoantibodies against gut epithelium in children with small intestinal enteropathy. *Lancet* 1982; i: 566–7.
26. Unsworth J, Hutchins P, Mitchell J, *et al.* Flat small intestinal mucosa and antibodies against the gut epithelium. *J Pediatr Gastroenterol Nutr* 1982; 1: 503–13.
27. Savilahti E, Pelkonen P, Holmberg C, Perkkio M, Unsworth J. Fatal unresponsive villous atrophy of the jejunum, connective tissue disease and diabetes in a girl with intestinal epithelial cell antibody. *J Pediatr Gastroenterol Nutr* 1989; 8: 259–65.
28. Seidman EG, Lacaille F, Russo P, Galeano N, Murphy G, Roy CC. Successful treatment of autoimmune enteropathy with cyclosporine. *J Pediatr* 1990; 117: 929–32.
29. Coletti RB, Guillot AP, Rosens, *et al.* Autoimmune enteropathy and nephropathy with circulating antiepithelial cell antibodies. *J Pediatr* 1991; 118: 858–64.
30. Jonas MM, Bell MD, Eidson MS, *et al.* Congenital diabetes mellitus and fatal secretory diarrhea in two infants. *J Pediatr Gastroenterol Nutr* 1991; 13: 415–25.
31. Goulet O, Habib R, Sadoun E, *et al.* Diarrhea and diabetes with antibodies (AAb) against gut epithelium in two infants [Abstract]. *J Pediatr Gastroenterol Nutr* 1991; 13: 330(A).
32. Habib R, Bezian A, Goulet O, Blanche S, Niaudet P. Atteinte rénale des entéropathies auto-immunes. *Ann Pediatr* 1993; 2: 103–7.
33. Catassi C, Mirakian R, Natalini G, *et al.* Unresponsive enteropathy associated with circulating enterocyte autoantibodies in a boy with common variable hypogammaglobulinemia and type 1 diabetes. *J Pediatr Gastroenterol Nutr* 1988; 7: 608–13.
34. Levy M. Autoimmune enteropathy anti-tubular basement membrane antibodies and glomerulonephritis. *J Pediatr* 1992; 120: 659.
35. Martin-Villa JM, Regueiro JR, De Luan D, *et al.* T-lymphocyte dysfunctions occurring together with apical gut epithelial cell antoantibodies. *Gastroenterology* 1991; 101: 390–7.
36. Coulthard M, Searle J, Patrick M, *et al.* Cyclosporin-responsive enteropathy and protracted diarrhea. *J Pediatr Gastroenterol Nutr* 1990; 10: 257–61.
37. Bousvaros A, Leichtner AM, Book L, *et al.* Treatment of pediatric autoimmune enteropathy with tacrolimus (FK506). *Gastroenterology* 1996; 111: 237–43.
38. Pearson RD, Swenson I, Schenk EA, Klish WJ, Brown MR. Fatal multisystem disease with immune enteropathy heralded by juvenile rheumatoid arthritis. *J Pediatr Gastroenterol Nutr* 1989; 8: 259–65.
39. Sanderson IR, Phillips AD, Spencer J, Walker-Smith JA. Response of autoimmune enteropathy to cyclosporin A therapy. *Gut* 1991; 32: 1421–6.
40. Kutlu T, Brousse N, Rambaud C, Ledeist F, Schmitz J, Cerf-Bensussan N. Number of T cell receptor (TCR) $\alpha\beta+$ but not of TCR $\gamma\delta+$ intraepiothelial lymphocytes correlates with the grade of villous atrophy in coeliac patients on a long term normal diet. *Gut* 1993; 34: 208–14.
41. Halstensen TS, Scott H, Brantzaeg P. Intraepithelial T cells of the TcRγ/δ + CD8$-$ and Vγ1/$\phi\gamma$1+ phenotypes are increased in coeliac disease. *Scand J Immunol* 1989; 30: 665–72.
42. Moore L, Xiaoning XU, Davidson G, Moore D, Carly M, Ferrante A. Autoimmune enteropathy with anti–goblet cell antibody. *Hum Pathol* 1995; 26: 1162–8.
43. Murch SH, Meadows N, Morgan G, Phillips AD, Walker-Smith JA. Severe enteropathy and immunodeficiency in interleukin-2 deficiency [Abstract]. *J Pediatr Gastroenterol Nutr* 1994; 19: 335.
44. MacDonald TT, Ferguson A. Hypersensitivy reactions in small intestine. III. The effect of allograft rejection and of graft-versus-host disease on epithelial cell kinetics. *Cell Tissue Kinetics* 1977; 10: 301–12.
45. Guy-Grand D, Vassali P. Gut injury in mouse graft-versus-host reaction. Study of its occurrence and mechanism. *J Clin Invest* 1986; 77: 1584–95.
46. MacDonald TT, Spencer J. Evidence that activated mucosal T cells play a role in the pathogenesis of enteropathy in human small intestine. *J Exp Med* 1988; 167: 1341–9.

47. Kumar V, Kono DH, Urban JL, Hood L. The T-cell repertoire and autoimmune diseases. *Annu Rev Immunol* 989; 7: 657–82.
48. Cerf-Bensussan N, Brousse N, Jarry A, *et al.* Role of *in vivo* activated T cells in the mechanisms of villous atrophy in humans: study of allograft rejection. *Digestion* 1990; 46 (suppl): 297–301.
49. Mirakian R, Locatelli M, Bottazzo GF. Disclosure of novel autoantigens in human autoimmunity. *Lancet* 1998; 352: 255–6.
50. Kobayashi I, Imamura K, Yamada M, *et al.* A 75 kDa autoantigen recognized by sera from patients with X-linked autoimmune enteropathy associated with nephropathy. *Clin Exp Immunol* 1998; 111: 527–31.
51. Kobayashi I, Nakanishi M, Okano M, Sakiyama Y, Matsumoto S. Combination therapy with tacrolimus and betamethasone for a patient with X-linked autoimmune enteropathy. *Eur J Pediatr* 1995; 154: 594–5.

DISCUSSION

Dr. Delvin: You showed us an electronmicrograph from a case of microvillous inclusion disease, in which I noticed the rather large secretory granules. As this disorder could be a trafficking disease of protein, lipid, or whatever, what is in those granules and what is the structure of the *cis-* or *trans-*Golgi apparatus in these cells? Are these particles or organelles completely disrupted as well?

Dr. Goulet: That is a difficult question. It is difficult to determine normality. The intracytoplasmic contents, including the Golgi apparatus and the mitochondria, are supposed to be normal. But because part of the microvillus comes from the Golgi apparatus, the assumption must be that it is not in fact normal. But no abnormality has ever been described. As to your first question, I do not know what the microvesicles in the cytoplasm contain.

Dr. Milla: If I just could comment on the secretory granules. Alan Phillips, working with John Walker-Smith, was the person who described those secretory granules, and to this day he does not know what they are. He did a number of investigations in patients with microvillous atrophy, trying to understand whether this was a trafficking defect or not, and was able to show very clearly that hydrolases were inserted into the apical membrane of enterocytes quite normally in these patients. In looking at the microvillous inclusions, they have alkaline phosphatase and hydrolases in them, so it seems very unlikely that this is a trafficking defect and more likely that portions of the apical membrane become unstable for some reason, and then form these vesicles. I think that Dr. Goulet has perhaps somewhat simplified the situation, and many patients do not fall into these neat categories. Examples in the literature show patients with microvillous atrophy who were documented as being quite normal shortly after birth. Then, some incident had occurred in which they developed a diarrheal illness, but biopsy initially showed a morphologically normal intestine. Some weeks later, however, the microvillous inclusions appeared. So, the situation is far from straightforward and the phenotypes seen may be quite distantly related to the underlying defect.

I would like to ask Dr. Goulet a question about tufting enteropathy: we have dubbed this condition "epithelial dysplasia," yet a marked inflammatory component exists in the lamina propria, and the patient's condition can be improved symptomatically if that inflammatory component is dealt with. Why is there an inflammatory component if this is an abnormality of cell-to-cell adhesion of the epithelia?

Dr. Goulet: In relation to your comment about oversimplification, I did mention that probably two or more forms of microvillous inclusion disease exist according to onset, with the earliest onset being related to the worse disease. The mild forms were well described and reported by Phillips and Schmitz in a paper in the *Journal of Pediatric Gastroenterology and Nutrition* (1). I accept that we probably miss some other forms of this disease.

As to your question, Walker-Smith's group demonstrated an inflammatory component in epithelial dysplasia or tufting enteropathy (2). Probably abnormal intestinal permeability occurs with uptake of bacterial products or food antigens, and so on; secondly, from the appearance of the abnormal epithelium, it seems likely that the homing of the intraepithelial lymphocytes and their number and function are disturbed. We can understand this association of an inflammatory process, and indeed Walker-Smith and his colleagues have shown that they can produce clinical improvement in these patients with FK506 or cyclosporine (2). However, this treatment did not resolve the villous atrophy or the underlying disease.

Dr. Zoppi: I would like to know if autoimmune enteropathy is more common in patients with congenital IgA deficiency.

Dr. Goulet: That is a good question. In the diagnosis of this disease, the most important criterion is to eliminate severe combined immune deficiency or combined immune deficiency. In some mild and very common immune deficiencies, particularly IgA deficiency, however, it is well known that there is an association with autoimmune processes. From our own patients and from a review of published reports, it is clear that IgA deficiency is not uncommon in autoimmune enteropathy. An association with IgG2 and IgG4 deficiency has also been described (3). To answer your question, yes, autoimmune enteropathy can be associated with mild immune deficiency, but that is probably not the only explanation, because many of the patients do not have any immune deficiency.

Dr. Seidman: Along those lines, it is worth mentioning the recent case published by Murch et al. wherein severe immune deficiency was associated with autoimmune enteropathy (4). That child had life-threatening infectious complications and, in fact, died of septic complications. We wrote an editorial about the logical paradox that autoimmunity is more common in the face of immune deficiency (5).

Dr. Nanthakumar: Has anybody looked at what happens in the proximal tubules of the kidney in microvillous inclusion disease?

Dr. Goulet: Dr. Lentze has looked at this, so maybe he will answer.

Dr. Lentze: We did look at the kidney. In two patients, we found a particular form of albumin excreted in the urine that was of different molecular weight from normal serum albumin, and Alan Phillips in London found the same protein in the urine of one of his patients. On genetic analysis, looking at whether this was a particular genetic defect, we could not find anything—it was just a pure polymorphism—but it certainly looks as though the kidney is involved. Morphologically, nobody has yet looked at the brush borders in the renal tubules, although it seems as if a particular defect might be in the kidney.

Dr. Marini: I believe that some cases of microvillous atrophy are associated with the hyper IgE syndrome. We have seen two familial cases of this syndrome in which diarrhea developed during fetal life. In both cases, the cause of the diarrhea was later found to be microvillous atrophy. I have a question. In cases wherein was seen an abnormality of the hair, was neutrophil function assessed? Normally, if a problem with brittle hair exists, neutrophil function is impaired, and the patients improve if given granulocyte-stimulating factor.

Dr. Goulet: I agree that the relationship between autoimmune enteropathy and hyper IgE syndrome is clearly defined. It probably involves immunologic mechanisms that are different from the ones I described. Diseases involving the development of epithelium are not known to be expressed during the fetal life except in some cases of microvillous atrophy. One case was described wherein distension of the colon was shown on prenatal echography, but no fetal diarrhea with hydramnios.

In answer to your question, T-cell function and neutrophil function are normal. It seems that this particular deficiency involves cooperation between T and B cells in the formation of antibodies, and the best way to asses that is to perform vaccination and assess the level of antibodies. The most important clinical problems in these patients are that they are small for gestational age without any catch-up, even on TPN, and that they have intractable diarrhea associated with villous atrophy.

Dr. Marini: From our very limited experience and from talking with others, our impression is that babies suffering from microvillous atrophy are more difficult to maintain on TPN than other conditions such as short gut syndrome.

Dr. Goulet: I absolutely agree. Patients with microvillous atrophy constitute the most difficult part of our daily work. Intestinal losses are often increased by increasing the amount of TPN, so it becomes a vicious circle. For that reason, these patients are in a very, very dangerous state, even on parenteral nutrition. So, as soon as the condition of the patient allows, we assess for intestinal transplantation.

Dr. Panagiotou-Angelakopoulou: Does any evidence show that impaired fatty acid metabolism plays a role in immune activation in autoimmune disease in humans? If so, do you think that one could reduce the activity of these disorders by regulating fatty acid balance?

Dr. Goulet: Polyunsaturated, long chain fatty acids do play a role in inducing peroxidation phenomena. However, I am not sure whether this is of such a degree that modulating fatty acid intake would help such severe conditions as autoimmune enteropathy. It could be an interesting therapeutic approach, but with rather a small chance of being successful.

Dr. Milla: You introduced a very important therapeutic advance in autoimmune enteropathy, which is bone marrow transplantation. Clearly, this is a difficult group of patients, and bone marrow transplantation carries a heavy clinical load. What criteria do you apply to these patients before submitting them to transplantation?

Dr. Goulet: I would need the following to be present: (a) severe clinical disease with fever, generally poor condition, severe protein loosing enteropathy, and so on; (b) very severe digestive disease with crypt abscesses, epithelial blunting, and so forth; and (c) serious extra-digestive tract involvement, such as diabetes and renal disease. We had a patient in for bone marrow transplant who developed diabetes during the hospital admission but before the transplant. It was challenging to perform the bone marrow transplant as we did not know what would happen to the diabetes. Fortunately, it reversed completely and the patient's condition is now normal. My conclusion about bone marrow transplantation is that we need to have the patient as early as possible. If we wait for a long time, doing many investigations to confirm worsening renal disease or diabetes, these patients eventually cease to be candidates for bone marrow transplantation.

REFERENCES

1. Philipps AD, Schmitz J. Familial microvillous atrophy: a clinicopathological survey of 23 cases. *J Pediatr Gastroenterol Nutr* 1992; 14: 380–96.
2. Murch S, Graham A, Vermault A, *et al.* Functionally significant secondary inflammation occurs in a primary epithelial enteropathy. *J Pediatr Gastroenterol Nutr* 1997; 24: 467.
3. Goulet O, Brousse N, Canioni D, *et al.* Syndrome of intractable diarrhea with persistent villous atrophy in early childhood: a clinicopatological survey of 47 cases. *J Pediatr Gastroenterol Nutr* 1998; 26: 151–61.
4. Murch SH, Fertleman CR, Rodrigues C, *et al.* Autoimmune enteropathy with distinct mucosal features in T-cell activation deficiency: the contribution of T cells to the mucosal lesion. *J Pediatr Gastroenterol Nutr* 1999; 28: 393–9.
5. Seidman EG, Hollander GA. Autoimmunity with immunodeficiency: a logical paradox. *J Pediatr Gastroenterol Nutr* 1999; 28: 377–9.

Gastrointestinal Functions, edited by Edgard E. Delvin and
Michael J. Lentze. Nestlé Nutrition Workshop Series, Pediatric
Program, Vol. 46, Nestec Ltd., Vevey/Lippincott Williams &
Wilkins, Philadelphia © 2001.

Inflammatory Bowel Disease and Related Models

Hans A. Büller

Department of Pediatrics, Sophia Children's Hospital, Rotterdam, The Netherlands

In the clinical setting, inflammatory bowel disease usually presents as either Crohn's disease or ulcerative colitis (1), and emerging consensus indicates that the underlying disorder, which is characterized by chronic inflammation of the gastrointestinal tract, is the endpoint of several, possibly many, distinct pathophysiologic processes. The true cause is unknown, but it seems clear that an intriguing interaction between *extrinsic factors* (e.g., the flora of the intestine, diet, or drug treatment) and *intrinsic factors*, particularly the genes involved in the immune response, plays an important role in the pathogenesis of the disease. The inflammation of the intestinal mucosa in inflammatory bowel disease is characterized by an influx of large numbers of neutrophils and macrophages that are recruited by chemokines and proinflammatory cytokines (2). The neutrophils and macrophages produce cytokines, eicosanoids, proteolytic enzymes, and free radicals that finally lead to tissue damage. The initiating events that give rise to this nonspecific inflammation remain elusive. However, consensus points to an aberrant activation of the mucosal immune system being a major pathogenic mechanism in inflammatory bowel disease. Although differences are seen between the immunologic abnormalities found in Crohn's disease and those found in ulcerative colitis, it appears that many of these abnormalities are common to both diseases.

As stated, intrinsic and extrinsic factors are involved in a yet unknown interaction resulting in inflammatory bowel disease. It will be the elucidation of these interactions in years to come that will help us understand the etiology. Furthermore, extensive epidemiologic human studies as well as animal studies provide ample evidence that inflammatory bowel disease qualifies as a complex genetic disorder, which is difficult to describe by means of simple mendelian models (3). More likely, several genes interact in different combinations with multiple environmental factors to produce distinct disease entities that share chronic intestinal inflammation as a common feature.

Clinicians have long known that a tremendous heterogeneity exists among patients with inflammatory bowel disease. Although these conditions can be divided on clinical and histopathologic grounds in two disease categories, ulcerative colitis and

Crohn's disease, in approximately 15% of the patients it is impossible to make this distinction. Where this is the case, the condition is called "indeterminate colitis" (4). The clinical course, prognosis, and efficacy of treatment seem to vary in the different disease groups, suggesting that distinct categories can be defined within the ulcerative colitis and Crohn's disease syndromes. Unraveling the heterogeneity and pathogenesis of inflammatory bowel disease will assist the clinician in making a proper diagnosis, in assessing prognosis, and in developing adequate therapeutic strategies.

For the clinician, inflammatory bowel disease presents either as a constellation of abdominal pain, diarrhea, poor appetite, and weight loss, or as a set of complaints encompassing rectal blood loss and frequent loose stools often accompanied by the urge to defecate and tenesmus (1,5). The latter symptoms suggest an inflammatory process in the colon but do not prove the existence of ulcerative colitis and, indeed, Crohn's disease may present as an ulcerative colitis-like syndrome. The presentation with abdominal pain and weight loss suggests an inflammatory process in the small intestine or proximal colon. Of particular importance in both presentations is the presence of extraintestinal manifestations, other systemic symptoms (e.g., fever and malaise), growth failure, and delayed puberty (2,6).

No single test exists that confidently confirms Crohn's disease or ulcerative colitis. The diagnosis is made on the basis of compatible clinical presentation and proper endoscopy with sufficient material from multiple sites for histologic examination. In every child suspected of having inflammatory bowel disease, a full colonoscopy and, when possible, ileoscopy are required. Gastroscopy should be performed if indicated by clinical features or symptoms. Visualization of the small intestine should preferably be performed by small bowel follow-through radiography. All other investigations are supportive but should not replace colonoscopy and small intestinal radiology and, with a low clinical threshold, upper gastrointestinal endoscopy. In most cases, differentiation of Crohn's disease from ulcerative colitis can be made on macroscopic and microscopic criteria (1,2,5,6).

ETIOLOGY

The causes of the chronic inflammatory bowel diseases are still unknown. It is of interest that the incidence of both diseases increases significantly in late childhood and adolescence. This raises the possibility that early events including viral infections may be associated with the later development of inflammatory bowel disease (2).

In recent years, considerable advances have been made in the treatment of this disorder, both in adults and in children (7). It is of the greatest importance to realize that an intestinal surface area of 5,000 m^2 is in intimate contact with the outside world. In this environment, a constant struggle occurs between tolerance and immune reactivity. It is remarkable that this contact between the outside world and delicate intestinal mucosa seems to run smoothly, and that inflammation is a relatively infrequent event. In this respect, the human immune system makes constant critical decisions about whether to react to an antigen or to suppress the immune response.

In the human intestine is a large pool of immunocompetent T cells that regulates these processes. It has become clear that most of the interactions between antigens and T cells, particularly those with ubiquitous antigen, lead to tolerance caused by induction of anergy or clonal deletion of the T cells (2). It is obvious that in inflammatory bowel disease this homeostasis is disturbed, probably through different immune pathways, resulting in mucosal inflammation. However, evidence now indicates that fundamental differences occur in the immunologic events and processes found in Crohn's disease and ulcerative colitis (2).

Crohn's disease is associated with chronic cell-mediated immunopathology. The inflammation is transmural, localized anywhere within the gastrointestinal tract, and with a predominance of activated CD4 + T lymphocytes and macrophages together with other inflammatory cells. Interestingly, noncaseating granulomas are thought to be pathognomonic; however, they are not found often, although they are seen (rarely) in ulcerative colitis.

In contrast with Crohn's disease, humoral immunopathology predominates in ulcerative colitis, and is associated with deposition of immune complexes and the presence of antineutrophil cytoplasmic antibodies (ANCA) (2). As in Crohn's disease, it has now become clear that CD4 + Th-1 cells are central in the pathogenesis (8). It has been shown that isolated lamina propria mononuclear cells from patients with Crohn's disease have the characteristics of Th-1 secretion pattern, including interleukin (IL)-2 and γ-interferon, in contrast with ulcerative colitis, which does not show this pattern (9). Ulcerative colitis is not primarily regarded as a condition of cell-mediated immunopathology but is characterized by neutrophil infiltration, epithelial damage, and autoantibody formation (2,9). The role of T-cell activation in ulcerative colitis is less well established than in Crohn's disease, although the disease process is consistent with a Th-2 pattern of cytokine production.

Clear infiltration of activated macrophages occurs in both conditions, and it is well accepted that macrophages play a critical role in their pathogenesis. These macrophages produce many cytokines, such as tumor necrosis factor α (TNF-α) and IL-1, found in tissues from patients with all types of inflammatory bowel disease (7,8).

We have come to realize that inflammatory bowel disease is not one disease. It is most probably the result of more than one factor or influence that, with the correct genetic background, leads to the disease (3,10). It is well known for its clinical heterogeneity and for individual differences in the efficacy of treatment. Currently, three main theories relate to the cause or pathogenesis of inflammatory bowel disease. First, specific pathogens may trigger the disease. In Crohn's disease, for example, measles virus, *Mycobacterium paratuberculosis*, or *Listeria monocytogenes*, and also *Helicobacter* spp., have been implicated. In ulcerative colitis, *Escherichia coli* may play a role. Second, a primary defect may result in increased permeability or defective healing that results in a constant antigenic drive from the luminal content of the intestine. This theory is controversial; it is likely that a secondary increase in permeability plays a role in determining the clinical course of inflammatory bowel disease. Third, an overly aggressive immune response to normal bacterial antigens may occur in genetically susceptible hosts. This theory is especially relevant to Crohn's disease: uptake of bacterial components leads to activation of mucosal immune cells; these then secrete proinflammatory cytokines, which are potent inducers of local inflammation.

Rather than relying on only one theory, it seems probable that a more complex approach is necessary to determine the causes of inflammatory bowel disease. This approach is based on careful clinical analysis as well as on experimental animal studies. In the pathogenesis of inflammatory bowel disease, we should separate a series of events that are not necessarily related. These events are (a) initiation, (b) potentiation, (c) acute inflammation, (d) antigenic drive plus genetic susceptibility, (e) immunoregulation, and finally (f) tissue damage and (g) disease. It is of the greatest importance to carefully delineate these different events as they are the basis for possible new treatments for inflammatory bowel disease.

The initiation phase is not well understood; infections, drugs (non-steroidal anti-inflammatory drugs [NSAIDs]), toxins, or other antigens may initiate the process (2). Some attention has been paid to a possible role of measles virus, especially in the context of the clear increase in the incidence of Crohn's disease that has occurred in the latter half of this century, coinciding with the measles vaccination program. Striking epidemiologic evidence indicates that Crohn's disease is frequent in individuals exposed to measles virus *in utero* (11).

In the second phase is found a potentiation by luminal bacteria or dietary factors that results in a constant antigenic drive causing acute inflammation. The most compelling evidence that normal resident bacteria are involved in the intestinal and systemic response in inflammatory bowel disease is the consistent demonstration that chronic gastrointestinal and joint inflammation is absent when experimental models of inflammatory bowel disease are induced in germ-free animals (12). It is this constant antigenic drive plus the genetic susceptibility that results in the perpetuation of the inflammation.

The genetic susceptibility is well known from twin studies and the familial clustering of cases of ulcerative colitis and, especially, of Crohn's disease (3,10). Indeed, a family history in a first degree relative is the most important risk factor for the development of inflammatory bowel disease. Interestingly, inflammatory bowel disease has very rarely been described in spouses. Of importance is the high rate of disease concordance for Crohn's disease among monozygotic compared with dizygotic twins (13). Linkage for either Crohn's disease or ulcerative colitis has occurred to chromosomes 1, 3, 7, 12, and 16. The identification of genes that may predispose to the development of inflammatory bowel disease is the subject of many studies (3,10). This gene hunting relies on association studies and linkage analysis in affected families. Regarding association studies, major histocompatibility complex (MHC) class II antigens, adhesion molecules such as intracellular adhesion molecule 1 (ICAM-1), TNF-α, and the IL-1 receptor antagonist have been reported. The linkage approach in sibling pairs with inflammatory bowel disease, however, is more successfully applied to the search for susceptibility genes. Under normal circumstances, a downregulation of this potentiation and acute inflammation occurs with tissue repair, but when this antigenic drive occurs in a person with genetic susceptibility an imbalance of the immune regulation will follow.

In the intestine, a delicate balance exists between proinflammation and immuno-suppression. Factors such as IL-1, TNF-α, IL-12, and γ interferon are all proinflam-matory cytokines, whereas IL-1 RA, TNF-α, IL-4, IL-10, IL-11, and transforming growth factor β (TGFβ) are important for immunosuppression. The possible role of these cytokines has been demonstrated in mice with knockout of genes involved in this immunoregulatory balance. For example, T-cell receptor, IL-2, and IL-10 genes have been knocked out, resulting in the development of inflammatory bowel disease (12).

It is this delicate balance, however, that provides us with the opportunity to inter-fere with new drug treatments. The restoration of the mucosa by downregulation of proinflammation or upregulation of immunosuppression will be the key to further development of adequate treatments for inflammatory bowel disease. It is now well established that the proinflammatory state leads to tissue damage with infiltration by polymorphonuclear neutrophils and macrophages. This inflammation causes a constant release of oxygen radicals, nitric oxide, and all the other components known to play a role in inflammation. The proinflammatory status with tissue damage finally leads to disease with the clinical symptoms of bloody diarrhea and pain.

Thus, it seems appropriate to suggest that inflammatory bowel disease results from a genetically conditioned susceptibility to immune-mediated bowel injury, which is triggered by one or more environmental factors. A major emphasis of recent inflammatory bowel disease research is aimed at understanding the imbalance in the regulatory cytokines that normally control and limit intestinal inflammation. Understanding the mechanisms involved in this chain of events—initiation, potentia-tion, acute inflammation, antigenic drive, genetic susceptibility, immunoregulation, tissue damage, and finally disease—provides us with new treatment options.

TREATMENT OPTIONS

Treatment of inflammatory bowel disease requires long-term and often lifelong therapy to control symptoms and prevent relapse. The choice of drugs is determined by disease category, severity, and extent, which can all be established by a proper diagnostic workup, as discussed (1,5,6). Optimal management of the patient with inflammatory bowel disease usually requires a combination of nutritional support, appropriate use of the different pharmacologic agents, and timely surgical interven-tion. Nutritional status and growth, sexual maturation, psychosocial adjustment to disease, and compliance with treatment should be monitored as carefully as the clinical signs and symptoms of disease activity (1,5,14,15).

As the success of management depends on the degree to which the patient and the family understand and participate in the treatment, they must be educated about the disease. The onset of disease comes at an especially vulnerable time (5). Less than 2% of all patients with inflammatory bowel disease present before the age of

10; however, 30% present between the ages of 10 and 19 years, a period of significant growth and development.

Of all the available treatments, only colectomy for ulcerative colitis is curative (16). However, pharmacologic treatment constitutes the mainstay of daily treatment in inflammatory bowel disease. It needs to be emphasized that almost all studies using a variety of drugs have shown the persistence of endoscopic lesions, despite resolution of symptoms and hematologic abnormalities (1,6).

As a result of recent developments in our understanding of the cause of inflammatory bowel disease, it seems appropriate that the treatment of these conditions in the near future should be a comprehensive approach consisting possibly of four components, based on the chain of events described above.

1. Reduce the antigenic drive, either by using antibiotics or by giving certain bacteria that can restore the gut flora or bacterial balance.
2. Influence the immune response using conservative treatment such as 5-aminosalicylic acid (5-ASA), steroids, and other immune-suppressive agents (e.g., azathioprine or methotrexate); also consider new options such as anti-TNF or IL-10.
3. Influence the mucosal barrier by giving healing agents and stimulating mucous production. No satisfactory treatment along these lines is currently available, but further research in this field is certainly necessary.
4. Especially in children, it is important to pay attention to nutrition. If necessary, enteral feeding should be given. Interesting new developments are possible with enteral feeds containing different combinations of proteins, fats, and carbohydrates as well as specific growth factors or cytokines (2).

A further challenge in the successful management of inflammatory bowel disease in children will be the need to design appropriate studies and include sufficient pediatric patients. Only in very few studies have patients been stratified on the basis of their disease characteristics. In pediatrics, medical treatment is also best validated in the setting of randomized, controlled trials.

New developments in inflammatory bowel disease treatment are tending to suggest a combination of treatments, where in the past only one or two drugs were used, such as 5-ASA or sulfasalazine in combination with steroids. Today, the treatment approach is aimed more at different levels of the pathogenesis. The concept now is that if two or three keys are needed to open a lock, do not try only one. The current treatment of inflammatory bowel disease is to start with a salicylate preparation (sulfasalazine or 5-ASA) in mild to moderate inflammatory bowel disease to obtain remission and achieve possible maintenance (1,5,6). 5-ASA is rapidly absorbed in the proximal small intestine. Therefore, delivery systems have been developed to facilitate its release in the distal small intestine or colon. The beneficial effect of 5-ASA on the mucosa of the intestine probably reflects the local bioavailability of the active drug. Only a few small trials have established its role in inflammatory bowel disease in children (1,5). Large scale studies of efficacy and optimal dosage of 5-ASA preparations for children are needed. Attention should be paid to its possible adjunctive role with other widely used drugs for treating inflammatory bowel disease.

A second option is corticosteroids (including topically acting agents), which are often needed to induce a remission in moderate to severe cases. No role for corticosteroids is seen in maintenance treatment of inflammatory bowel disease. Despite the availability of new and novel drugs, corticosteroids remain the mainstay of the acute treatment of inflammatory bowel disease. To obtain remission, however, it is important to give steroids for a sufficient length of time and in adequate dosage, if necessary intravenously. It has been established that alternate day dosage is associated with fewer side effects and allows linear growth to continue (1,5,6,16). No relationship has been established between steroid dose and clinical response in pediatric patients. The maximal dose used varies from 40 to 60 mg/d.

The third line of pharmacologic agents used in the treatment of inflammatory bowel disease includes the immunomodulators (5,6,17,18), including azathioprine, 6-mercaptopurine (6-MP), methotrexate, and cyclosporine. They are all used in moderate to severe inflammatory bowel disease, especially in steroid-dependent patients or in refractory disease. Cyclosporine is used only in acute severe disease, particularly ulcerative colitis to postpone surgery (1,5). A possible role is seen for azathioprine, 6-MP, and methotrexate in maintenance therapy (17). It is of interest that azathioprine and 6-MP have been in use for more than 20 years and have been shown to be relatively safe and effective. In the clinical setting, either azathioprine or 6-MP has been used when repeated (two or more) attempts to taper off steroids have failed. Unfortunately, the clinical effects of these agents are slow to take effect, 6 weeks or more, and sometimes for as long as 6 months (average 3–4 months). Most of the studies with these two drugs have been performed in patients with Crohn's disease. Data on the efficacy of azathioprine or 6-MP in ulcerative colitis are more limited and reflect primarily uncontrolled experience or small trials (16,17). From experience with Crohn's disease, however, it seems fair to assume that these immunosuppressive agents will help control the inflammatory process in ulcerative colitis, but because of their slow onset of action they are not useful in acute management. The results of clinical trials suggest that these drugs are effective in maintaining remission in both Crohn's disease and ulcerative colitis. (17).

Methotrexate has also been shown to be effective in refractory cases of Crohn's disease (18), but this remains to be established in pediatric studies. Similarly, the role of methotrexate as maintenance therapy needs pediatric evaluation, but the reports from adult studies look promising.

Cyclosporine should not be considered as a routine therapeutic option for inflammatory bowel disease. Its current value is as an alternative to colectomy in patients with severe ulcerative colitis unresponsive to parenteral steroids (1,5,6). The initial success has not been repeated in follow-up studies. Studies with cyclosporine in refractory Crohn's disease have been disappointing. In addition, the initial enthusiasm has been dampened by potential drug toxicity and by a tendency for disease recurrence with cessation of cyclosporine treatment.

The fourth type of treatment, and possibly the first line of nonpharmacologic therapy in inflammatory bowel disease, is by nutrition, which may be used as initial treatment or as supportive therapy. Nutrition has been shown to be more effective in Crohn's disease than in ulcerative colitis (1,6). As mentioned, malnutrition is a well-recognized complication of inflammatory bowel disease, especially in Crohn's disease. Approximately 30% to 40% of children diagnosed with inflammatory bowel disease show growth retardation or malnutrition (5,6). The combination of optimal treatment of intestinal inflammation and the provision of adequate nutrition are of paramount importance in the management of young patients with inflammatory bowel disease. The beneficial effects of supplementary enteral nutrition on linear growths are well documented.

The efficacy of exclusive enteral nutrition as primary treatment for active Crohn's disease is controversial. The mode of action is a matter of debate, but elimination of dietary antigens, overall nutritional repletion, and alteration of intestinal microbial flora have all been suggested. No support is found for the view that elemental diets are more effective than polymeric formulations (1). In the case of pediatric patients, keep in mind that enteral nutrition may be of therapeutic benefit even if its efficacy does not equal that of corticosteroids.

Surgery may play an important role in the treatment of inflammatory bowel disease (1,5,6,16), primarily when pharmacologic and nutritional approaches have failed, especially in severely growth retarded children. However, surgery also plays a role in longstanding disease wherein an increased incidence is seen of metaplasia and cancer. In Crohn's disease, surgery is important in treating the complications of the disease, whereas in ulcerative colitis it is ultimately curative. In Crohn's disease refractory to all medical or nutritional treatment, intestinal resection often results in a significant asymptomatic interval. However, the identification of macroscopic disease after resection, in most cases within a few months or years after surgery, emphasizes that surgery is not curative in Crohn's disease. As mentioned, although in most cases medical management is successful in controlling ulcerative colitis and prolonged remissions are possible, a cure can be obtained only through surgical excision. The current availability of techniques to restore adequate transanal defecation after colectomy makes accepting this operation much easier for the patient.

Finally, biologicals are the new drugs in our repertoire. These are genetically engineered compounds to block or counteract specific mediators of inflammation such as anti-TNF chimeric monoclonal antibodies, recombinant IL-10, or ICAM-1 blockers (7,19–24). It is apparent that initiation and perpetuation of mucosal inflammation is associated with an imbalance of proinflammatory and anti-inflammatory cytokines produced within the intestinal mucosa. Proinflammatory cytokines (TNF-α, IL-11 and IL-12) and anti-inflammatory cytokines (IL-10, IL-11 and TGF-β) have been identified as therapeutic options. Increased production of proinflammatory cytokines is a dominant feature in T-lymphocyte–dependent models of inflammatory bowel disease that are considered relevant to Crohn's disease. The initial observations in genetically manipulated mice showed that altered mucosal production of a single cytokine can cause inflammatory bowel disease. The importance of anti-inflammatory mechanisms is emphasized by the observation that the mere inactivation of a single anti-inflammatory cytokine gene, for example IL-10 or TGF-β, causes intestinal inflammation because of increased secretion of proinflammatory cytokines (7). Thus, normal function of the intestinal mucosa requires a balanced production of pro- and anti-inflammatory cytokines (7). With this improved understanding of the immune system, a new family of agents—often referred to as biologicals—is being developed. Biologic agents include antibody-based therapies, recombinant proteins, gene therapy, and nucleic acid-based therapies.

Evidence now indicates a hierarchy of cytokines and that specific targeting of a single cytokine can be beneficial in the clinical setting (7,20,22). In this respect, we discuss the results of only the human clinical trials using anti-TNF-α antibody and recombinant human IL-10 and ICAM-1 inhibition. The other approaches will be mentioned only briefly.

Animal studies, as well as human biopsies, have shown the central role of TNF-α in T-cell dependent intestinal inflammation. The first human study in patients with Crohn's disease using anti-TNF monoclonal antibody was performed by Van Dullemen et al. (19), who showed that giving this antibody was safe and effective. A double-blind, placebo-controlled trial by Targan et al. showed that chimeric monoclonal antibody cA2 to TNF-α in patients with Crohn's disease was effective in moderate to severely affected, treatment-resistant patients (20). The striking finding was that one single infusion was sufficient and lasted on average for 4 months. The therapeutic effect occurs rapidly and is associated with a significant reduction in intestinal inflammation (19–21). The mechanism involved in the apoptosis occurring after binding of antibody to cells that express TNF-α on their surface is a fascinating new field of research. A multicenter study with a single infusion with a murine-human anti-TNF-α monoclonal antibody in the treatment of children with active Crohn's disease has recently been completed (Baldassano, et al., in preparation). The results show that this compound is active in children, and results are comparable with those in the adult study.

In a double-blind, placebo-controlled study by Van Deventer et al., IL-10 was given as a daily bolus infusion over 1 week to adult patients with refractory Crohn's disease (22). The patients who were treated showed a clear clinical effect of the IL-10 infusion, with no major side effects.

These studies show the effect of either inhibiting a proinflammatory cytokine or providing a cytokine needed to counteract inflammation. It is of interest that most studies so far have involved patients with Crohn's disease, although TNF-α neutralizing antibodies appear to be effective in ulcerative colitis (7). This same antibody was also effective in cotton-top tamarins, the only spontaneously occurring model of ulcerative colitis in a large animal. Thus, antibodies or other inhibitors of inflammatory mediators may be similarly beneficial in human patients with ulcerative colitis.

Another human study was performed using an antisense phosphorothioate oligodeoxy nucleotide (ISIS 2302), which inhibits ICAM-1 expression (24). ICAM-1 plays an important role in the trafficking and activation of leukocytes and is constitutively expressed at low levels on vascular endothelial cells and some leukocytes. It is upregulated in response to proinflammatory mediators. The results of this antisense oligonucleotide given intravenously during a 4-week period were encouraging and this treatment appeared to be safe. Larger trials are needed.

Thus, cytokine-based therapeutic interventions are coming of age, with anti-TNF-α showing efficacy in controlled trials. In addition, IL-10 and inhibition of ICAM-1 are promising and provide an exciting outlook for future cytokine and mediator-oriented treatments for inflammatory bowel disease.

Summarizing the recent developments in our approach in the treatment of inflammatory bowel disease, it is obvious that, apart from the conventional treatment with 5-ASA and steroids, immunomodulators such as azathioprine and 6-MP are widely used, especially in Crohn's disease, but also in ulcerative colitis. Cyclosporine has become the drug of choice in severe ulcerative colitis where a short-term effect is needed (1,5,6), although no long-term benefit has been shown. For patients who still need to grow, the development of topically acting glucocortisteroids, especially for ileocolonic Crohn's disease, is of importance. Studies are under way to prove that these are associated with a decrease in side effects in comparison with systemic steroids. These new, topically acting steroids, however, are now only of value in the initial treatment of Crohn's disease and do not seem to play a role in maintaining remission. Immunomodulatory treatment with anticytokines is an exciting development. The first studies in adults have been published on the use of anti-TNF monoclonal antibodies and several other (anti-) cytokines or mediators, and a study in children has recently been finished. This seems a very promising approach in active severe Crohn's disease, and repeated administration of TNF blocking agents may play a role in maintenance therapy. Future options in the treatment of inflammatory bowel disease are clearly widening and their development is essential for controlling a chronic disease that effects children for the rest of their lives. The complete control of the inflammation should be our final goal in the absence of curative treatment.

ANIMAL MODELS

Above, attention was paid to the immunologic imbalance that induces intestinal inflammation in response to luminal flora and possibly other factors. Experimental animal models have led to a more detailed understanding of the different components of the immune pathways involved in chronic inflammation of the intestine. Some mouse strains, for example, are more susceptible to the induction of colitis than others, clearly indicating the role of the genetic background.

Experimental animal models allow us to analyze early events, and to delineate mediators of inflammation and genes that determine susceptibility in ways that are not feasible in humans (12). Particularly in mice, genetic factors can be studied by gene targeting and gene disruption.

Chronic inflammatory bowel disease can be induced in experimental animals to increase our understanding of nonspecific inflammatory mechanisms. However, most of these models look at one particular factor and do not allow us to study the complex interactions seen in humans. A model with a high degree of homology to many forms of human inflammatory bowel disease, especially ulcerative colitis, is the spontaneous colitis that develops in cotton-top tamarins. Unfortunately, this species is endangered and very difficult to handle (12).

It is obvious that not one animal model is ideal for inflammatory bowel disease. Such a model should have a defined genetic background and a well-characterized immunologic system. Furthermore, the inflammation should occur spontaneously without the use of chemicals or genetic manipulation. In addition, these animals should show a pathology very similar to the human counterpart, and the inflammation should preferably be controlled by the common therapeutic agents in daily use in human patients with inflammatory bowel disease.

Clear advantages are seen in the use of animal models. For example, it allows controlled manipulation of the luminal flora and components of the diet, and even immunologic and genetic manipulations. Thus far, four types of animal model exist. As discussed briefly, the most intriguing is the spontaneous model. Then, the immunologic model wherein certain populations of purified T cells given to mice are able to elicit certain disease characteristics and, thus, mediate chronic inflammation (25,26). The two remaining animal models can be divided in exogenous and genetic models. In the exogenous models, the colitis is induced using chemicals such as acetic acid or trinitrobenzene sulfonic acid. Many other chemicals are used to obtain transient inflammation of the intestine, as review by Elson et al. (12). Genetic models are discussed below.

In the remainder of this chapter, focus is first on spontaneous models such as the cotton-top tamarin and the mouse C3H/HeJ Bir substrain (12,27) and then on the relevant genetic models.

Spontaneous Models

The cotton-top tamarin is found in Colombia. In captivity, these animals develop a spontaneous colitis that behaves much like ulcerative colitis. It begins with periodic excacerbations of acute colitis, with diarrhea and weight loss. At an older age, these animals have a high risk of developing adenocarcinoma of the colon. The process of inflammation is similar to ulcerative colitis, with inflammation of a chronic nature, together with acute inflammation, neutrophil infiltration, crypt abscesses, and mucin depletion (12). In the chronic state, plasma cells, lymphocytes, and macrophages are diffusely present in the mucosa.

Interestingly, the inflammation can be treated with sulfasalazine. The cause of this disease in cotton-top tamarins is unknown, but stress or climate may play a role as it does not seem to occur in the wild. This animal forms a very interesting model, as the disease closely resembles human inflammatory bowel disease; furthermore, novel therapeutic drugs, the influence of neurohumoral factors, and the molecular basis of the dysplasia-cancer sequence in chronic colitis can be studied. The disadvantage of the cotton-top tamarins is their size and the costs involved in breeding them.

It is obvious that genetically defined strains of inbred laboratory mice circumvent these problems. The mouse, as described by Sundberg et al. and named C3H/HeJ

Bir (27), spontaneously develops colitis. This strain was developed using mice with clinical symptoms of inflammatory bowel disease. The substrain develops colitis mainly in the cecum and right colon at the time of weaning. Interestingly, most abnormalities disappear when the mouse becomes an adult, although the disease can recur sporadically in animals older than 1 year. In contrast, small lesions around the anorectum are common throughout life. The histopathology of the colonic disease is characterized by acute and chronic inflammation with crypt abscesses, ulceration, and submucosal hyperplasia and scarring. Extensive investigation for possible pathogens has been negative and genetic analysis suggested that the disease is inherited as a quantitative trait (12,27).

Mutant Mice Models

Several models of intestinal inflammation in mutant mice are known. Functional inactivation of genes leading to grossly impaired T-cell function (e.g., IL-2 and the T-cell receptor knockouts) results in spontaneous inflammation of the intestine (28,29).

The IL-10 knockout mice show a normal lymphocyte development and antibody response; later in life, however, these mice develop chronic intestinal inflammation (30), which can be prevented but not cured by administration of IL-10 (31). The knockout model of IL-2 is interesting, because IL-2 is important in promoting growth and expansion of T cells, differentiation of B cells, and activation of macrophages and NK (natural killer) cells. The colitis that develops, which is dependent on exposure to bacteria, resembles ulcerative colitis with continuous mucosal inflammation (12,28). In contrast, the IL-10 knockout mouse develops inflammation in the small and large intestine that is more Crohn's-like, with regional variability and transmural pathology. Also, in the IL-10 knockout mouse the development of inflammation does not occur in a germ-free environment (30). The lack of IL-2 provides an enhanced Th-2 response, whereas the lack of IL-10 enhances the Th-1 response as a pathogenic mechanism.

Disruption of the T-cell receptor (TCR) α also leads to colitis (29). In contrast with the IL-2 and IL-10 model, these mice are symptom-free for the first 3 to 4 months and then developed a chronic and acute type of continuous inflammation in the colon, with pathology resembling ulcerative colitis. Bacteria seem to play no role in the development of this inflammation (12,29).

Similar models using IL-7 transgenic mice have resulted in the development of chronic colitis (32). IL-7 is a potent regulatory factor for proliferation of intestinal mucosal lymphocytes expressing functional IL-7 receptor. The animals developed chronic colitis at 4 to 12 weeks of age, with histopathologic similarity to ulcerative colitis. Interestingly, the IL-7 was to be found increased in the colonic mucosal lymphocytes and not in the colonic epithelial cells (32). Another interesting finding was observed in mice lacking TNF-AU–rich elements (33). In these mutant mice, the disruption of this element in the mouse genome resulted in chronic inflammatory arthritis and Crohn's-like inflammatory bowel disease. The TNF-AU–rich element is important in TNF metabolism and expression, thus indicating that this dysregulation might play a role in the development of analogous disease in humans (33).

All these genetically manipulated models involve a wide range of cytokines and cytokine mediators. It seems likely that in the near future further understanding of the mechanisms involved in inflammatory bowel disease will emerge from careful analysis of new and old mutant animal studies.

REFERENCES

1. Griffiths AM. Inflammatory bowel disease. *Adolescent Medicine* 1995; 6: 351–68.
2. MacDonald TT, Murch SH. Aetiology and pathogenesis of chronic inflammatory bowel disease. In: Walker-Smith JA, MacDonald TT, eds. Chronic inflammatory bowel disease in childhood. *Baillieres Clin Gastroenterol* 1994; 8: 1–34.
3. Yang H, Rotter JI. Genetic aspects of idiopathic inflammatory bowel disease. In: Kirschner JB, Shorter RG, eds. *Inflammatory bowel disease*. Baltimore: Williams & Wilkins, 1995: 301–31.
4. Offerhaus GJA, Drillenburg P, Ten Kate FJH, Van Dullemen HM, Tytgat GNJ. What is indeterminate colitis? In: Tytgat GNJ, Bartelsman JFWM, Van Deventer SJH, eds. *Inflammatory bowel disease*. Dordrecht: Kluwer, 1995: 145–9.
5. Grand RJ, Ramakrishna Y, Calenda KA. Therapeutic strategies for pediatric Crohn disease. *Clin Invest Med* 1996; 19: 373–80.
6. Cohen MB, Seidman E, Winter H, *et al.* Controversies in pediatric inflammatory bowel disease. *Inflamm Bowel Dis* 1998; 4: 203–27.
7. Van Deventer SJH. Cytokines and cytokine-based therapies. *Curr Opin Gastroenterol* 1998; 14: 317–21.
8. Romagnani P, Annunzialo F, Baccari MC, Parronchi P. T cells and cytokines in Crohn's disease. *Curr Opin Immunol* 1997; 9: 793–9.
9. Mullin GE, Lazenby AJ, Harris ML, Bayless TM, James SP. Increased interleukin-2 mRNA in the intestinal mucosal lesions of Crohn's disease but not ulcerative colitis. *Gastroenterology* 1992; 102: 1620–6.
10. Dignass A, Goebbel H. Genetics of inflammatory bowel disease. *Curr Opin Gastroenterol* 1995; 11: 292–7.
11. Ekbom A, Daszak P, Kraaz W, Wakefield AJ. Crohn's disease following in-utero measles virus exposure. *Lancet* 1996; 348: 515–17.
12. Elson CO, Sartor RB, Tennyson GS, Riddell RH. Experimental models of inflammatory bowel disease. *Gastroenterology* 1995; 109: 1344–67.
13. Tysk C, Lindberg E, Jarnerot G, Floderus-Myrhed B. Ulcerative colitis and Crohn's disease in an unselected population of mono- and dizygotic twins. *Gut* 1988; 29: 990–6.
14. Gokhale R, Favus M, Karrison T, Sutton M, Rich B, Kirschner B. Bone mineral density assessment in children with inflammatory bowel disease. *Gastroenterology* 1998; 114: 902–11.
15. MacPhee M, Hoffenberg E, Feranchak A. Quality-of-life factors in adolescent inflammatory bowel disease. *Inflamm Bowel Dis* 1998; 1: 6–11.
16. Hyams J, Davis P, Grancher K, Lerer T, Justinich C, Markowitz J. Clinical outcome of ulcerative colitis in children. *J Pediatr* 1996; 129: 81–8.
17. Kirschner BS. Safety of azathioprine and 6-mercaptopurine in pediatric patients with IBD. *Gastroenterology* 1998; 115: 813–21.
18. Feagan BG, Rochon J, Fedorak RN. Methotrexate for the treatment of Crohn's disease. *N Engl J Med* 1995; 332: 292–7.
19. Van Dullemen H, van Deventer S, Hommes D, *et al.* Treatment of Crohn's disease with anti-tumor necrosis factor chimeric monoclonal antibody (cA2). *Gastroenterology* 1995; 109: 129–35.
20. Targan S, Hanauer S, van Deventer S, *et al.* A short term study of chimeric monoclonal antibody cA2 to tumor necrosis factor α for Crohn's disease. N Engl J Med 1997; 337: 1029–35.
21. Stack W, Mann S, Roy A, *et al.* Randomised controlled trial of CDP571 antibody to tumour necrosis factor-α in Crohn's disease. *Lancet* 1997; 349: 521–4.
22. Van Deventer SJH, Elson C, Fedorak R. Multiple doses if intravenous interleukin 10 in steroid refractory Crohn's disease. *Gastroenterology* 1997; 113: 383–9.

23. Bank S, Sninsky C, Robinson M. *et al.* Safety and activity evaluation of rhIL-11 in subjects with active Crohn's disease [Abstract]. *Gastroenterology* 1997; 112: A927.
24. Yacyshyn B, Bowen-Yacyshyn M, Jewell L, *et al.* A placebo-controlled trial of ICAM-1 antisense oligonucleatide in the treatment of Crohn's disease. *Gastroenterology* 1998; 114: 1133–42.
25. Morrisey PJ, Charrier K, Braddy S, Liggitt D, Watson JD. CD4 + cells that express high levels of CD45RB induce wasting disease when transferred into congenic severe combined immunodeficient mice. Disease development is prevented by co-transfer of purified CD4 + T cells. *J Exp Med* 1993; 178: 237–44.
26. Cong Y, Brandwein SL, McCabe RP, *et al.* CD4 + T cells reactive to enteric bacterial antigens in spontaneously colitic C3H/HeJBir mice: increased T helper cell type 1 response and ability to transfer disease. *J Exp Med* 1998; 187: 655–64.
27. Sundberg JP, Elson CO, Bedigian H, Birkenmeier EH. Spontaneous, heritable colitis in a new substrain of C3H/HeJ mice. *Gastroenterology* 1994; 107: 1726–35.
28. Kundig TM, Schorle H, Bachmann MF, Hentgartner H, Zinkernagel RM, Horak I. Immune responses in interleukin-2-deficient mice. *Science* 1993; 262: 1059–61.
29. Mombaerts P, Mizoguchi E, Grusby MJ, Glimcher LH, Bhan AK, Tonegawa S. Spontaneous development of inflammatory bowel disease in T cell receptor mutant mice. *Cell* 1993; 75: 274–82.
30. Kuhn R, Lohler J, Rennick D, Rajewski K, Muller W. Interleukin-10-deficient mice develop chronic enterocolitis. *Cell* 1993; 75: 263–74.
31. Berg DJ, Davidson N, Kuhn R, *et al.* Enterocolitis and colon cancer in interleukin-10-deficient mice are associated with aberrant cytokine production and CD4(+) TH1-like responses. *J Clin Invest* 1996; 98: 1010–20.
32. Watanabe M, Ueno Y, Yajima T, *et al.* Interleukin 7 transgenic mice develop chronic colitis with decreased interleukin 7 protein accumulation in the colonic mucosa. *J Exp Med* 1998; 187: 389–402.
33. Kontoyiannis D, Pasparikis M, Pizarro TT, Cominelli F, Kollias G. Impaired on/off regulation of TNF biosynthesis in mice lacking TNF AU-rich elements: implications for joint and gut-associated immunopathologies. *Immunity* 1999; 10: 387–98.

DISCUSSION

Dr. Brandtzaeg: I would like to make a comment on your choice of model. I am not sure that I would agree that the spontaneous models have taught us most about inflammatory bowel disease, because disease in them is just as mysterious as the disease in the human. We still do not know why animals or humans get these diseases. In the immunologic models, on the other hand, where the immune system is manipulated, either by mutating genes or introducing genes, we know exactly what is wrong with the animals as a background. The real lesson from those experiments, I believe, is that it is always distally in the intestine where the first lesions occur. When imbalance occurs in the immune system in any way, the individual can remain reasonably healthy except in the colon. That shows that the most important defense function we have in the body is to defend that last part of mucosa. That has been a tremendous lesson, I think.

Dr. Büller: I tend to agree with you, although I believe the immunologic studies, particularly those in the SCID mice, are somewhat down the chain of events. I prefer the spontaneous models because they allow us to look at initiating events. That is what we have to focus on, because otherwise we will find ourselves making all kinds of different knockouts of something that is downstream from where the disease started. I would love to see research being focused in the direction of the initiation of the disease.

Dr. Brandtzaeg: I believe that the spontaneous models may take just as long to unravel as it will take to unravel the disease in humans. Also, I believe the cotton-top tamarins can give you a nasty bite!

Dr. Sherman: I agree that spontaneous models of colitis will provide new information, but for a different reason. Jim Fox et al., at MIT, have found that cotton-top tamarins have a novel strain of *Helicobacter* spp. in the colon. If this *Helicobacter* infection is treated, the animals do not develop colitis in captivity (1).

Dr. Black: Would you comment a little more on the role of nutrition in the treatment of inflammatory bowel disease? Could this be primary, or is it always secondary to drug treatment?

Dr. Büller: I should have mentioned that we are in the process now of looking at the nutritional aspects of the primary treatment of inflammatory bowel disease. Some exciting results were seen in using nutrition together with growth factors as primary therapy (2). We will probably start to use nutritional therapy, either as initial treatment or as supportive treatment, in difficult cases. Kirschner also showed that nutrition can be used to overcome growth retardation (3). So, for pediatricians nutrition is essential. I am glad you made that comment, because I think we need to stress that.

Dr. Issenman: Would you elaborate on the interplay between nutritional factors and bacterial factors? I noticed you split them in your discussion.

Dr. Büller: I split them because I do not know enough about them. I would separate them on the basis that the bacterial flora approach is to isolate the good bacterial factors (e.g., the lactobacilli) and administer them in the hope of improving gut function, whereas the nutritional approach is to provide an antigenic drive that can be influenced in a completely different way, with a monoprotein base or the addition of specific growth factors. Maybe they will merge eventually, because any beneficial factors that the bacteria provide for the mucosa may perhaps be added to nutritional therapy, TGF-β, for example.

Dr. Spolidoro: What is your opinion on Walker-Smith's studies using a casein-based, lactose-free diet as the initial treatment of inflammatory bowel disease, without drugs (4,5)?

Dr. Büller: I think Walker-Smith should be complimented for sticking to that therapy while most of the rest of Europe was trying new drugs. Do not forget, as many as 50 drugs are now on the market to treat inflammatory bowel disease. Nutrition has been overlooked for too long. I believe that pediatricians should be actively looking at nutrition. I have been working with Walker-Smith on the design of a study to evaluate the use of a defined formula for initial treatment of patients with inflammatory bowel disease. He is still the person who really believes in this, together with a few other researchers in the United Kingdom. In mainland Europe, this has not been the trend, although we may be changing our minds.

Dr. Panagiotou-Angelakopoulou: It has been shown that essential fatty acids can inhibit natural cytotoxicity, which is altered in ulcerative colitis. They can also inhibit the synthesis of cytokines and the production of leukotriene B_1 and thromboxane. On that basis do you think they have a role in the treatment of ulcerative colitis or Crohn's disease?

Dr. Büller: To be blunt, these are among those 50 drugs already on the market! What I have tried to show with these chains of events is that intervention is at the lower end of the chain, and that has generally been disappointing. In looking critically at the studies that have been done, these agents have some positive effects but they never achieve the status of definitive therapy.

Dr. Marini: Is the incidence of inflammatory bowel disease influenced by breastfeeding in infancy?

Dr. Büller: Maybe Dr. Koletzko can answer that?

Dr. Koletzko: During my time in Toronto, we performed a study in patients with Crohn's disease and ulcerative colitis, using healthy siblings as controls for environmental and genetic factors. In Crohn's disease, we found that breastfeeding was protective, irrespective of duration, with an odds ratio of 3.5, when possible confounders were taken into account.

Dr. Goulet: My question is about the use of anti-TNF antibody. We know that the main criterion for inclusion in the study was severe refractory Crohn's disease, without regard to age, disease duration, localization, and so on. Did you look retrospectively in either the adult or the pediatric study at predictive factors for failure or success of anti-TNF therapy? It is likely that age and disease duration will modify the immunologic profile and, with the same histologic pattern, different immune profiles emerge. Have you any idea whether the selection of patients according to their immune profile or disease duration influenced the success or failure of anti-TNF therapy?

Dr. Büller: That is a very good question. Dr. Braegger was also involved in those studies and maybe he can comment, but I do not think this was studied. It seemed that it either worked or it did not work, but I do not think we took account of the clinical background.

Dr. Braegger: I do not think we can answer these questions at the moment as we have only investigated 21 patients. We need more data before we can analyze the results in that way.

Dr. Roy: What does epidemiology tell us? The rising prevalence in continental Europe of inflammatory bowel disease is particularly worrying. Back in the 1970s, I presented a series of about 200 patients from one Canadian hospital, which at the time was more than all the known patients in the whole of France. Now, the disease is quite prevalent in France.

Dr. Büller: The incidence is also increasing in North America. We do not know why, which is exactly why we have to look carefully at children at that initial stage to find out what is happening then.

Dr. Alpers: I do not know why it is increasing. The issue of increased detection certainly does not explain it all. In parts of the United States, we are also seeing it much more in blacks now than previously.

Dr. Lyonnet: Some genetic studies have been biased, because the severe forms of these disorders are more likely to be detected. How carefully have you looked for asymptomatic bowel disorders in the parents of affected children?

Dr. Büller: That has been the criticism of this whole aspect of genetic anticipation. We have no definite answer. Those studies should be repeated to see if genetic anticipation really exists, but I tend to believe such is the case because it has been shown to play a role in other diseases. I think we should have ongoing research to try to answer that question.

Dr. Delvin: In relation to genetic anticipation, it is worth considering the research that has been done on other diseases completely outside the field of gastroenterology—for example the fragile X syndrome and autism. Genetic sequences have been found in children with these conditions that are multiple repeats, and the longer the repeat, the more severe the condition (6). Once the genetic background of a disease is known, molecular genetics may help determine whether genetic anticipation exists.

Dr. Lyonnet: To follow up on that comment: the diseases you are referring to are all triplet expansion disorders. If, from the clinical background, one could be fairly sure that genetic anticipation exists, it would be a good to look for amplification of triplets in those patients. The amplification in the genome could be detected in such patients, whatever the gene. Maybe those strategies could be applied to inflammatory bowel disease.

Dr. Büller: I think that work is ongoing.

Dr. Ghoos: Please say something about the use of growth factors or polyamines.

Dr. Büller: We went through a long phase in pediatric nutrition research looking at all kinds of fatty acids. I am glad to report that the hype is subsiding now and we are coming down to earth over the importance of these. Unfortunately, a new hype may be emerging, which is adding in all these different polyamines or growth factors or whatever you want to call them. I am a little more optimistic about adding TGF-β. For example, Fell et al. showed, at the level of messenger RNA, that all kinds of cytokines in the mucosa are influenced when TGF-β is given (2). I would like to emphasize again that these critical studies have to be done in patients. We will not know the answer from animal models or *in vitro* studies. Those studies are being done now, and pediatricians should realize that whenever they have a patient they should enter that patient into a study rather than treating randomly. Look at budesonide and anti-TNF use in the United States: these are being used by a lot of pediatricians I know, without one patient being entered into a study. We should press pharmaceutical companies to help us do proper studies.

Dr. Brandtzaeg: First a comment on TNF-α antibody therapy. We need to be aware of the fact that TNF-α has many attack points in the gut, so it is not strange that very individual reactions occur. We do not know what we are doing usually. TNF-α can reduce apoptosis of T cells, activation of a metalloproteinases, activation of endothelial cells, and epithelial permeability.

Dr. Büller: If a medical student 10 years ago had said that giving a single infusion of one antibody to one cytokine would make a disease disappear, I think that student would have been sent out of the room and told to restudy immunology. But, now this has happened. One infusion is given to the patient and, in those who respond, the effect lasts for at least 2 or 3 months. It has always has amazed me that effective therapy can be just round the corner. I agree, we have to be very careful and follow up these patients, but to have that possibility now is a tremendous step forward.

Dr. Brandtzaeg: I am not playing it down. It is magic how it works, and especially how long it works. I just wanted to say that individual variation occurs, which will take some time to understand. And other antibodies are found that are more specific now, such as the antibody to α4β7, the so-called ''homing molecule'': rumor from clinical trial has it that this is also magic. At least with that agent, we know what we are doing—we are blocking the emigration of activated B and T cells into the gut.

Dr. Büller: How do you explain the fact that giving more IL-10 is counterproductive?

Dr. Brandtzaeg: I cannot explain that. It is a very tricky multifactorial cytokine, that is all I can say.

If we go back to the 1950s, psychiatrists were very concerned with this field: they explained everything about inflammatory bowel disease. Then, they were overruled by the immunologists. Now, however, we are in a phase where we are learning about the interaction between the neuroendocrine system and the immune system, the brain–gut axis, so now psychiatrists are again examining this area. Many psychological and psychiatric studies are going on right now in adult inflammatory bowel disease. I would like your comment on this newly blossoming activity.

Dr. Büller: A beautiful study is being done in Sweden looking at children with inflammatory bowel disease, and a carefully selected control group with tension headache, diabetes, and healthy controls. They found that 60% of the children with inflammatory bowel disease had positive DSM III criteria for psychiatric illness, of which 15% were severe (7). Their nice control group makes you believe there is something to this study. When all the genes are known, we will know if a depression gene is close to where we think the ulcerative colitis or Crohn's disease gene is. In pediatrics, I believe one has to be very careful not to overlook the psychiatric aspects of disease. Adult physicians are used to this, but pediatricians tend to hold the view that by treating the inflammatory bowel disease, the psychiatric aspects will go away.

Dr. Lionetti: Many papers have been published that appear to show that budesonide is as effective as conventional steroids in moderate Crohn's disease, but clinicians say it does not work very well. My personal experience with four children is a bit disappointing. What is your personal experience?

Dr. Büller: We are now in the midst of a multicenter European study on budesonide, but not enough patients have been enrolled, because the drug is being used everywhere without proper assessment. This is very sad. We need those studies to answer questions about comparative efficacy, which was built into the study: one arm is budesonide, the other is steroids. If we can enter enough patients into the study, we could answer your question. From my own experience, no great difference was seen between budesonide and steroids; however, the study was designed to look at side effects and we really need to know if budesonide is a better drug than steroids from that point of view too. We also need to know about effects on growth.

Dr. Seidman: With respect to the theory of permeability in the pathogenesis of inflammatory bowel disease, most of the available data suggest that permeability is a secondary phenomenon rather than a primary one, at least from a pediatric perspective. Although nearly half of the studies show that permeability is a factor in family members, the other half show it is not!

Returning to a previous discussion on contamination in early life, the theory goes that infections that induce defenses in the gut in infancy and childhood may turn out to be protective against inflammatory bowel disease later on, whereas if a child grows up in a society where hygiene is so good that very little enteric infection occurs early in life, then perhaps that child is more susceptible to inflammatory bowel disease. In looking at our population here in Montreal, we have children born in Canada who come from countries where inflammatory bowel disease is unheard of, yet here they develop those diseases fairly commonly.

You raised some philosophically interesting points about animal models. One thing that always surprises me is that we go to great lengths to knock out genes from the immune system in animals, but in fact we have very good human knockout models that we have not tried to understand sufficiently. An example would be chronic granulomatous disease or CD11/CD18 leukocyte adhesion molecule deficiency, and a number of others. What has always impressed me is that most of the Crohn's-like illnesses we see that are caused by congenital inborn errors of the immune system relate to neutrophil dysfunction, and nobody is really looking at neutrophil function any more in inflammatory bowel disease—everybody is fixated on the effector cell, which is most probably a CD4+ T cell. However, perhaps normal neutrophil function prevents inflammatory bowel disease, which has not really been examined enough in these patients.

REFERENCES

1. Fox J. A novel urease-negative *Helicobacter* species associated with colitis and typhlitis in IL-10-deficient mice. *Infect Immun* 1999; 67: 1757–62.
2. Fell JME, Hollis A, Paintin M. Normalisation of mucosal cytokine mRNA in association with clinical improvement in children with Crohn's disease treated with polymeric diet [Abstract]. *J Pediatr Gastroenterol Nutr* 1998; 26: 544.
3. Kirschner BS. Growth and development in IBD. *Acta Paediatr Scand* 1990; (suppl 366): 98–104.
4. Heuschkel RB, Walker-Smith JA. Enteral nutrition in inflammatory bowel disease of childhood. *JPEN* 1999; 23: (suppl) S29–32.
5. Walker-Smith JA. Mucosal healing in Crohn's disease. *Gastroenterology* 1998; 114: 419–20.
6. Rousseau F, Rouillard P, Morel ML, Khandjian EW, Morgan K. 1998 Prevalence of carriers of premutation-size alleles of the FMRI gene—and implications for the population genetics of the fragile X syndrome. *Am J Hum Genet* 1995; 57(5): 1006–18.
7. Engstrom I, Lindguist BL. Inflammatory bowel disease in children and adolescents: a somatic and psychiatric investigation. *Acta Paediatr Scand* 1991; 80: 640–7.

Gastrointestinal Functions, edited by Edgard E. Delvin and Michael J. Lentze. Nestlé Nutrition Workshop Series, Pediatric Program, Vol. 46, Nestec Ltd., Vevey/Lippincott Williams & Wilkins, Philadelphia © 2001.

Genetics of Gut Mobility Disorders

The Model of Hirschsprung's Disease

Stanislas Lyonnet, J. Amiel, R. Salomon, T. Attié, R. Touraine, J. Steffann, A. Pelet, C. Nihoul-Fékété, M. Vekemans, A. Munnich

Département de Génétique et Unité INSERM U-393, Hôpital Necker-Enfants Malades, Paris, France

Recent advance in the molecular genetics of Hirschsprung's disease have confirmed the complex genetic basis of this congenital disorder. In particular, after the demonstration of mutations of the *RET* proto-oncogene in a significant proportion of both familial and sporadic cases, additional genes have been identified as responsible for colonic aganglionosis in humans and rodents. These findings originated from the study of knockout mouse models and naturally occurring rodent models of Hirschsprung's disease (*Piebald Lethal*, *Lethal Spotted*, and *Dominant Megacolon* in mice, *Spotting Lethal* in rats), which were shown to carry homozygous mutations at the endothelin-B receptor (*EDNRB*), the endothelin 3 (*EDN3*), or the *SOX10* genes. Finally, genes encoding the ligands (*GNDF* and neurturin in particular) and coreceptors of the *RET* proto-oncogene, as well as genes involved in the endothelin signaling pathway such as the endothelin-converting enzyme 1 gene, represent additional candidates for Hirschsprung's disease.

Several genes appear to be involved in determining the genetic forms of Hirschsprung's disease, whether isolated or syndromic. Moreover, the same genes and probably additional loci are likely to play a role in determining different degrees of severity and the sex-dependent penetrance of Hirschsprung's disease in humans. Thus, this disease is an interesting model of a congenital malformation, and dissection of its genetic cause may provide a unique opportunity to distinguish between a polygenic and a genetically heterogeneous disease, thereby helping to understand other complex disorders and congenital malformations hitherto considered multifactorial in origin. Finally, the study of the molecular basis of Hirschsprung's disease is also a step toward understanding the developmental genetics of the enteric nervous system, providing support for the role of the tyrosine kinase and endothelin signaling pathways in the development of neural crest derived enteric neurons in the human.

TABLE 1. *Human and mouse genes and loci involved in Hirschsprung's disease predisposition*

Genes (disease loci)	Humans				Mice		
	Phenotype	Inheritance	Chromosomal assignment	Natural mutants	Knockouts	Inheritance	Chromosomal assignment
RET (HSCR1)	HSCR	AD	10q11.2	—	*RET-/-* Megacolon Kidney abnormalities	AR	6
EDNRB (HSCR2)	HSCR+WS HSCR	AR? AD?	13q22	*Piebald lethal (s^l)* Megacolon Color spotting	*EDNRB-/-* Megacolon Color spotting	AR	14
EDN3 (HSCR3)	HSCR+WS HSCR	AR? AD?	20q13.2–q13.3	*Lethal spotting (ls)* Megacolon Color spotting	*EDN3-/-* Megacolon Color spotting	AR	2
SOX10	HSCR+WS	AD	22q13	*Dominant megacolon (Dom)* Megacolon Color spotting	?	AD	15

The mode of inheritance of the disease traits are indicated.
Natural and targeted mouse mutants are indicated with their resulting phenotypes. AD, autosomal dominant; AR, autosomal recessive.

304

THE GENETIC BASIS OF HIRSCHSPRUNG'S DISEASE

Hirschsprung's disease is a congenital disorder of the intestinal innervation affecting about 1 of 5,000 live births. Genetic factors in Hirschsprung's disease are suggested by several observations (1,2): (a) the increased risk in siblings of affected individuals (4%) as compared with the population incidence; (b) the unbalanced sex ratio (male-to-female ratio 4:1); (c) its association with other genetic diseases, including malformation syndromes and chromosomal anomalies (multiple endocrine neoplasia [MEN] type 2, Waarderburg syndrome, Smith-Lemli-Opitz syndrome, trisomy 21, interstitial deletion or chromosomal rearrangements involving either chromosome 10 or chromosome 13); and (d) the existence of several animal models of colonic aganglionosis showing specific mendelian modes of inheritance.

The high proportion of sporadic cases (80% to 90%), the variable expressivity (different extent of the aganglionic tract among related patients), and the incomplete, sex-dependent penetrance are suggestive of both a complex pattern of inheritance (multifactorial disease), and involvement of more than one gene (genetic heterogeneity) in the pathogenesis of Hirschsprung's disease (2).

On the basis of these observations, segregation analysis performed on different sets of patients and families suggested different modes of inheritance, apparently depending on the length of the aganglionic tract. In particular, an autosomal dominant mode of inheritance with incomplete penetrance was more likely in long segment Hirschsprung's disease, and an autosomal recessive or multifactorial mode of inheritance was more likely in short segment disease (Table 1).

THE *RET* PROTO-ONCOGENE IS RESPONSIBLE FOR AN AUTOSOMAL DOMINANT FORM OF HIRSCHSPRUNG'S DISEASE

Mapping a Major Locus for Hirschsprung's Disease to Chromosome 10q

The first step toward understanding the molecular basis of Hirschsprung's disease, as well as the nature of its genetic transmission, was the observation that a young female patient with total colonic aganglionosis (TCA) carried a *de novo* interstitial deletion of chromosome 10: 46,XX,del10q11.21-q21.2 (3). Following the hypothesis that a major gene responsible for Hirschsprung's disease had to be present in the DNA portion encompassing the deletion, human–hamster somatic cell hybrids retaining the deleted and the nondeleted chromosome 10 were produced from lymphocytes of the patient with TCA, using an immunomagnetic-positive selection method. The availability of these two somatic cell hybrids allowed mapping of a series of chromosome 10–specific polymorphic markers, either inside or outside the deletion.

Using seven polymorphic DNA markers (microsatellites) thus mapped within the deletion, a genetic linkage analysis was performed in 15 families with Hirschsprung's disease. The results of this study confirmed that, in all these families, a gene responsible for Hirschsprung's disease was located on chromosome 10 in close linkage with a particular group of microsatellites (4). At the same time, another study, performed by analyzing five independent Hirschsprung pedigrees, confirmed genetic linkage to the proximal portion of chromosome 10q (5).

Refinement of the genetic and physical maps of the proximal portion of the long arm of chromosome 10 was possible because of the following factors. (a) One or more genes responsible for familial medullary thyroid carcinoma (FMTC), MEN type 2A (MEN2A), and type 2B (MEN2B) had been previously mapped to the same chromosomal region and, consequently, several new highly polymorphic markers were developed. (b) Two additional interstitial deletions of chromosome 10q associated with Hirschsprung's disease were observed. Characterization of the smallest region of overlap (SRO) among these three deletions of chromosome 10 carried by the corresponding cell hybrids obtained by immunomagnetic selection allowed us to narrow the candidate Hirschsprung's disease region to an interval of less than 250 kilobase (kb). The *RET* proto-oncogene was the only cloned gene known to be located in this interval (6).

Identification and Distribution of Mutations of the *RET* Proto-Oncogene in Hirschsprung's Disease Patients

To test the *RET* proto-oncogene as a candidate gene for Hirschsprung's disease, a strategy was devised to detect point mutations of this gene coding sequence in Hirschsprung's disease patients (7,8). In particular, starting from the published complementary DNA (cDNA) sequence and by using a polymerase chain reaction (PCR)-based approach, the exon–intron structure of this gene was reconstructed. The intronic sequences flanking the 5′ and 3′ of each of its 20 exons were used to design primers and to amplify each exon, which was then subjected to single strand conformational polymorphism (SSCP) analysis.

Since then, missense and nonsense mutations, few-base-pair deletions or insertions, and intronic mutations of the proto-oncogene have been identified in patients with Hirschsprung's disease by several different groups (7–14)—although in different proportions in familial and sporadic cases—as well as in the long segment and short segment forms of the disease. Thus far, 64 mutations have been reported among the 281 patients with Hirschsprung's disease analyzed (22.8%) (7–14). Of these mutations, 27 were identified among Hirschsprung's disease pedigrees, and 37 among sporadic cases. Moreover, 44 of 103 mutations (42.7%) caused the long form of Hirschsprung's disease, whereas 15 of 100 (15%) were responsible for the short form. The remaining 5 of 78 mutations (6.4%) were identified in patients with unspecified forms of Hirschsprung's disease.

As opposed to what was observed in MEN2A and MEN2B patients (detailed below) where mutations localized in exons 10, 11, 13, 14, 15, and 16 of the *RET* proto-oncogene occurred in 97% and almost 100% of the patients, respectively, only a limited proportion of familial and sporadic cases of Hirschsprung's disease were found to carry a *RET* mutation. Such percentages have been estimated with broad ranges; however, based on the largest nonbiased series reported so far, we might estimate that a *RET* mutation has been found in nearly 35% to 50% and 8% to 15% of familial and sporadic cases, respectively.

Moreover, as exclusion of linkage between *RET* and autosomal dominant Hirschsprung's disease could be proved in very few of the families or extended pedigrees analyzed so far in different laboratories (either short or long segment disease), and as the frequency of mutations found in families with Hirschsprung's disease with an apparent autosomal dominant mode of inheritance is still low, it has to be hypothesized that not all *RET* mutations have been detected in the patients studied. Although denaturing gradient gel electrophoresis (DGGE) analysis, recently applied to the search for *RET* mutations, has apparently increased the rate of mutation detection, a proportion of unidentified mutations might still be located in the promoter region or in the 3′ untranslated region of *RET*, corresponding to sequences not yet analyzed for mutations in patients with Hirschsprung's disease. Alternatively, another gene closely linked to *RET* might harbor Hirschsprung's disease mutations. A further explanation of this inconsistency might reside in the recurrence, in families with unrelated *RET* Hirschsprung's, of apparently innocuous *RET* nucleotide substitutions, the possible subtle effects of which on the splice process, for instance, may play a precausative role in determining the disease phenotype. This intriguing view involves a wider role of *RET* in Hirschsprung's disease pathogenesis and the contemporary action of several other genes, as detailed later in the chapter.

Genotype-Phenotype Correlation

A breakdown of patients with Hirschsprung's disease studied in different laboratories may yield a possible explanation for the different rates of mutation detection reported. Indeed, the high proportion of patients with long segment Hirschsprung's disease (44 of 80) studied by Attié et al. (13) may account for their apparently higher efficiency in detecting mutations, as 76% (25 of 33) were found in patients with this form of the disease. A similar result was observed in the series of 121 patients studied in the Genoa laboratory, in which 17 of 23 mutations (74%) were identified among patients with long segment Hirschsprung's disease (11,14); accordingly, the proportion of *RET* mutations identified in long segment disease is identical in both series of patients, at 57%. Finally, it may not be coincidental that all heterozygous large deletions of *RET* reported thus far were associated with long segment Hirschsprung's disease and that the two cytogenetically visible deletions were observed in patients with TCA and small bowel involvement.

Parental Origin of De Novo Hirschsprung's Disease Mutations

We carried out a study to identify the parental origin of *de novo* mutations in Hirschsprung's disease. In contrast to the observation made in MEN2B patients, in whom *de novo* mutations almost always occur in the paternal chromosome, we showed that both maternal and paternal alleles were involved in the occurrence of *de novo* Hirschsprung's disease mutations. However, a larger series of cases has to be studied to draw more significant conclusions.

Hypothesis on the Pathogenesis of the *RET*-Dependent Hirschsprung's Disease Cases

Several animal studies indicate that *RET* is expressed in various cell lineages derived from the neural crests, in the developing peripheral and central nervous system, and at different stages of kidney organogenesis (15). In the human, *RET* expression has also been shown in subsets of enteric ganglion cells (16) as well as in tumors of neural crest origin (e.g., neuroblastomas, medullary thyroid carcinomas, and pheochromocytomas). Finally, the targeted disruption of the *RET* proto-oncogene causes total intestinal aganglionosis and renal agenesis in homozygous mutant mice (17). These data suggest that the *RET* proto-oncogene plays a role in the control of proliferation, differentiation, migration, or commitment of subsets of neural crest cells.

Analysis of the localization and *in vitro* expression of the mutations within the different domains of the *RET* proto-oncogene, carried out in several different neuro-cristopathies, has opened the way to an understanding of how this gene, when mutated, can trigger either a proliferative or an inactivating response. In particular, although the mutations present in MEN2 patients are clustered in specific domains of the gene, those present in cases of Hirschsprung's disease are scattered all over the gene. Moreover, for a few of the Hirschsprung-determining mutations, a loss of function effect has been demonstrated (18,19), whereas a common gain of function effect has similarly been shown in the MEN2A, MEN2B, MTC, and FMTC mutations tested so far (20).

Point mutations in one of five cysteines of the extracellular domain of the *RET* proto-oncogene (codons 609, 611, 618, 620 in exon 10, and 634 in exon 11) are found in patients with either MEN2A, FMTC, or MEN2A and in localized cutaneous lichen amyloidosis. In a small proportion of FMTC families, three germline *RET* mutations have been described in exons 13 (Glu768Asp), 14 (Leu804Val), and 15 (Ser891Ala) within the intracellular domain of *RET*. On the other hand, a unique mutation changing the highly conserved methionine 918 of the catalytic core region of the tyrosine kinase domain (exon 16) into threonine is present in almost all MEN 2B patients, whereas the remainder carries an Ala883Phe mutation of exon 15. These latter mutations seem to activate *RET* as a dominant transforming gene through a gain of function mechanism that is not yet completely understood.

On the other hand, the functional loss of one copy of *RET* is involved in determining an autosomal dominant form of Hirschsprung's disease. However, possible additional mechanisms have to be invoked to explain the pathogenesis of some peculiar "*RET*-dependent" Hirschsprung cases, including those carrying missense mutations in the cysteine residues 609 and 620 without any clinical symptoms of MEN2A or MTC (21). Moreover, pedigrees have been reported with the cosegregation of Hirschsprung's disease with either MEN2A or FMTC and, in some of these, a documented germline mutation in cysteine 609, 618, or 620 cosegregated with the disease phenotypes (22,23). A possible explanation to the coexistence of such opposed phenotypes within the same family and in single individuals has recently been proposed by Takahashi et al., who found that these mutations can induce the *Ret* homodimers responsible for tumorigenesis of thyroid C cells, as well as result in impairment of the *Ret* cell surface expression responsible for Hirschsprung's disease (24).

GENETIC HETEROGENEITY OF HIRSCHSPRUNG'S DISEASE

Animal Models and the Endothelin Pathway Genes

Among different hypotheses already discussed, the low detection rate of *RET* mutations in patients with Hirschsprung's disease has also led to the postulate that one or more additional Hirschsprung genes exist. The availability of animal models of Hirschsprung's disease has played a crucial role in identifying some of these genes (25). As shown in the Table, three murine models and one rat model were known, the corresponding defects of which did not map on chromosomal regions homologous to human chromosome 10q (mouse chromosome 6 and rat chromosome 4). In addition, in the *Piebald Lethal* (s^l), *Lethal Spotting* (*ls*), *Dominant Megacolon* (*Dom*) mice, and in the *Spotting Lethal* (*sl*) rat, aganglionic megacolon is always associated with pigmentation defects.

Identification of novel human Hirschsprung's disease genes was achieved after targeted disruptions of the *EDNRB*, and the *EDN3* genes were shown to result in megacolon and white spotting of the coat in the mouse (26,27). The genetic defects carried by the s^l and *ls* mouse strains were already known to map in the same chromosomal regions where these two candidate genes have been located (28). Screening for mutation in these two loci showed deletion of the entire *EDNRB* gene and a missense point mutation of the *EDN3* gene in the s^l and the *ls* mice, respectively (29). More recently, a 301 base pair (bp) interstitial deletion of the *EDNRB* gene was identified in the *sl* rat strain. In these rodent models, the presence of a null *EDNRB* allele does not seem to determine the length of the aganglionic segment. Therefore, the action of *EDNRB* mutations might be modulated by a number of possible epistatic factors or modifier genes, which would determine different degrees of penetrance or variable expressivity of the aganglionic megacolon. The presence of genes capable of modifying the phenotype of the s^l mouse strain has recently been demonstrated in the mouse genome, and six genetic modifier loci of the mutation piebald spotting were identified on mouse chromosomes 2, 5, 7, 8, 10, and 13.

These observations have been useful in disclosing additional aspects of the genetics of Hirschsprung's disease in the human. In particular, a missense W276C mutation of the *EDNRB* gene has been characterized in a large Mennonite pedigree where Hirschsprung's disease was apparently inherited as a recessive trait and where low penetrant pigmentary defects were also observed. In contrast to the recessive,

fully penetrant defects in rodent models, this human mutation is neither fully dominant nor fully recessive, being present in 74% of the homozygotes and in 21% of
the heterozygotes. As the W276C mutation affects the residual activity of *EDNRB*,
this might explain the dosage effect of this mutation and its incomplete penetrance.
However, the requirement of additional predisposing genes for the development of
megacolon in heterozygotes is suggested in this kindred by the identification of a
possible modifier locus on human chromosome 21. Finally, the high heterogeneity
of the human genetic background might explain the wide discrepancy observed
between human Hirschsprung's disease and the corresponding rodent models of
intestinal aganglionosis, both in the mode of inheritance and in the severity of the
disease phenotype. Additional novel mutations of the *EDNRB* gene have been reported in sporadic Hirschsprung's disease cases (30) and in a family with recurrence
of Hirschsprung's disease and Waardenburg syndrome (31), thus indicating that
these mutations are responsible for a small but significant proportion of patients
with aganglionic megacolon.

In the light of the finding in the *ls* mouse strain, several patients with Hirschsprung's disease have been screened for *EDN3* mutations. To our knowledge, very
few *EDN3* mutations have been characterized so far, but they include a sporadic
case of Hirschsprung's disease associated with deafness and pigmentary anomalies
in a patient in whom a homozygous frameshift mutation of the *EDN3* gene coding
sequence resulted in the complete absence of mature *EDN3* (32,33).

Finally, the molecular defect underlying the *Dominant Megacolon (Dom)* mouse
model of Hirschsprung's disease has been identified (34). In particular, a 1-bp insertion of *Sox10*, an *Sry*-related transcription factor expressed during embryonic development, has been shown to be responsible for the disease phenotype that recurs in this
mouse strain, which is characterized by intestinal aganglionosis and white spotting in
the coat (I,L). Mutation search in patients with Hirschsprung's disease has revealed
that the involvement of this gene is restricted to those patients who also show pigmentary defects or deafness, or both (the Shah-Waardenburg syndrome or type 4 Waardenburg syndrome).

Possible Role of the *RET* Ligands (*GDNF*) and Neurturin (NTH), and *RET* Co-Receptors (GFR-α Family)

The recent identification of *RET* ligands—the glial cell line-derived neutrophic
factor (*GDNF*), neurturin, artemin, and persephin—has provided a further Hirschsprung's disease candidate gene to be tested in those patients not showing mutations in
any other gene. It turns out that several co-receptors (membrane-bound glycoproteic
molecules) are required to activate the tyrosine kinase activity of *RET* as part of a
ligand complex including the co-receptor *GFRα-1*. In addition to *GDNF*, *RET* was
shown to have at least three additional ligands—neurturin, artemin, and persephin—which, as with *GDNF*, act in combination with co-receptors to activate *RET*,
GFRα-2, *GFRα-3*, and *GFRα-4* for neurturin, artemin, and persephin, respectively.

The production of *GDNF* knockout mice, showing intestinal aganglionosis and renal agenesis or dysgenesis, has played a fundamental role in this discovery. However, the hope that many Hirschsprung cases showing no mutation of the *RET* gene could be explained by the presence of *GDNF* or neurturin mutations was illusory, because only a few nucleotide changes of the *GDNF* sequence have been found; indeed, most of these are associated with *RET* mutations, suggesting that *GDNF* mutations alone are not sufficient to impair normal intestinal innervation (35). Along the same lines, so far only one family with a neurturin gene mutation has been identified, in which a *RET* variant was also cosegregating, suggesting that both mutations were required to predispose to the very severe Hirschsprung phenotype in this family (long segment aganglionosis) (36). The recent demonstration of the lack of any *GFRα-1* mutation in large sets of patients with Hirschsprung's disease has strengthened the conclusion that mutations of the *RET* ligand complex have little if any effect on the pathogenesis of intestinal aganglionosis. The large family of co-receptors that has finally been identified, including *GFRα-3* and *GFRα-4*, is suggestive that *RET* might represent a signal transducer common to several different pathways, probably directing migration or differentiation of different subtypes of neural crest cell lineages.

HIRSCHSPRUNG'S DISEASE AS A MODEL COMPLEX GENETIC DISEASE: A RECONCILING HYPOTHESIS

In addition to these data on the molecular genetics of Hirschsprung's disease, recent observations concerning the association of mutations affecting different genes in the same patient strongly indicate that more than one gene, each adding a variable contribution, is involved in the final Hirschsprung phenotype. Therefore, a re-examination of those *RET* alleles considered initially to be private variants or rare polymorphisms is required to assess their possible role in the pathogenesis of Hirschsprung's disease. A genetic linkage study has confirmed this hypothesis, localizing in addition a new susceptibility Hirschsprung's disease gene on 9q34.

The knowledge that Hirschsprung's disease is a complex genetic disease will allow us in the future to reconstruct the gene network that directs the development of the intestinal innervation, to distinguish the contribution of each Hirschsprung gene to this network, and to identify new Hirschsprung candidate genes that may play a minor role in the phenotypic expression of the defect by modifying the effect of the known major Hirschsprung genes.

GENETIC COUNSELING

Determining the risk of recurrence of Hirschsprung's disease and, thus, the possibility of providing proper genetic counseling, presents the same difficulties as in any other multigenic or multifactorial condition.

Regarding families with Hirschsprung's disease with a known *RET* mutation, a classic pattern of autosomal-dominant inheritance could be proposed. However, although a future offspring has a 50% risk of inheriting a mutant allele, neither the penetrance nor the expression (length of aganglionic segment) of the trait could be predicted on a rational basis. Moreover, preliminary data, based on the study of 17 families with Hirschsprung's disease, indicate that the penetrance of the *RET* mutation is sex dependent (72% and 51% in male and female cases, respectively).

These data make genetic counseling very difficult and, in our opinion, make the proposed prenatal diagnosis of Hirschsprung's disease impossible. In addition, genetic counseling issues have to take into account the great improvements that have occurred in the surgical management of Hirschsprung's disease during recent decades.

With respect to clinical issues, several families with Hirschsprung's disease have been reported with mutations at one of the critical cysteine residues of exons 10 and 11 of the extracellular domain of *RET*, known to predispose to MEN2A. The main clinical implication of this observation is that a subgroup of patients with Hirschsprung's disease is at risk for MEN2A, or at least for MTC. In view of the wide range of age of onset of these tumors, such a risk cannot be discounted. This raises the problem of lifelong monitoring of the patient and of explaining the hypothetical oncologic risk to the family, bearing in mind that the calcitonin test has a false-positive rate of 5% to 10%.

As already anticipated, segregation analysis had shown that Hirschsprung's disease is a heterogeneous genetic disorder. Accordingly, the detection of mutations of the *EDNRB* and *EDN3* genes in sporadic patients or in small families suggests that dysfunction or loss of function of the endothelin system is involved in some cases. On the basis of these data, it is advisable, in the absence of *RET* mutations, to search for *EDNRB* and *EDN3* mutations.

Finally, in most cases of Hirschsprung's disease, it is not yet possible to define a true recurrence risk. In these cases, genetic counseling can be still empirically based on the length of the aganglionic tract and the sex of the probands, using estimates provided by Passarge (37) and Badner et al. (2).

CONCLUSIONS

A molecular approach to Hirschsprung's disease has shown that a coordinated series of several embryonic steps is required for the normal development of the enteric nervous system. In particular, the normal expression of the *RET* proto-oncogene probably represents a crucial step. The endothelin system also plays a role in the development of the intestinal innervation. In addition, other factors or proteins may well be involved in the development of Hirschsprung's disease, such as the *RET* ligand, the product of the human homologue of the murine *Dom* gene, namely the *SOX10* protein, and finally endothelin converting-enzyme 1 (ECE 1).

Moreover, a series of modifier genes seems to play a role in determining the Hirschsprung's disease phenotype (incomplete penetrance), the variable degree of severity of the disease (variable expression), and the sex-dependent recurrence. Some of these genes may be identified through a genetic study of large Hirschsprung pedigrees and animal models.

In all, these observations support the view that the inheritance of Hirschsprung's disease is multifactorial, as has already been postulated. Owing to this complex pattern of inheritance and to the large number of genes involved, genetic counseling is still difficult in this condition and is largely based on empiric risks.

ACKNOWLEDGMENTS

We thank the families with Hirschsprung's disease for their constant help, all the surgeons and pediatricians who referred patients and biological material to us, and the colleagues who have been involved with us in elucidating part of the molecular bases of Hirschsprung's disease, in particular in the United States (A. Chakravarti, S. Bolk, M. Angrist), in Canada (L. Mulligan), in Italy (G. Romeo, I. Ceccherini, G. Martuciello, A. Puliti), in France (M. Gossens, V. Pingault), and in The Netherlands (C. Buys, R. Hofstra).

REFERENCES

1. Garver KL, Law JC, Garver B. Hirschsprung disease: a genetic study. *Clin Genet* 1985; 28: 503–8.
2. Badner JA, Sieber WK, Garver KL, Chakravarti A. A genetic study of Hirschsprung disease. *Am J Hum Genet* 1990; 46: 568–80.
3. Martucciello G, Bicocchi MP, Dodero P, *et al.* Total colonic aganglionosis associated with interstitial deletion of the long arm of chromosome 10. *Pediatr Surg Int* 1992; 7: 308–10.
4. Lyonnet S, Bolino A, Pelet A, *et al.* A gene for Hirschsprung disease maps to the proximal long arm of chromosome 10. *Nat Genet* 1993; 4: 346–50.
5. Angrist M, Kauffman E, Slaugenhaupt SA, *et al.* A gene for Hirschsprung disease (megacolon) in the pericentromeric region of human chromosome 10. *Nat Genet* 1993; 4: 351–6.
6. Takahashi M, Buma Y, Iwamoto T, Inaguma Y, Ikeda H, Hiai H. Cloning and expression of the *ret* proto-oncogene encoding a tyrosine kinase with two potential transmembrane domains. *Oncogene* 1988; 3: 571–8.
7. Romeo G, Ronchetto P, Yin L, *et al.* Point mutations affecting the tyrosine kinase domain of the *RET* proto-oncogene in Hirschsprung's disease. *Nature* 1994; 367: 377–8.
8. Edery P, Lyonnet S, Mulligan LM, *et al.* Mutations of the *RET* proto-oncogene in Hirschsprung's disease. *Nature* 1994; 367: 378–9.
9. Pelet A, Attié T, Goulet O, *et al.* De-novo mutations of *RET* proto-oncogene in Hirschsprung's disease. *Lancet* 1994; 344: 1769–70.
10. Edery P, Pelet A, Mulligan LM, *et al.* Long segment and short segment familial Hirschsprung's disease: variable clinical expression at the *RET* locus. *J Med Genet* 1994; 31: 602–6.
11. Yin L, Barone V, Seri M, *et al.* Heterogeneity and low detection rate of *RET* mutations in Hirschsprung disease. *Eur J Hum Genet* 1994; 2: 272–80.
12. Angrist M, Bolk S, Thiel B, *et al.* Mutation analysis of the *RET* receptor tyrosine kinase in Hirschsprung disease. *Hum Mol Genet* 1995; 4: 821–30.
13. Attié T, Pelet A, Edery P, *et al.* Diversity of *RET* proto-oncogene mutations in familial and sporadic Hirschsprung disease. *Hum Mol Genet* 1995; 4: 1381–6.
14. Pasini B, Ceccherini I, Romeo G. *RET* mutations in human disease. *Trends Genet* 1996; 12: 138–44.
15. Pachnis V, Mankoo B, Costantini F. Expression of *ret* proto-oncogene during mouse embryogenesis. *Development* 1993; 119: 1005–17.
16. Martucciello G, Favre A, Takahashi M, Jasonni V. Immunohistochemical localization of *Ret* protein in Hirschsprung disease. *J Pediatr Surg* 1995; 30: 1–3.
17. Schuchardt A, D'Agati V, Larsson-Blomberg L, Costantini F, Pachnis V. Defects in the kidney and enteric nervous system of mice lacking the tyrosine kinase receptor *Ret*. *Nature* 1994; 367: 380–3.
18. Pasini B, Borrello MG, Greco A, *et al.* Loss of function effect of *RET* mutations causing Hirschsprung disease. *Nat Genet* 1995; 10: 35–40.

19. Pelet A, Geneste O, Edery P, *et al.* Various mechanisms cause *RET*-mediated signaling defects in Hirschsprung disease. *J Clin Invest* 1998; 101: 1415–23.
20. Santoro M, Carlomagno F, Romano A, *et al.* Activation of *RET* as dominant transforming gene by germline mutations of MEN2A and MEN2B. *Science* 1995; 267: 381–3.
21. Mulligan LM, Eng C, Attié T, *et al.* Diverse phenotypes associated with exon 10 mutations of the *RET* proto-oncogene. *Hum Mol Genet* 1994; 3: 2163–7.
22. Edery P, Eng C, Munnich A, Lyonnet S. *RET* in human development and oncogenesis. *Bioessays* 1997; 19: 389–95.
23. Caron P, Attié T, David D, *et al.* C618R mutation in exon 10 of the *RET* proto-oncogene in a kindred with multiple endocrine neoplasia type 2A and Hirschsprung's disease. *J Clin Endocrinol Metab* 1996; 81: 2731–3.
24. Takahashi M, Iwashita T, Santoro M, Lyonnet S, Lenoir GM, Billaud M. Co-segregation of MEN2 and Hirschsprung's disease: the same mutation of *RET* with both gain and loss-of-function? *Hum Mutat* 1999; 13: 331–6.
25. Cass DT, Zhang AL, Morthope J. Aganglionosis in rodents. *J Pediatr Surg* 1992; 27: 351–6.
26. Hosoda K, Hammer RE, Richardson JA, *et al.* Targeted and natural (Piebald-Lethal) mutations of endothelin-B receptor gene produce megacolon associated with spotted coat colon in mice. *Cell* 1994; 79: 1267–76.
27. Baynash AG, Hosoda K, Giaid A, *et al.* Interaction of endothelin-3 with endothelin-B receptor is essential for development of epidermal melanocytes and enteric neurons. *Cell* 1994; 79: 1277–85.
28. Puffenberger EG, Kauffman ER, Bolk S, *et al.* Identity-by-descent and association mapping of a recessive gene for Hirschsprung disease on human chromosome 13q22. *Hum Mol Genet* 1994; 3: 1217–25.
29. Puffenberger EG, Hosoda K, Washington SS, *et al.* A missense mutation of the endothelin-B receptor gene in multigenic Hirschsprung disease. *Cell* 1994; 79: 1257–66.
30. Amiel J, Attié T, Jan D, *et al.* Heterozygous *EDNRB* mutations in isolated Hirschsprung disease. *Hum Mol Genet* 1996; 5: 355–7.
31. Attié T, Till M, Amiel J, *et al.* Mutation of the endothelin receptor B gene in Waardenburg-Hirschsprung's disease. *Hum Mol Genet* 1995; 4: 2407–9.
32. Edery P, Attié T, Amiel J, *et al.* Mutation of the endothelin 3 gene in the Waardenburg-Hirschsprung disease (Shah-Waardenburg syndrome). *Nat Genet* 1996; 12: 442–4.
33. Bidaud C, Salomon R, Van Camp G, *et al.* Endothelin-3 gene mutations in isolated and syndromic Hirschsprung disease. *Eur J Hum Genet* 1997; 5: 247–51.
34. Pingault V, Bondurand N, Kuhlbrodt K, *et al.* SOX10 mutations in patients with Waardenburg-Hirschsprung disease. *Nat Genet* 1998; 18: 171–3.
35. Salomon R, Attié T, Pelet A, *et al.* Germline mutations of the ligand, GDNF, are not sufficient to cause Hirschsprung disease. *Nat Genet* 1996; 14: 345–7.
36. Doray B, Salomon R, Amiel J, *et al.* Mutation of the *RET* ligand neurturin supports multigenic inheritance in Hirschsprung disease. *Hum Mol Genet* 1998; 7: 1449–52.
37. Passarge E. The gastrointestinal tract. In: Harper PS. *Practical genetic counselling*, 3rd ed. Chichester: John Wright, 1988: 227–35.

DISCUSSION

Dr. Nanthakumar: You have not explained the biased sex ratio.

Dr. Lyonnet: No significant association was found between any marker on the X chromosome and susceptibility to Hirschsprung's disease. So, I have no clear explanation for the sex bias. It may be that it is a postgenetic effect; for example, a hormonal or developmental effect that might influence the penetrance of each of these loci, so resulting in increased susceptibility in males.

Dr. Lentze: The increased prevalence of Hirschsprung's disease with trisomy 21 is something which should be of interest to geneticists. What is there on chromosome 21 that influences the prevalence of this condition?

Dr. Lyonnet: I wish I knew. We looked to see whether these patients have the classic non-disjunction type of chromosome 21 at the first meiosis event, and they do; no difference is seen in the origin of the trisomy between those with Hirschsprung's disease and those without. The other rare cases we came across are patients with partial trisomy 21 resulting from an unbalanced translocation inherited from a balanced parent. Those patients have only trisomy for the most distal part of chromosome 21, 21q23, which is the minimal region for Down's syndrome, and two of these had Hirschsprung's disease. Unfortunately, the mapping of the partial trisomic region does not match up in these two patients. So, we have no clear explanation for the association, although it is obviously important.

Dr. Milla: It is good to see how the multigenic theory is slowly progressing. You mentioned environment and, in looking at other multigenic disorders (e.g., venous thrombosis), clearly other events are going to result in the initiation of the pathologic process. For this type of disorder, that is likely to be very early in embryogenesis. Do you have any insight into what those environmental events might be?

Dr. Lyonnet: Not a single one that is worth mentioning! People who study the developing gut say that the length of the intestine is not the same in males as in females. Hormonal factors also need to be studied. Vascular factors have been evoked, but I know of no evidence that interrupting arteries would result in abnormal migration of neurons. Finally, hyperthermia during pregnancy has been suggested to predispose to Hirschsprung's disease but that has not been proved.

Dr. Milla: I think vascularization comes a bit late to be involved.

Dr. Delvin: Regarding the sex ratio, might the extra facilitating factor or chromosomal site go unnoticed because of lyonization? This cannot happen in the male, so it might explain the imbalance to the two sexes.

Dr. Lyonnet: X chromosome inactivation would be the explanation if some additional females had been shown to have Hirschsprung's disease on the basis of skewed inactivation, so I do not think this would be a good explanation. Another suggestion that has been made is mitochondrial DNA; in that case, however, it is not the sex of the child that is concerned, but the sex of the parents transmitting the disorder.

Dr. Roy: Do we know anything about the development of neural crest cell migration in constipation?

Dr. Lyonnet: We have not studied that. The approach of the geneticist is very brutal and derives from the phenotypic description provided in the gastroenterology clinics. What we could eventually study, for example, would be families or series of patients with particularly severe and well-documented constipation. However, we have not studied any such patients as yet. We have various families with *RET* gene mutation where some family members, grandparents for example, are constipated. In one family, Hirschsprung's disease is clearly seen in two siblings and in the father, and the grandmother also says that she is very constipated, but we do not know whether they all have Hirschsprung's disease or the so-called "ultrashort segment."

Dr. Goulet: In your study of affected siblings, did you classify the cases according to whether they had long segment or short segment disease?

Dr. Lyonnet: The sibling pair pools get much closer to what is observed in sporadic sets of patients—roughly 80% short segment and 20% long segment, as compared with previous studies in multigenerational families wherein was seen a clear increase in long segment disease, which is not the most frequent disorder overall. So, these sibling pair studies get much closer to what is observed in the general population.

Dr. Lentze: I would like to ask you about another kind of neurointestinal disease, not Hirschsprung's—the so-called "neurointestinal dysplasia." I am currently treating a pair of siblings, a girl and a boy, who both have neurointestinal dysplasia by the classic microscopic definition. Is there any advance in terms of the genetics of this disease? That information would help tremendously.

Dr. Lyonnet: I am aware of one study by the group in Genoa, Italy, of a family with neurointestinal dysplasia showing that *RET* was unlikely to play a role. I am not aware of any further testing of candidate genes in that kindred. A second, unpublished study had similar results. For us to make progress in that direction, we need another set of affected sibling pairs, or good ideas on chromosomal anomalies or candidate genes to be found in such patients.

Dr. Milla: Various studies have attempted to find genetic defects in familial cases with the phenotypic abnormality called intestinal neuronal dysplasia. People have looked at *RET* endothelin and *GDNF*, and anecdotally nobody has found any abnormality. The only light on the horizon is a mouse knockout model of *Hox* 11.1 or *Enx*, in which hypoplasia of enteric ganglia is seen above an aganglionic area. The real difficulty about intestinal neuronal dysplasia is that the appearance described by histopathologists on human biopsy material can be produced by various different factors, including inflammation in the bowel. So, it is difficult to understand what individual cases mean, and the ones that are meaningful are those wherein more than one family member is affected.

Dr. Mäki: When looking at sibling pair studies in other diseases, I am struck by the fact that when the study is repeated the results often do not confirm the locus found on the first study. Are other people studying the same thing and do you think they will find other regions in other chromosomes?

Dr. Lyonnet: What you imply is true and happens sometimes, for instance, in common disorders such as psychiatric diseases or hypertension. What makes me believe scientifically in these data is not whether they can be confirmed or not, but that the inheritance factor in Hirschsprung's disease is so very high, as I showed with lambda factor. It is likely, from segregation analysis, that genetic factors play a very important role in this disease, much more important than in autoimmune disorders such as lupus erythematosus or rheumatoid arthritis, or immune disorders that clearly show familial aggregations. I believe that pyloric stenosis follows a similar pattern of complex inheritance, as everyone has encountered several sibships and distantly related patients.

Gastrointestinal Functions, edited by Edgard E. Delvin and
Michael J. Lentze. Nestlé Nutrition Workshop Series, Pediatric
Program, Vol. 46, Nestec Ltd., Vevey/Lippincott Williams &
Wilkins, Philadelphia © 2001.

Conclusions

Michael J. Lentze, Edgard E. Delvin

We have the difficult and demanding task of summarizing what has been covered for the past 3 days. We will highlight some of the points that have been made, and pose a few questions about future developments.

During the first day, we learned a lot about the influence of homeobox genes in the development of the gut. It was elegantly shown that many of these genes have a profound influence on the development and regionalization of the intestine from proximal to distal; for instance, homeobox gene C4 is responsible for the proximal region, C8 perhaps for the gastric region, and D12 and D13 for the caudal region. What we do not know is how this all works, what signals these genes, what gene products are being produced in terms of doing the signaling, and their interrelationship with the various gut compartments.

We heard that CDX2 is a very important homeobox gene. For instance, CDX2 influences sucrase–isomaltase, and we had an elegant talk about sucrase-isomaltase and lactase. We learned that *Hox* C11 influences the regulation of lactase–phlorizin hydrolase, whereas *Hox* C4, *Hox* C8, and *Hox* D12 and D13 affect other parts of the gut. In his coverage of motility, Professor Peter Milla stimulated us to think about the development of these important genes, and what kind of influence they have, not only in normal development but also in disease. We do not know much about the underlying molecular physiology; thus, in the future, we need to gain an understanding of the physiologic events that lead to regionalization, differentiation, or forming an organ at the right place, so we do not have the stomach at the end of our intestine and *vice versa*. Organ formation is a finely regulated process, and molecular physiology will play a major role in exploring how it is achieved.

We heard stimulating talks about structure–function interrelations. Professor Nicholas Wright related how the assembly of intestinal cells is achieved, and what determines apical versus basolateral, or the differentiation steps between stem, absorptive, goblet, and endocrine cells, and their clonality. We now have an understanding of the basic mechanism. What we do not know is how the balance between all these cells is achieved, so that we produce the right number of goblet cells, endocrine cells, or absorptive cells. And what if something goes wrong? What happens in celiac disease or in other intestinal or colonic diseases? These are events we are beginning to understand in the normal intestine, but we are still some way from understanding what happens to them in disease. The role of the extracellular matrix, which has a profound effect on the differentiation of intestinal cells, was outlined elegantly.

What we did not discuss is how apoptosis is achieved between crypt and villus cells: the fine balance between production or reproduction from stem cells and loss of absorptive cells from the villus. An interrelationship must exist between the two, and it is absolutely necessary to understand how apoptosis of the villus cells is achieved in relationship to the production rate of intestinal cells in the crypts. This is for the future. The fine balance that exists is profoundly disturbed in many of the diseases we have discussed such as celiac disease, inflammatory bowel disease, and of course in cancer. To study structure–function relationships is becoming ever more important in trying to understand the pathogenesis of the diseases facing us. Perhaps, this may also lead to a better understanding of why, for instance, villus cells cannot be made in celiac disease.

The other important organ in the intestine is the immune system, the gut-associated lymphoid tissue, which is as important as the absorptive cells and other specialized cells of the intestine. In his elegant presentation, Professor Per Brandtzaeg discussed homeostasis of the intestinal mucosa. We know a lot about the role of intestinal mucosal defense, but the questions remains: how is it triggered? When do we achieve it? Is it better to swim in the Ganges early, or is it better later on? What happens to people who do not have the chance to swim in the Ganges? Can we do something to their immune system to prevent, for instance, the triggering of TH2 to TH1 reactions, which can lead to inflammatory bowel disease, allergy, or other immune reactions? So, the adaptive mechanism of mucosal immunity over time—which means achieving mucosal immunity in early life—has profound effects on the risk of later disease. In Western societies, where hygiene standard is high, we learn that the cost of these high standards is the development of a much higher rate of allergy than that experience by populations where such standards have not yet been achieved. The only reasonable explanation seems to be that adaptive mechanisms of mucosal immunity in early life play a much larger role than we had anticipated. Can we influence this by other measures—therapeutic or nutritional, or by prebiotics or probiotics? We do not yet know.

We only touched lightly on the subject of oral tolerance. But oral tolerance is as important as the adaptive mechanisms of mucosal immunity in later life. Many studies have shown that if certain antigens are fed to people with chronic arthritis, they have fewer lesions and less arthritis than when not fed on these particular antigens. The same is true for diabetic mice, mice with ulcerative colitis, and so on. So, we believe there will be great developments in the future toward achieving oral tolerance from the viewpoint of disease reduction. Of course, this is also relevant to autoimmune enteropathy. The important clinical burden this represents in pediatric gastroenterology will keep us wondering for many years about the nature of this disease and about how we can treat it. At present, whatever we do, 50% of affected infants are still going to die.

A subject that was purposely avoided, but which we think should now be mentioned, is the fact that the intestinal stem cell is a fantastic target for future gene therapy, because it is relatively easy to access: when the target cell is known, whatever is needed can be given orally. Then, not only can we treat mutations of intestinal diseases such as enzyme deficiencies, transporter deficiencies, and so on, but we may find this approach useful for targeting extraintestinal disease; it might even lead to the cure of some of the severe metabolic diseases of other organs, for example phenylketonuria, tyrosinemia, maple syrup urine disease, congenital lactic acidosis, and many others. So, a potential exists in the intestinal stem cells to act as a target for future gene therapy that could help patients, not only with intestinal disease, but also with many other diseases.

We cannot summarize all the presentations, but the interrelationship between basic scientifically oriented presentations and clinical presentations was a feature of this workshop, and gave us all a perspective on where the field is going, what we can expect in the future, and how this all relates to our clinical practice. We believe we have been presented with a good mixture of basic science and clinical gastroenterology, and the discussions showed just how much general interest this generated.

Subject Index

References followed by "f" indicate figures; those followed by "t" denote tables.